HYPOTHERMIA
in Biology and in Medicine

Vojin Popovic, D.Sc.

Professor of Physiology
Emory University School of Medicine
Atlanta, Georgia

Pava Popovic, D.Sc.

Senior Research Associate
Emory University School of Medicine
Atlanta, Georgia

GRUNE & STRATTON, INC.
A Subsidiary of Harcourt Brace Jovanovich, Publishers
New York San Francisco London

Library of Congress Cataloging in Publication Data

Popovic, Vojin, 1922-
Hypothermia in biology and in medicine.

Includes bibliographies.
1. Cold—Therapeutic use. 2. Cryosurgery.
3. Hypothermia, Induced. I. Popovic, Pava, joint author. II. Title. [DNLM: 1. Hypothermia.
2. Hypothermia, Induced. WO350 P829h]
RM863.P63 615'.8329 74-19380
ISBN 0-8089-0853-7

Grune & Stratton, Inc.
111 Fifth Avenue
New York, New York 10003

Library of Congress Catalog Card Number 74-19380
International Standard Book Number 0-8089-0853-7
Printed in the United States of America

To Our Parents

Contents

Preface

The goal of this book is to create a reference source that includes most of the recent literature in the field of hypothermia. The authors hope that this text will stimulate further research efforts in this field. The book includes an abundance of data from animal experimentation and from clinical practice. It is hoped that this text will contribute to a better understanding of the basic physiological principles of hypothermia as well as to support and to clarify the work in clinical research.

The long history of sustained effort to find out what hypothermia encompasses has produced many contradictions. It is still unknown why a profoundly cooled animal, or a patient, can survive only a few hours at low body temperature while hibernators live for weeks or months. Other problems remain unsolved and many physiological mechanisms are still poorly understood. It appears now that the great mass of collected information might soon fall into a meaningful form. But at present, this has not been done. Therefore, this book does not provide a clear-cut answer to what is the physiology of hypothermia. Instead, it outlines major experimental and clinical findings accumulated during the last 10 to 20 years.

One thing apparent to the experimental scientist and to the clinician is the protective role of hypothermia, often observed in situations that might endanger life. This protective role was chosen as the binding thread for the presentation of this text.

It is hoped that students and workers in the field will find this monograph useful. We hope that researchers and clinicians in the field of biological cooling will be interested in using this comprehensive text on hypothermia and related fields.

Hypothermia deals with the body in its entirety. Although the hypothermic organism might benefit momentarily from the protective effects of a decreased body temperature, it is striving to restore comfortable normothermia. If in this text the organism appears to be divided into organs and organ systems, it is only because such an artificial division might help the reader to find a particular item of interest.

The Bibliography in this monograph (at the end of each chapter) covers the physiological aspects of life at low temperature. Though the authors of this book are not clinicians, they have also drawn material from the tremendous progress made in the applied sciences, medical, veterinary, agricultural, and others. In many instances the applied scientists have been pioneers in the field of hypothermia, innovating technqiues and new approaches often before all of the intricate mechanisms of cooling were understood. Therefore, the clinical and other literature in the applied sciences is discussed here in detail.

Contributions made in English, French, Italian, and German are referred to in each Bibliography in their original language. The Bibliography in other languages is translated. The references cited conclude with 1972 except in some instances when even more recent literature was available.

Introduction

"It is always best to start from the beginning."
THE STRAWMAN, FROM THE WIZARD OF OZ.

GENERAL

The search for the prolongation of life by lowering the body temperature, cheating death by profound cooling, has intrigued biologists and laymen for centuries. This fascination with the idea of extending life can be found in novels, many folktales, philosophies, and religions. Immortality at any cost, by selling the soul or by freezing the body, has been the refrain heard throughout recorded time. Recently new discoveries have rekindled that dream. Cells can be frozen to a temperature approaching absolute zero where life can be suspended for a seemingly indefinite duration and can be resuscitated at will by rewarming. Semen and blood, once frozen, can be kept alive, not only for hours or days but for months or years. From a dream came reality, for hypothermia is now used in clinical work. Cooling the body of a homeotherm or of a patient to a temperature of 5 to 10 C, a temperature that was thought lethal only 20 years ago, permits an interruption of the circulation for 1 or 2 hours by deep hypothermia and new operative procedures. The creation of a "bloodless field" has facilitated surgical procedures. It has been found that hypothermia elicits a protective role in many biologically harmful situations. Cooling also separates many intricately intertwined physiological processes that cannot be easily studied collectively. These are some of the reasons that hypothermia was used and studied in the past, is being used now, and will be in the future.

One might say that hypothermia is one of the oldest fields of physiology, having been studied for centuries. Aristotle was fascinated by the profound cooling observed in hibernation; he mistook hibernation for dying and the subsequent arousal as a resuscitation brought on by spring. Hypothermia has been studied by the French physiologist Magandie (early nineteenth century) through his student Claude Bernard (the "father of physiology"), then his pupil Dastre (late nineteenth century), later his pupil Giaja, and their large European schools. Giaja inspired the authors of this book who were fascinated by the intricacies of cold physiology from their early student days. Almost every physiologist in the past has worked in the field of hypothermia, and each of them contributed new facts about physiological processes at decreased temperatures. More important, that acquired knowledge has helped them to have an increased understanding of the physiology of normal temperatures.

Despite the voluminous collection of data, postulation of a comprehensive theory about hypothermia is evolving slowly. The reason that some investigators in the field feel overwhelmed is the quantity of unrelated and sometimes contradictory data and the great variability of experimental designs and complex clinical situations. If one accepts the idea that hypothermia is the entire physiology repeated at several levels of lowered temperature, and that physiology at a normal temperature is still only a large mosaic with many missing parts, then one understands why the greatest adventures in cold physiology are still ahead of us.

DEFINITION

The body temperature of a homeotherm (mammals and birds only) fluctuates during the day and night, reaching a peak and a valley during a 24-hour period. The decrease in body temperature that occurs in diurnal animals and man during the night is usually 1 or 2 C lower than the peak value. In some species this difference could be even larger. Hypothermia does not encompass these circadian rhythms of body temperature. Hypothermia is the condition produced by deep cooling from external cold, drugs, or failure of the temperature-regulating mechanism, which brings a profound decrease in the body temperature. The winter cooling of poikilotherms (cold-blooded animals), the entering of winter torpor by hibernators, or the cooling of a harvested organ for transplantation should not be called hypothermia, though the last case is widely accepted.

The physiological changes caused by cooling in a homeotherm depend on the depth and on the duration of hypothermia. According to depth, the hypothermic state can be characterized as shallow or mild hypothermia (to 30–32 C), moderate hypothermia (to 22–25 C), profound or deep hypothermia (to 0–8 C), supercooling (−2 to −8 C), and freezing. The duration of hypothermia is determined as acute (few hours), prolonged (several hours), or chronic (days or weeks).

COOLING TECHNIQUES

The cooling techniques used today in experimental and clinical situations could be divided into two classes, surface and internal (core) cooling. Surface-cooling techniques encompass cooling a frigore (exposure to external cold only), hypercapnic hypoxic technique (progressive decrease in pO_2 and progressive increase in pCO_2 in the inspired air with exposure to a moderate environmental cold), and helium-oxygen cooling. Core cooling includes the extracorporeal cooling of blood or the cooling of a body cavity with ice-cold saline. Localized brain, lung, gastric, peritoneal, colonic, leg, or arm cooling techniques sometimes produce a generalized core cooling.

When the rest of the body is simultaneously warmed, the cooling of an organ might be profound, close to the freezing point in this case. The protective effect of hypothermia is exerted only to that particular organ. This preferential or localized cooling was found to be useful in clinical situations. Differential hypothermia designates the cooling of the entire body or the cooling of an organ combined with a localized warming (microwave or ultrasound) of a specific detailed area of this organ. These techniques are discussed in appropriate chapters of the text.

During the initial phase of the "fight or flight" mechanism (mild hypothermia) one often finds increases in some of the physiological processes (O_2 consumption, respiration, some kidney functions, cardiac output, learning, etc.). The second phase of progressive cooling (moderate hypothermia) is characterized by a continuous diminution of the physiological processes. The third phase (profound hypothermia) is a state of general depression which changes many of the basic physiological functions (''vital functions''). This phase is the one in which physiological dissociations are observed; for instance, when the critical temperature for the cessation of respiration is reached, the other functions are diminished, though basically unchanged until their critical points are reached. During supercooling all physiological processes are depressed to such a degree that they are difficult to detect. During the freezing phase they are almost abolished.

Insufficient knowledge of the fundamental physiological changes created by hypothermia, combined with the large variability of experimental conditions (various levels of body temperature, varieties of animal species, lengths of hypothermic exposure, types of patients) confuses the picture further. Uniformity of experimental conditions is the only answer to this problem. It is important to remember that hypothermia does not heal, but only extends the time the clinician may use for his procedures.

DURATION OF SAFE HYPOTHERMIA AND CAUSE OF DEATH

Hypothermia is protective in many physiologically detrimental situations. This protective role of hypothermia is created by a decrease in the metabolic rate, and is more pronounced in profound hypothermia. Unfortunately, the survival time of mammals, rather long in shallow hypothermia, is greatly shortened when the body temperature is profoundly decreased. Ultimately, the deeper the cooling that is achieved, the shorter the safe survival of the cooled animals becomes. While human patients and animals can survive for weeks at a body temperature lowered only by a few degrees, the cooling of experimental animals to a body temperature of 24 C shortens the period of safe survival to 24 hours. Cooling of the animals to a temperature of 15 C narrows the survival time to 5 or 6 hours. At a body temperature close to the freezing point, the safe survival time is 1 to 2 hours. Though the reasons for the limited survival time in deep hypothermia are still not understood, it seems that an inadequate tissue perfusion is the major factor. Perhaps a failure in the coordination of physiological functions is critical at the time of biological death. Alternatively, enzymatic systems of the cell may be irreversibly changed after functioning for a lengthy period at a low level. It is possible that hypothermic episodes lead to an alteration of the membrane permeability of cells, an accumulation of reduced intracellular intermediates, consequently choking to death those cells and tissues that regulate vital bodily functions.

1

Freezing (Cryobiology)

"Vivre, c'est mourir un peu."

INTRODUCTION

Cryobiology deals with the biological and medical phenomena occurring at temperatures below 0 C.

Homeotherms, mammals and birds, cannot survive the freezing of their entire body. However, some of the frozen tissues, the skin, and the blood, can be returned to their normal functions after thawing. When cryoprotective substances are used the isolated mammalian cells can withstand freezing even better. The beneficial effects produced by cryoprotective agents are due to the dehydration of the cells and the decrease in the amount of free water that can freeze at a low temperature. Although the physiology, anatomy, and pathology of freezing are not well understood, the science of cryobiology appears to be like a tree bringing fruits much before it maturated.

Even in this early stage of development cryobiology has become of practical importance. Since the discovery of the protective effects of glycerol, cells and tissues have been successfully frozen and used for clinical applications and for use in agriculture. The number of researchers in the field of cryobiology has grown rapidly during the last decade. In 1965 the Society for Cryobiology was formed. It covers scientific advances through its journal *Cryobi-*

ology and organizes conferences. The meetings of the American Cancer Society in 1964 and NASA in 1968 dealt with related topics. Various monographs have been published. Some of the outstanding monographs are *Cryobiology* by Meryman[258]; "Freezing and Drying of Biological Materials" by St. Whitelock, et al[380]; *Recent Research in Freezing and Drying* by Parkes and Smith[282]; "Biological Effects of Freezing and Supercooling" by Smith.[367]

Freezing seems to offer unusual possibilities for the long-term storage of organs, and thereby the establishment of organ banks. Freezing reduces the danger from irradiation.[119] At the present time, however, the techniques of freezing and thawing are still inadequate. They only permit the successful freezing of some cells and of some tissues. Most of the tissues and organs taken from an organism can neither withstand freezing or thawing injury nor the combination of both. Problems associated with cell injury are produced during freezing and thawing, and probably to a lesser degree during storage while frozen. Unfortunately, these processes are not well understood. Until a few years ago ice-crystal formation and the mechanical damage to cells during freezing were thought to be the main causes of death to cells. Later it was suggested that the hyperosmolarity caused by water loss during freezing was the main cause of the freezing injury. Recently the old hypothesis of ice-crystal formation has found its proponents once again. This shift in the search of new theories might well be explained by the lack of sufficient experimental evidence supporting one theory or the other.

Controlled freezing, the cooling of all cells within an organ following their optimal rate, appears to be the major problem during freezing. It probably differs from one organ to another. Controlled thawing should be applied also to the rewarming process. Temperatures of the frozen material should be kept very low and probably constant for the duration of storage. Mammalian cells usually must be treated with certain chemicals or drugs, known as cryoprotectants, prior to freezing below −3 C if significant numbers are to be viable after thawing.[181] Cryoprotection is accomplished by the use of such diverse compounds as glycerol, dimethyl sulfoxide (DMSO), dextran, some electrolytes, and nearly 50 other agents.[181]

MECHANICAL EFFECTS OF FREEZING

Some investigators believe that the mechanical injury induced by ice-crystal formation during the freezing procedure is the cause of damage and death to the cell.[359] When ice formation is prevented, no freezing damage in smooth muscle cells cooled to −78 C is observed.[102] While some animal cells can be recovered after freezing and extracellular ice formation, the intracellular ice crystals damage the cell irreversibly. There are very few exceptions to this rule.[319,345] Mouse skin, some tumor cells, and human spermatozoa survive the formation of intracellular ice. It is unresolved as to whether a rapid or a slow freezing is more detrimental to the cells.[377] However, it is quite clear that the rate at which the cells are cooled to subzero temperatures is vitally important for the low-temperature preservation of cells, tissues, and organs (Fig. 1-1).[189,211]

Rapid freezing and the storage at low temperatures produce very small ice crystals. Subsequent thawing must also be fast to keep the damage at a low level.[259] Better preservation of human epithelial cells is observed when cryoprotectants are used, when the cells are thawed rapidly, and when the storage is maintained at lower (−70 C) rather than at higher (−20 C) temperatures.[335] However, slow freezing damages the unprotected fertilized eggs of rabbits less than rapid freezing. It appears that a controlled rate of freezing using cryoprotectants is significantly better than rapid freezing by the immersion in liquid nitrogen.[387] This also applies to the thawing process[389] which should be correspondingly controlled to achieve good results (uniform heating of all tissues with a determinate rate). In some cases (bovine spermatozoa, various microorganisms) rapid cooling is extremely damaging even when freezing does not take place. This is called thermal or cold shock and it is thought to be induced either by changes in the intracellular cement which holds together the lipoprotein layers of cell membranes or by increased permeability of the cell membranes.[310]

BIOCHEMICAL CONSEQUENCES OF FREEZING

Besides the formation of ice crystals (extracellular and intracellular), dehydration and the increased cell solute concentration cause injury to the frozen cell.[241,257] These alterations might even be the main cause of cell death by freezing. There are exceptions; for instance, red blood cells easily withstand a loss of 80 percent of their water content during freezing to a temperature of −3 C.[241] Skin cells are also exceptions. After a partial freezing to temperatures of −1 or −2 C, and after losing 50 percent of their body water, hamsters can be revived and their skin does not suffer from frostbite.[363,364] In

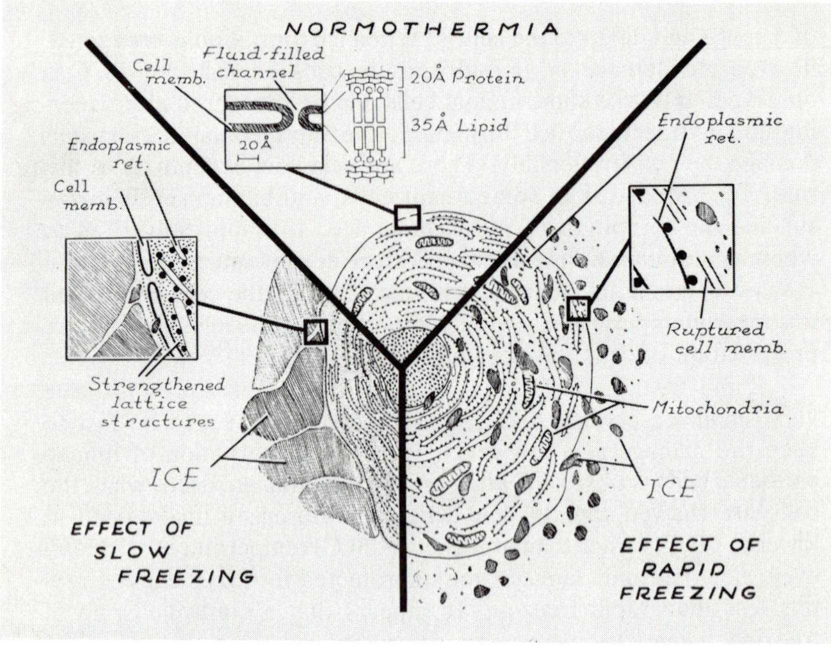

Fig. 1-1. Effects of slow or rapid freezing on an idealized cell. A composite drawing of a normal cell subjected to slow or rapid freezing. Note the molecular sandwich of the cell membrane with its fluid-filled channels in normothermia. Membranes of mitochondria and endoplasmic reticulum are also lipoprotein sandwiches similar to the cell membrane. Water drawn from the cell during slow freezing contributes to massive extracellular ice. Water remaining in the cell as lattices and clathrates serves to strengthen protein membranes as shown in the detail. Occasionally an extracellular ice crystal will cause denaturation and disruption of a protein structure. A cell rapidly frozen is subjected to a tremendous number of extremely small ice crystals, both intra- and extracellularly, which tend to utilize the bound water of proteins and thus denature them.[189]

addition to the dehydration and increased salt concentration, freezing changes the pH of the cells and causes a disturbance to the so-called structured water in the cell. Lovelock[221] proposed that denaturation of the lipid–protein complex might be the cause of freezing injury. Extremely fast cooling, 100 C/sec, does not induce ice-crystal formation in suspended cells or even in embryonic organs. It offers exciting possibilities once this method is applicable for the freezing of large pieces of excised tissues, whole organs, or the entire animal. Rinfret[320] used this same method to cool blood rapidly in metal containers submersed in liquid nitrogen so that no red blood cell was farther than approximately 1 mm from the wall. Red blood cells survive ultrarapid freezing (thousands of degrees per minute),[326,327] but neither this nor the previously mentioned techniques can be used for organized tissues and organs.

Very little is known about the biochemical activities in frozen tissues and organs. Methods have been developed that permit the determination of the CO_2 content of frozen tissues.[302]

CRYOPROTECTIVE SUBSTANCES

When cryoprotective substances are added to the blood or to the cells and tissues during freezing, the percentage of the water that can freeze is decreased. For example, one can point out that 1 mole of glycerol, the first cryoprotectant discovered, binds 3 moles of water and prevents them from freezing. Glycerol and other cryoprotectants prevent lethal injury during freezing by forming firm hydrogen or coordinate bonds to water.[161] The concentration of salts during the freezing process does not increase as much as it would without the addition of cryoprotectants.

Rostand[324] was the first to use glycerol to protect spermatozoa during freezing. Before him several investigators used various sugars to protect spermatozoa. In 1949 Polge et al[301] rediscovered glycerol and developed new techniques, new theories, and new approaches for the use of cryoprotectants not only for spermatozoa but also for red blood cells[360] as well as for other cells and tissues. Dimethyl sulfoxide (DMSO) also shows cryoprotective effects. The cryoprotective nature of DMSO was discovered by Lovelock and Bishop.[223] DMSO penetrates the cell much faster than glycerol and hence for many cells, tissues, and organs, DMSO has become the preferred protective agent. Aside from its cryoprotective property, DMSO has many other desirable pharmacological qualities: local analgesic, antiinflammatory, bacteriostatic, diuretic[167]; in many traumatic conditions[169]; radioprotective property.[119,125] These properties made DMSO one of the "wonder drugs" of the 1960s. The biological effects of DMSO were discussed in depth at a recent conference organized by the New York Academy of Sciences and published in a separate issue of the Adademy.[406] It was suggested that the common link between the cryoprotective and the radioprotective effects of various agents is based on the modification of the water content in cells.[24]

The pharmacological properties of DMSO have been studied extensively.[5,6,29,62,152,181,277–279,396] The DMSO has a rapid turnover rate.[95,195] In adult guinea pigs, injected with 2 ml of 50 percent DMSO^{14}C, the drug was found mostly in the interstitial fluid and along the cell membranes outside the cells while practically no ^{14}C-labeled DMSO was detected inside the cell.[231,232] The embedding of DMSO in hypothermic animals is decreased by a factor of 2 as compared to normothermic animals. DMSO when administered to rats is embedded faster in the soft tissues and shows a higher concentration in these cells but it also disappears from them rapidly. Hard tissues retain DMSO longer than soft tissues.[95] However, after protecting cells, tissues, and organs during the freezing procedure and during storage, glycerol or DMSO must be removed gradually during rewarming. Removal of the cryoprotectants is necessary because of their possible toxicity at normal body temperatures. Preserved cells and tissues containing cryoprotectors cannot be used for clinical applications. The removal of cryoprotective agents is a long and expensive process, though considerable advances have been made recently.

Karow and Webb,[188] working on isolated rat hearts, were the first to observe that cryoprotectant toxicity increases not only with concentration but also with temperature. Cool solutions of cryoprotectants are much less toxic than warm solutions, as confirmed by many investigators working with a variety of models.[60,103,155,235,274,369] The reason cells can tolerate higher cryoprotectant concentrations in cool solutions is because the rate of diffusion is slower and therefore the effective concentration is reduced.[180]

In order to study the toxicity of cryoprotective substances perfused isolated rabbit ear techniques were employed.[139] DMSO is superior to glycerol for the freezing of kidney cells at temperatures which are rather low[306] but not during shallow freezing.[270] Many experimental animals show a fairly good tolerance toward DMSO. On the other hand, this agent has a teratogenic action on chick embryos and, in a high concentration, even on the mammalian fetus.[74] Frozen mouse eggs can be fertilized and the normal embryonic development takes place in the presence of glycerol.[349]

Additionally, cryoprotectants seem to have a pseudotoxic effect on excitable tissue such as muscle and nerve. In contrast to true toxicity, the pseudotoxic effect is an inhibition of excitable phenomena reversible by washing the cryoprotectant from the tissues. This effect, first described by Karow et al[186] on cardiac muscle, is seen here as a reversible negative inotropic and negative chronotropic effect. The effect has been confirmed.[154] The isolated guinea pig uterus and intestine[101] exhibit a reversible reduction of contractility after treatment with the cryoprotectants DMSO, glycerol, methyl formamide, dimethyl formamide, methyl acetamide, and dimethyl acetamide. The frog sciatic nerve exhibits a reversible reduction of conduction velocity after treatment with glycerol or DMSO.[307,334] Pseudotoxic phenomena probably represent the similar effect of each of the cryoprotectants on the cell membrane, a common site of cryoinjury.

Although some large molecular compounds of cryoprotective agents enter the cells either with difficulty or not at all (nonpenetrating cryoprotectants), they still protect the cells from freezing and thawing injuries[318] in both rapid and slow cooling. Polyvinylpyrrolidone (PVP), despite its low molecular weight, protects frozen rate bone marrow in a concentration of only 20 percent.[293] Polyvinylpyrrolidone has a smaller cryoprotective effect than DMSO but also a more stable one.[291] Some investigators have suggested that the action of nonpenetrating cryoprotectants is based on the external coating of the cells by polymers or on the reduction in colloid osmotic swelling.[104] The technique commonly used today to remove cryoprotectants consists of successive resuspension of the thawed cells in a liquid media that has increasingly smaller concentrations of the cryoprotective chemicals. The sudden resuspension of cells in a medium free of the cryoprotectants is often deleterious. For the thawed organs, dialyzing systems should be used before the temperature of the organ is increased above 3 to 4 C. Properties of cryoprotectants have been discussed at some length by Doebbler,[96] Karow,[181] and other investigators.

Summary

Mechanisms for the action of cryoprotectants have not been found as yet. They have become even more enigmatic since it was discovered that some of these chemicals do not enter the cell at all.

Some investigators have suggested that their action is based on the external coating of the cells by polymers.

RESISTANCE IN NATURE TO FREEZING INJURY

Many viruses and bacteria are resistant to freezing even without cryoprotectants. Spores, because of their very low water content, easily withstand freezing. Some larvae survive freezing to a temperature of −26 C, with a loss of most body water.[337] Nematodes precooled to a temperature of −30 C easily survive deep freezing in liquid oxygen.[14] More complex organisms are less resistant to freezing injury but can survive a supercooling lasting from 2 hours (bats) and 12 hours (baby ground squirrels) to 48 hours (insects).[171,304]

Among the first reported experiments in freezing were those that Reaumur performed on insects.[315] Some insects retain motility in a supercooled state at a temperature of −10 C.[13] The amazing ability of many insects to withstand low temperatures during the winter months can be attributed to supercooling, not freezing.[403] Some insects even need subzero temperatures to complete their life cycle.[365] Cold adaptation observed during the winter months increases the resistance of the insects to freezing injury.[217,371] This ability of some insects to survive freezing can be attributed to a naturally occurring high concentration of glycerol (4% fresh body weight)[16,17,19,333] which appears in their bodies before the advent of winter. In these insects, ice crystals were formed in the body cavities and in some of the tissues.[18] This protective action of some agents against freezing, which insects have been taking advantage of for hundreds of centuries, has been stumbled upon by man only recently when he accidentally discovered the cryoprotective effect of glycerol.

Some invertebrates, as well as fish, can survive cold temperatures during the winter months either by becoming supercooled or by osmoconcentration.[338]

Umminger[391] has recently shown that killifish (*Fundulus heteroclitus*) develop hyperglycemia when supercooled. With no additional glucose source, these supercooled fish can survive for 50 days, but when this hyperglycemic state is maintained by the addition of glucose to the water, the fish live for up to 80 days at the same temperature. Similar to this finding, young rats, supercooled to a body temperature of −3 C, can survive circulatory arrest lasting for 1 hour,[305] while newborn ground squirrels, which later in life can withstand low temperature of hibernation with ease, may be recovered after 11 hours of clinical death.[304]

FREEZING OF ENZYMES

The effects of freezing and thawing on purified enzymes[76,255] or on proteins[289] are poorly understood. The loss of enzyme activity after freezing is probably caused by the dissociation of subunits of the molecules of enzymes during freezing, by lowering of the pH, and by increasing the concentration of salts. This is why enzymes that have many subunits are probably damaged more by freezing than enzymes which consist merely of one or of a few subunits. It is possible that during the thawing process the unusual reassociation of subunits and the interaction at wrong positions occur and abnormal polymers are formed. These polymers have a very small catalytic potential. Ethylene glycol, DMSO, glycerol, and polyvinylpyrrolidone protect the enzymes during freezing. The mechanisms of this protection are not understood.[25]

While some of the enzymes are very sensitive to freezing, others are not, as for instance, various dehydrogenases examined in the tissues of Hedera helix.[374] It is possible that in the case of cold-sensitive enzymes some metabolic pathways in the frozen cells are changed leading to an accumulation of products harmful to the cell. It is also possible that the dynamic relationship between proteins and the structured water which occupies pores and micelles in the cell membrane is disrupted during freezing and that this might result in damage to the cell. One enzyme that is inactivated, at least to some degree, during freezing is lactic dehydrogenase. It "leaches" out from the frozen sperm cells into the seminal plasma.[308]

FREEZING OF CELL CONSTITUENTS

Freezing of mammalian cell nuclei was studied by Stowell et al.[376] The cell nuclei are protected better by ultrarapid cooling than by slow cooling. Slow freezing, which preserves the viability of whole cells better, forms large intranuclear ice crystals in the nucleoplasma and damages the nuclei more than fast freezing. Ultrarapid freezing and ultrarapid thawing do not induce any damage to the nuclei. Other cytoplasmic organelles and other subcellular systems withstand slow freezing and rapid thawing better than the nuclei. This is especially true when cryoprotective agents are used. The freezing of cells to −192 C does not induce breakage of the double helix of DNA.[350] It appears that thc plasma mcmbrane is especially sensitive to freezing and thawing injury, and might represent the limiting factor in cell survival.[149]

PRESERVATION OF ANIMAL CELL SUSPENSIONS

Recent advances in the cryobiology of cell suspensions are numerous. Today, it is known that viruses, bacteriophages, and fungi can survive storage in liquid nitrogen.[77,240,254] Viruses can survive the freezing and storage at a temperature of −70 C for many years but they perish much faster at a temperature of −20 C.[344] Yeast cells,[245] many microorganisms,[271] and sea urchin egg cells[15] also survive freezing. It cannot be predicted which cells will survive freezing. Some cells that appear to be badly distorted in their structure do survive and become viable after thawing, whereas other cells that do not show any damage histologically are dead after thawing. It is interesting to note that some cells can survive freezing under conditions in which some of their isolated enzymes do not survive.

The intracellular ice (which damages the cell) is formed by inoculation from the extracellular ice crystals. Contraction of the freezing-resistant cells during water loss does not lead to a fatal injury and such cells can regain a normal appearance and activity after thawing. Freezing injury to the suspended cells appears to be the result of disorganization of the protoplasmic structure of the cell surface, possibly by a drastic dehydration of the water layer surrounding the protoplasmic surface.

FREEZING OF SPERMATOZOA

Investigators attempted to freeze spermatozoa as early as the eighteenth centrury. Sporadically they have continued to be attracted to this problem. The discovery of cryoprotective substances has opened the way for the successful freezing of spermatozoa. This has proved to be not only of theoretical interest but also of practical importance.[301] In the United States more than 4 million dairy cattle are bred each year with frozen semen. Though today, one knows more about the freezing of bovine spermatozoa than of any other cells (with the possible exception of erythrocytes), it is still difficult to explain why the semen of one bull is more resistant to freezing injury than semen of another bull.[300] The bull spermatozoa are usually frozen and kept in liquid nitrogen. DMSO protects the spermatozoa from freezing injury too, but it appears more toxic at higher temperatures.[346] The spermatozoa of other animals[107] and man[65] can be successfully frozen also. Glycerol is often used for the preservation of bovine[301,348] and human spermatozoa. The liquid scintillation method using ^{45}Ca appears to be a reliable method for evaluating freeze–thaw injury to spermatozoa.[386] Sherman discusses the problem of the clinical use of frozen human spermatozoa in one of his numerous papers, with emphasis on the possible genetic alterations induced by freezing and by storage in the frozen state.[347]

STORAGE OF FROZEN TUMOR CELLS

The first report of tumor cells that survived freezing and thawing was published 70 years ago. It appears that the process of slow freezing and rapid rewarming damages the tumor cells less than rapid freezing and slow rewarming. Glycerol protects tumor cells during freezing,[335] a fact which is today widely used by tumor researchers for long-term (1–7 years) preservation of transplantable tumors.[147,383] Cultured L1210 lymphocytic leukemia cells were frozen and stored in liquid nitrogen up to 1 year and were recultured directly without an intermediate passage in mice. There was no significant change in the population doubling time of 16 hours, and the cells retained their ability to induce leukemia in DBA/2 mice.[100] DMSO is more convenient as a cryoprotective agent than glycerol because of its much faster passage through cell membranes (3–5 minutes at room temperature as compared to 60 minutes for glycerol).[48]

FREEZING AND LONG-TERM PRESERVATION OF BLOOD

At the beginning of this centruy Landsteiner discovered the existence of different blood groups in man and created the rationale for compatible blood transfusions. Citrate was introduced in 1914 as an anticoagulant. Presently, it is still widely used for practical purposes in blood banks. When blood is stored in a refrigerator, the enzyme content of the red blood cell diminishes continuously. It is believed that the decrease in hexokinase activity is the main factor for the aging of red blood cells.[209] Even with the best techniques available, the progressive loss in viability of the stored red blood cells is rather high. The changes observed in the stored, cooled (but not frozen) blood are of chemical and biological nature. After a 3-week freezing storage, 25 percent of the red blood cells are lost during the initial 24 hours after transfusion. Besides the aging process, "storage lesion" is a factor in the deterioration of red blood cells preserved at temperatures between 4 and 10 C. The lowest temperature at which blood can be kept unfrozen is −3 C.

That freezing might preserve blood for extended periods of time, making it "young" for years, was suggested 100 years ago. Unfortunately, the first experiments in this field showed that hemolysis was always present after freezing and thawing of the red blood cells. The amount of ice formed in blood frozen at a temperature of −2 C is 75 percent. The amount increases up to 92 percent at a temperature of −8 C. Further cooling to −25 C does not change this percentage.[228] Early experiments in 1951 showed that short-term freezing (3 hours) did not appreciably decrease the survival of transfused red blood cells.[262] The freezing process at near-zero temperatures damages the red blood cells mechanically and produces hemolysis.[272] Recent investigations have shown that ultrarapid freezing is successful for the preservation of blood. However, the layers of blood to be frozen cannot be larger than a few millimeters. Even in the case of frozen blood kept at a temperature slightly below the freezing point, the safe period for its preservation is still only 3 weeks. During slow freezing the ice crystals are formed outside the red blood cells. The crystals grow, withdrawing the water from the cells as well as from the suspending medium until all the water that can be frozen is removed and the red blood cells collapse. During fast freezing, ice crystals are formed both outside and inside the cells. These intracellular crystals cause irreversible damage to cells. Over 15 years ago Lovelock[219] suggested that the principal damaging effect associated with freezing is the change in the concentration of electrolytes present inside and outside of the cell, though the destructive action of exposure to a concentrated salt solution is not instantaneous. Cryoprotectants do diminish this effect; they protect blood[360] and other tissues and cells. The protective action of glycerol is associated with smaller concentration of electrolytes within the cell during freezing.[220] Before the blood can be used for a transfusion it is important for the cryoprotectants to be removed because of their toxicity.

Even after 44 months of storage in glycerol at −79 C, human red blood cells can be used clinically.[148] Red blood cells stored at −196 C[328] can survive the transfusion. But a higher temperature of storage in the frozen state is detrimental to the survival of red blood cells.[263] Several factors (temperature, ice-crystal formation, concentration of solutes, etc.) determine the amount of the red blood cells that can survive freezing.[242] Even a small concentration of glycerol protects the red blood cells during rapid freezing.[4] There are species differences; i.e., glycerol protects rabbit blood but not sheep or ox blood.[49] Noradrenalin appears to increase the amount of glycerol found in the plasma.[56,138] This observation may be of practical interest for a larger embedding of cryoprotectants in living cells and tissues before freezing. DMSO protects the red blood cells adequately.[159] Lactose and dextrose have been used also as cryoprotective agents for blood.[379] Dextrose, sucrose, and polyvinylpyrrolidone[290,292] exert protective roles similar to that of glycerol and DMSO, the rate of cooling being the determining factor for the percentage of surviving red blood cells.[312] The PVP does not need to be removed from blood before use.[318] Low cooling velocities appear to be more beneficial with glycerol and DMSO,[313] whereas sucrose and dextrose protect the red blood cells better during rapid freezing.[314] Technological advances show that as much as 90 percent of the red blood cells (protected by glycerol 14% v/v) survive the freezing injury.[328] Current methods for processing frozen red blood cells, and a discussion on their safety factors, efficiency, and applicability for civilian and military use were reported recently.[393,394]

Japanese experience[172] with the preservation of glycerol-protected packed red blood cells shows results similar to those found in the United States. Transfusion of the frozen and subsequently thawed blood does not bring any unfavorable reactions. Unfortunately, it appears that the freezing of blood cannot fully prevent posttransfusion hepatitis.[172] Dutch experience with the freezing and preservation of blood shows equally good results.[202]

Recently Huggins[160] developed a new technique permitting the freezing of large quantities of blood, thereby opening the possibility for the clinical application of frozen human blood. Huggins successfully used the frozen blood protected by glycerol or DMSO for repeated transfusions in patients. The frozen blood was kept in disposable plastic bags at a temperature of −85 C, while the thawing was done at a temperature of 40 C. The cryoprotectants as well as the white blood cells and some of the red blood cells destroyed by freezing, had to be washed out before transfusion.[392] Huggins[160] observed additional beneficial effects in patients with acquired hemolytic anemia after transfusions of frozen blood. The mechanism of this unusual acceptance of frozen red blood cells in patients with hemolytic anemia is not yet understood. If this observation is substantiated, the administration of frozen blood might become a new therapeutic approach in the treatment of this disease.

Frozen blood was used, though not on a large scale, in Vietnam. Forty-three patients received a total of 307 units of frozen blood at Danang, South Vietnam.[394] No significant difference was observed in the patients who received frozen red cells as compared to the patients who received nonfrozen cells. The plasma hemoglobin, bilirubin, platelet counts, urine hemoglobin, and serum creatinine after the transfusions were the same in both groups of patients. Valeri[394] discussed the indications for the use of frozen blood and pointed to the minimal logistic problems in supplying the frozen red cells to wounded soldiers or civilians.

Besides other factors, the extent of the freezing injury depends on the rate of freezing.[264,314] While rapid freezing of blood per se is better than slow freezing, the presence of glycerol protects the blood even during slow cooling.[208] For most of the cells the least injurious rate of freezing is 1 C/min, but the erythrocytes can tolerate a much faster rate of freezing. The storage temperature is important also to preserve the viability of frozen blood. Nevertheless, even under optimal situations the enzyme activity of the blood decreases and the aging process of the blood continues, though at a much slower pace than at a temperature of 4 C. After a 3-year storage the activity of the enzyme aldolase of the frozen blood is decreased to 50 percent. The sugar-protected erythrocytes kept at a temperature of −93 C survive better than when they are preserved at higher temperatures.[378] It appears that for most tissues and cells the safest storage temperature is the temperature of liquid nitrogen, −197 C,[201] and that a controlled cooling and warming is critical for the success of cell survival.[88]

Freezing of leukocytes (10% DMSO) has recently received major emphasis because of the eventual application in the supportive management of leukopenic patients.[75] Lethally irradiated guinea pigs can survive when infused with an adequate amount of homologous peripheral frozen blood leukocytes.[296]

Lymphocytes stored with DMSO at a temperature of −196 C survive freezing and can be used clinically.[22,202] For liquid nitrogen storage, ethylene glycol with dialysis after thawing gives optimum results.[162] Effective preservation of leukocytes[330] can be obtained by freezing with either DMSO or glycerol. The temperature of liquid nitrogen appears to be a suitable storage temperature.[327]

On the basis of experimental observations, Malinin[233] suggested that human PMN cannot withstand freezing in the presence of DMSO, and that the primary site of cryoinjury is the nucleus, and not the cytoplasm.

The long-term freezing preservation of platelets is of practical importance (as, for instance, in severe thrombocytopenia)[28] because the platelets perish after a few hours during a 4 C storage. It appears that DMSO protects the platelets during freezing[164] even when the freezing lasts 24 hours or longer.[116] The platelet numbers in preparations containing 1 M dimethyl sulfoxide and stored at −70 C for 8 days were not significantly different from those of the control suspensions.[134] Although experimentation in platelet freezing is still in its infancy, early results suggest the possibility of a meaningful improvement in the near future.

Blood serum can be successfully frozen.[92] When kept in this state at a temperature of −130 C for 3 years, it remains practically unchanged.[93] As shown during World War II plasma can be freeze-dried[133] for subsequent intravenous infusion. Current processing of plasma is based on the experience gained at that time.

It should be mentioned also that splenic cells, protected by 10 percent DMSO, have been frozen for 52 days and after thawing produced the same immunological activity as fresh cells.[137]

FREEZING OF ORGANIZED TISSUES AND ORGANS

Freezing of Bone Marrow

The complex tissue of bone marrow survives freezing with cryoprotective agents.[21,23,64,291] When cryoprotective substances are omitted, cell destruction of bone marrow becomes apparent. Successful freezing of bone marrow has aroused much interest because of the possibility of treating the hematopoietic system of man after radiation injury. Radiation protection of mice with bone marrow and spleen preserved at below freezing temperatures using polyvinylpyrrolidone was reported by Persidsky and Richards.[292]

The bone marrow is obtained by multiple aspiration (15–20 punctures) from the sternum and iliac bone. After sieving, the marrow is centrifuged and cooled in a 15 percent glycerol solution to 79 C.[288] Mouse bone marrow is well protected during freezing with glycerol.[388] DMSO adequately protects human bone marrow during freezing[135,284] and so does polyvinylpyrrolidone.[206] Lethally irradiated mice survive when injected with fresh or frozen bone marrow,[105] either isologous or homologous.[165] A storage temperature of −196 C appears to be better than one of −79 C.[285] Storage temperature of −100 C and DMSO preserve hematopoietic stem cells. These cells undergo self-renewal after being injected into lethally irradiated mice.[273]

Malinin et al[234] have shown that bone marrow frozen with glycerol and stored in liquid nitrogen (−120 to −196 C) was largely intact after 3-year storage.

Whole bone preservation by freezing is possible also,[61] though the cells of the bone graft die during freezing or freeze-drying. Frozen and devitalized bone is slowly resorbed and simultaneously replaced with new bone, a long-lasting healing process.[99] It appears, however, that replacement with frozen homographs is much slower than with fresh ones. However, it is not necessary for a bone graft to possess viable cells in order to stimulate bone repair on the part of the host. On account of the quoted observations, efforts in the field of bone freezing have been directed more toward preserving the osseous matrix than the viable cells.

By using a slow rate of cooling, Bartlett and Reade[35] successfully stored developing teeth in liquid nitrogen for periods of up to 3 months.

Freezing of Whole Organs

Few organs have been successfully frozen with cryoprotective agents. The hearts of 2-day-old chick embryos frozen in liquid nitrogen with 30 percent ethylene glycol resumed rhythmic activity after thawing.[128] Chicken embryos, frozen without cryoprotective agents, contract spontaneously when transplanted into the anterior chamber of rats' eyes. A small number of isolated heart muscle cells (8%) resume beating after freezing storage without cryoprotective substances.[339]

As Karow has shown in his experiments, a rat heart with cryoprotective agents can be frozen in vitro to a temperature of −20 C and kept at this temperature for 20 minutes before thawing. Spontaneous cardiac contraction after thawing was observed in 80 percent of the cases when slow cooling and 15 percent DMSO in Ringer solution were used.[186] The hearts that survived freezing had diminished contractile strengths and heart rates.[354] Longer storage or higher storage temperature decreases the probability of resuscitation.[190] Long-lasting freezing storage or higher concentrations of DMSO (30%) proved toxic[179] and the hearts failed to recover.[184] It should be pointed out that in this last case the rat hearts did not undergo the freezing process despite the temperature. On the other hand, it appears that some other organs have been supercooled without freezing and remained viable.

Hearts frozen to a temperature of −20 C without cryoprotectants do not survive freezing.[353]

Thus it appears that the concentration, the duration of exposure, and the temperature of administered cryoprotective agents determine the toxicity for isolated frozen hearts.[182,183] In order to keep a rat's heart perfused with blood until the moment of freezing a special Plexiglas device was recently developed with modified Wollenberger tongs.[213] There is indication that metabolic inhibitors such as magnesium sulfate which protect normothermic or slightly hypothermic hearts from anoxia[404] might be used in the future for the same purpose to protect hearts during freezing. Unfortunately, at least for the moment, the hearts of laboratory animals bigger than rats seem to be too large for successful freezing and thawing.[185,226,311] The difficulties found by workers in this field demonstrate the seriousness of the problems encountered in freezing large solid organs.[53,236] It has been suggested that the long-term preservation of the heart and other solid organs can be accomplished only by uniform freezing and uniform thawing. Supercooling, cooling without freezing, might be another approach when short-lasting preservation of hearts is needed.[168]

Unlike whole hearts, major blood vessels are remarkably resistant to freezing in vitro.[157] Despite the fact that the viability of the blood vessels is lost after freezing and thawing, they can still be used. The nonviable collagenous and elastic tissues of the wall permit functions of the wall structure as a blood conduit until regrowth and repair from healthy unfrozen areas occur.[114,151] The main advantage of this technique is that it permits the storage of arterial grafts, frozen and kept at room temperature.

There is no change in the small blood vessels in the rabbit ear frozen to a temperature of −10 C and thawed in vivo. The circulatory changes of large blood vessels in the ear observed after thawing might be associated with endogenous substances liberated or activated during freezing injury.[316]

However, microcirculation in cheek pouch of the golden hamster was profoundly changed after freezing and thawing. Momentary vasoconstriction was followed with progressive vasodilation, hyperemia, and eventual stasis. The arrest of circulation following freezing persisted throughtout a period of 24 hours and was confirmed by thrombosis of microvessels as observed by histological examination of the hamster's cheek pouch.[414]

Frozen skin homografts were found to be viable after supercooling[109,187] or freezing. A good protective effect has been demonstrated with ethylene glycol (30%) although DMSO is also effective.[30,199] Human skin protected by 30 percent glycerol and then frozen grows in a plasma clot culture like fresh skin.[26] Rewarming after profound cooling and supercooling of mouse skin does not change the oxygen consumption of the tissues although brief freezing decreases it appreciably.[109] The ears of rabbits can tolerate exposure to a temperature of −180 C for merely a few seconds. Longer exposure damages the ears permanently.[200]

Freeze-dried fascia lata can be used clinically with the same results as fresh tissue.[385]

The functional survival of smooth muscle cooled to −79 C is greatly improved by increasing the concentration of DMSO during cooling to prevent freezing[98] and by decreasing the concentration of the cryoprotectant during rewarming to avoid toxicity.[102] Attempts were also made to freeze dog lungs rapidly in situ.[120] In this case the ice-crystal formation was submicroscopic. A study with a light microscope indicated a good histological preservation of lung tissue.[373]

While kidney cells may be frozen and thawed with a high degree of success,[2] the whole kidneys of dogs were frozen and thawed with only partial success. After 10 to 30 minutes of freezing and after reimplantation of the kidneys in the right iliac fossa, 9 dogs in a group of 14 (after contralateral nephrectomy) had some renal functions.[268] Similar results were obtained by Halasz and co-workers.[140,141] Rapid freezing and rapid thawing can be performed when the kidneys of rats are used in situ. A freezing process of only a few seconds does not permanently damage the kidneys even in the absence of cryoprotectants.[66] The freezing process of the larger dog kidneys is much slower. It requires 2 to 5 hours for the temperature in the center of a large kidney to reach −180 C.[166] The freezing of large kidneys can be made faster and more uniform by perfusing the renal artery with liquid nitrogen.[336] In addition the potentially harmful long thawing time can be shortened by combining warm immersion as soon as possible with a warm perfusion.[375] It appears that a concentration of DMSO higher than 15 percent might offer solutions for more successful freezing of whole kidneys. The process of elimination of the cryoprotective substances after thawing and before rewarming the kidneys to a normal temperature is a considerable one, but it must be performed to avoid the overhydration of cells and edema.[67] At a normal body temperature glycerol is completely absorbed by the kidneys.[203] Even during the deglycerolization of the kidneys one still observes a large accumulation of edema fluid. The level of edema is decreased as the glycerol concentration of the kidneys becomes lower.[67] The water content of isolated kidneys is changed also when DMSO is added to the perfusate.[287] It is likely that the prolonged thawing periods are more destructive to the organs than the fast and well-controlled freezing.[236] The thawing of frozen kidneys by electrical conduction methods might offer some improvements, but this method is still in an early developmental phase.[193] The same applies to shortwave diathermy, the results of which have been unfavorable up to now.[210] In order to simplify the present complicated techniques (reimplantation of kidneys, problems of homograft rejection, etc.) to assess the viability of kidneys after freezing and thawing, new biochemical and histological methods for an evaluation of cellular damage in kidneys have been developed recently.[1,38,39,390]

Thermoelectric modules for encompassing canine kidneys were constructed a few years ago. They permit faster freezing of the kidney, reducing the time from 1 or 2 hours to 12 minutes.[218] Though the cooling device developed for this purpose is still crude for a controlled and uniform freezing, it still offers some advantages over the old techniques. These advantages include the application of a better control of the storage temperature, an easy adaptation for hyperbaric oxygen, and a combination with microwave heating. This technique has kept hypothermic though not frozen kidneys viable after a storage of 18 hours.

Because of the difficulties in preserving kidneys by freezing, supercooling them with DMSO has been attempted. After the reimplantation of the supercooled but not frozen kidneys of dogs, some functions like urine secretion were observed but no long-term survivals ever occurred.[230] Better results including the survival of dogs for 1 year were obtained when the supercooling of the kidney was done under 3 atmospheres of pure oxygen. However, the contralateral nephrectomy was performed in this case 3 weeks after the reimplantation of the supercooled kidney and the supercooling lasted merely 24 hours.[329] As was mentioned earlier, the hypothermic perfusion keeps the kidneys viable for periods twice as long as the kidneys that have been supercooled. Microwave heating, which would permit a fast and more uniform rewarming of the frozen kidneys and other solid organs, was attempted recently,[142] though the results were unsatisfactory on account of thermal runaway. This problem may be overcome with the construction of better microwave systems. It appears that the technique of low-frequency microwave heating offers at the present time more hope than any other one for controlled and uniform rewarming of organs.

Experiments of rapid thawing and of rapid perfusion of frozen dog livers have been reported. In these experiments the livers were pretreated with 33 percent glycerol and stored for a short time at a temperature of −20 C. The viability of thawed livers was proved by clearance studies and by their oxygen consumption after thawing.[265] Unfortunately, it has been shown that freezing of mouse livers destroys 50 percent of succinate-cytochrome C reductase system.[106]

In 1967 Hamilton and Lehr[143] demonstrated that the small intestine survives after 7 days of storage at −196 C. Bowel segments protected by DMSO or glycerol were successfully frozen using cold helium intraarterially and cold nitrogen intraluminally.[136]

Pieces of the parathyroid gland frozen rapidly and stored at a temperature of liquid nitrogen, show weak evidence of activity after implantation in parathyroidectomized animals. When the pieces of parathyroid glands were frozen in 15 percent glycerol, to a temperature of −195 C, the activity of the implants remained strong even after 75 days of freezing, and the serum calcium level of the parathyroidectomized recipients was found to be at the normal value. As in some cases described earlier, a more profound cooling (to a temperature of −195 C) provided better and longer protection, up to 125 days.[331,332] In another group of experiments pieces of thyroid tissue protected by DMSO after 14 days of storage at a temperature of −196 C were autotransplanted into the cerebral cortex. Histological examination 6 to 12 weeks after autotransplantation showed apparent viability of the transplanted tissue.[355] Survival of adrenocortical tissue of rats after freezing was also observed.[281]

Ovarian tissue probably can be successfully frozen with 15 percent (v/v) glycerol. Rat uterine horns, protected with glycerol[215] or with DMSO,[73] as well as the dog ureter[33] were frozen in liquid nitrogen equally well. The increased net weight of the tissue after thawing is associated with osmotic shock during the glycerol removal, while the loss of potassium and gain of sodium is associated with the freezing process itself. The dose–response curve to serotonin and acetylcholine of the thawed horns remained unchanged.[73]

Peripheral nerves excised from several species of Alaskan mammals continue to conduct impulses even when supercooled to a temperature of −6 C.[260] DMSO in 5 or 10 percent concentration offers significant cryoprotection for up to a 2 hours exposure to the frozen ventral nerves of Homarus.[20] Freezing pieces of the superior cervical ganglia of rats at a temperature of −76 C was unsuccessful without, but successful with 15 percent glycerol.[283] The transmitted action potentials of the ganglion were well preserved.[303] On the other hand, Suda et al[381] have found that excised cat brain protected with glycerol and frozen for 76 days shows electrical activity after thawing.

Corneal epithelium protected by glycerol during freezing and corneal endothelium protected by DMSO develop clear grafts in 75 percent of cases when the full-thickness transplants are implanted in the eyes of rabbits.[267] The rate of freezing (controlled freezing) seems to be very important for the favorable freezing of corneal tissue. Once the optimal freezing curves and the optimal concentration of the protective agents are determined, 100 percent survival of human endothelial corneal cells is observed.[72] Frozen corneas are used today in clinical practice. Completely satisfactory transplanted corneal grafts, both homo and hetero, were achieved after freezing with cryoprotective substances. Good results in transplantation of lamellar grafts frozen with glycerol were also reported. Good functional corneal grafts in human patients were described after the entire eye was soaked before freezing in 15 percent glycerol for 1 hour. Before successful transplantation donor eyes can be kept at a temperature of −79 C for 10 to 30 days.[266]

An apparatus for the simultaneous programmed control of DMSO concentration and temperature in organ perfusion was recently developed[286] which might overcome some of the present difficulties during controlled freezing of organs. Several attempts have been made to cool and freeze organized tissues to −79 C without permitting the concentration of electrolytes to increase above the normal level.[9] This method when fully developed might be of importance for useful freezing of organs.

It has been found that whole organs which have been frozen can be better transplanted than whole fresh organs. This might be of extreme importance for the development of future trends in organ transplantation. Whole rat adrenals and aortic segments can be better transplanted after freezing than when they are fresh. After transplantation the frozen adrenals show a decreased lymphocytic infiltration into the graft, a decreased host response, and an increased regenerative activity of the adrenal cortical cells and of the vascular endothelium. The reactions of the connective tissue are diminished if the connective tissue is frozen before transplantation. Vascularization of the transplanted renal tissue of rats is much improved after freezing of the graft in liquid nitrogen.[170] Immunological reactions of skin homografts are also decreased after freezing.

Surgical techniques during the past 20 years have progressed greatly and now permit transplantation of whole organs, including kidneys, lungs, spleens, and hearts. Immunological hazards after transplantation might be reduced by irradiation, by toxic drugs, and maybe even by freezing. The scarcity of organs is already the major limiting factor for success in the promising field of organ transplantation. It is likely that freezing may make available an unlimited number of organs for transplantation. For this purpose close collaboration of investigators in surgery, immunology, cryobiology, and other disciplines is needed.

Summary

On the basis of the information presented here it appears that the most promising approach for long-term preservation of whole organs is the use of controlled freezing, by means of the Peltier effect[97] combined with the highest tolerable concentrations of cryoprotective agents. The storage temperature should be rather low, probably as low as −190 C. The thawing should be fast and controlled employing low-frequency microwave heating. Effective removal of cryoprotective agents with the aid of dialyzing systems during the rewarming should be performed. Another possibility for successful freezing of organs might be a slow initial freezing which will induce "seeding" of microscopic ice crystals throughout the organ at temperatures of −5 to −15 C. This should be followed by a sudden rapid cooling of organs down to a temperature of −76 C or lower.[405]

FREEZING OF WHOLE MAMMALS

It appears that even in those instances when cells can be recovered after freezing, the percentage of recovery is never complete. In the case of organ systems or whole organisms and their functional relationships, recovery from freezing is not possible at the present time. The techniques which are adequate for single cells to be recovered from freezing are not applicable to complex organ systems or whole organisms. Speaking of freezing of whole organisms, Meryman[258] says the fact that "visions in the past have come true is no guarantee that all science fiction is but prologue to fact." The opinion of the authors of this book is that in the not too distant future successful freezing of complex organ systems and of small mammals will be accomplished. What is needed at the moment are new techniques and new approaches that will open new promising pathways.

The fact that artifically cooled young animals tolerate the same degree of deep body cooling for much longer periods than adult animals and the fact that adult hibernators are able to survive deep hypothermia longer than artifically cooled nonhibernators suggested

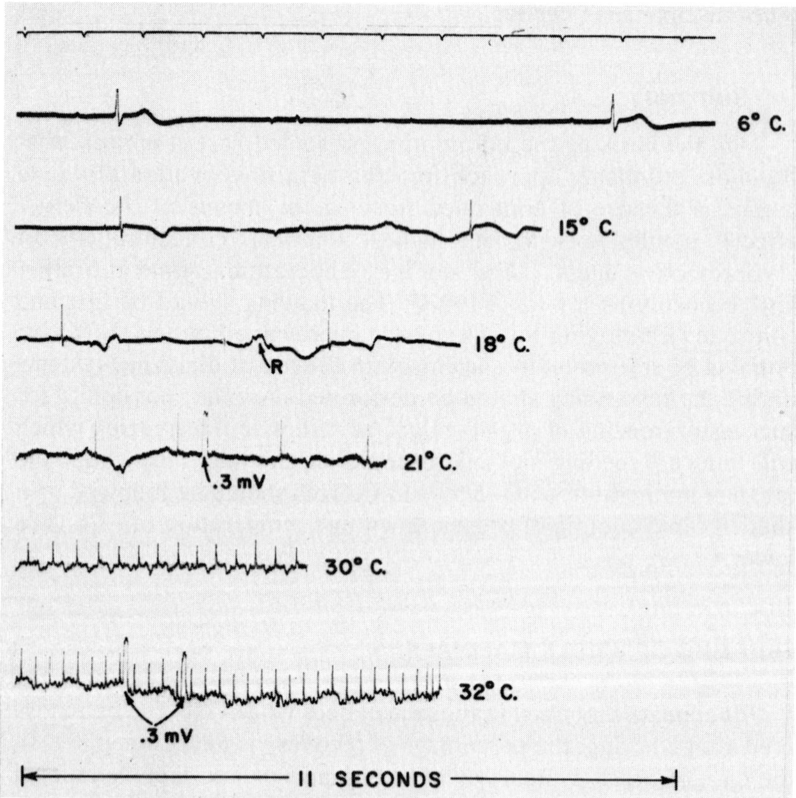

Fig. 1-2. Electrocardiogram of a 3.9-gm newborn ground squirrel during rewarming. Before rewarming the animal was kept 5 hours at a body temperature of −4 C. Top tracing shows the timed interval in seconds. Temperatures refer to the esophageal ones. First respiration (R) observed is at the body temperature of 18 C. Electrical calibration (0.3 mv) is included in the fourth and sixth tracing.

the idea that baby hibernators might survive a supercooling state better than any other group of mammals. The work of Popovic and Popovic proved that this is the case.[304] Newborn ground squirrels cooled to a body temperature of −3 to −4 C survived heart standstill longer than was previously thought possible for any mammal (Figs. 1-2 and 1-3).[304] Although there was not detectable electrical activity of their hearts, the animals were revived after having been in a supercooled state for 11 hours at a body temperature of −4 C. Deeper cooling to −8 C shortened the survival time to 5 hours. This fact may be explained by a probable increase of ice crystals already formed in the animal's body. The newborn gound squirrels survived only a short freezing exposure. Despite the fact that some of the animals seemed to be frozen, it is not certain that any of the surviving ground squirrels were completely frozen. When the temperature of the freezing medium was decreased to −70 C and the body temperature of the animals decreased to −15 to −35 C, the animals did not recover, but nevertheless showed some electrical cardiac activity during the rewarming period. The mechanism of this highly developed resistance to supercooling of the newborn ground squirrels is not clear. When baby rats were cooled to the same body temperature of −4 to −8 C, they did not survive, although their hearts resumed beating during rewarming. Baby rats survived 1 hour of supercooling at temperatures ranging from −1 to −3 C.[305]

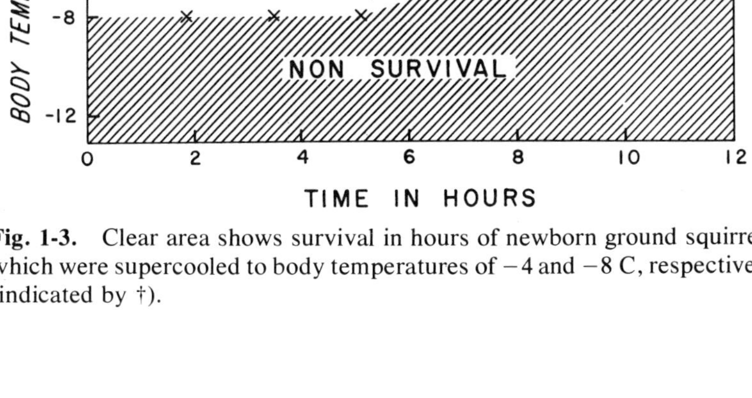

Fig. 1-3. Clear area shows survival in hours of newborn ground squirrels which were supercooled to body temperatures of −4 and −8 C, respectively (indicated by †).

Attempts to freeze the entire bodies of large experimental animals have been completely unsuccessful, whereas partial freezing of small laboratory animals was possible in a few cases.[7,8,224,361–364,366,368] Artificially cooled hibernators withstood the partial freezing better than nonhibernators.[364] This difference might be attributed to a faster reestablishment of the interrupted circulation observed in hibernators.[229] It appears that for this purpose fast rewarming from partial freezing might be beneficial and that microwave heating may offer better possibilities than other methods.[222]

Quite recently Mazur and co-workers made a breakthrough in the freezing of whole animals.[408] Mouse embryos survived freezing to −196 C. Survival required slow cooling (0.3 to 2 C/min). Depending on the specific rates used, 50 to 70 percent of more than 2500 frozen and thawed early embryos developed into blastocysts in culture after storage at −196 C for up to 8 days. When approximately 1000 of the survivors, including some frozen to −269 C (4 K), were transferred into foster mothers, 65 percent of the recipients became pregnant. More than 40 percent of the embryos in these pregnant mice gave rise to normal, living full-term fetuses or newborn mice.

Summary

Obviously, before entering into any clinical application of freezing, it would be well advised to look back and to evaluate the successes of freezing preservations. They are few but still impressive: blood, corneas, and sperm have been successfully frozen and there are some indications that successful freezing of whole organs may not be too far away.

FROSTBITE

Local cold injury by freezing peripheral tissues produces frostbites. Ninety-two thousand cases of frostbite were reported during World War II and 5000 during the Korean War. The clinical manifestations of frostbite are well known.[51] Trench foot often develops in soldiers who have their feet exposed for long periods of time to damp and cold but not necessarily a freezing environment.

Frostbite induces three types of vascular changes: arterial spasm, arteriovenous shunting, and arterial occlusions which are observed only in severe frostbite.[237] As the consequence of these vascular changes, tissue edema, blistering necrosis, and subsequent gangrene are seen. There are investigators who believe, however, that frostbite necrosis is induced by the direct effect of cold on the tissue and therefore represents a true thermal injury.

It appears that the vascular lesions due to frostbite embrace both endothelial injury with adherence of the formed blood elements, stasis, and thrombosis as well as an increased permeability of the capillaries with tissue edema. The first part of the problem might be solved, at least partially, by the administration of heparin.[31]

The amount of ice formed in the tissues depends mainly on the external temperature.[43] In experiments on the amputated feet of mice an external temperature of −2 C induced a 30 percent ice formation, while a temperature of −10 C increased the amount of ice formed to 50 percent.[227]

Immobility due to alcoholic stupor or peripheral vascular insufficiency increases the susceptibility to frostbite. Double freezing (freezing–thawing–freezing) produces in mice more tissue loss than a single freezing exposure.[261] Rapid thawing after experimental frostbite has been demonstrated to be more beneficial than a slow one.[145] However, the authors of some textbooks of surgery still suggest that a very gradual rewarming is the best treatment.[27]

The edema induced during freezing can be used for the determination of the degree of freezing injury according to Persidsky et al.[294]

Cold acclimation decreases the danger of experimental frostbite in rabbits[351] but hyperbaric oxygenation is not of value in reducing tissue loss in experimental and probably in clinical frostbite.[115]

Also low-molecular-weight dextran markedly improves the tissue survival after freezing injury. Unfortunately, dextran is effective if administered before, but not after, freezing.[269]

The rate of healing after frostbite was significantly improved after regional sympathectomy, as shown by Shumacker and other investigators.[94,123,124,237,357,358] It appears, however, that sympathectomy affects the vascular spasm only and does not help in the case of arterial occlusion produced by severe frostbite.[237]

Summary

The physiology and pathology of frostbite were once extensively studied. Today the interest has decreased except perhaps for

Russian investigators. Though most investigators believe that frostbite is not a direct thermal consequence of the exposure of cells and tissues to cold, some investigators disagree with this view. Frostbite induces vascular changes in various degrees according to the length of exposure, the external temperature, and the physiological conditions of the exposed organism. Rapid rewarming or thawing might be beneficial for a speedy recovery from frostbite damage, though most textbooks of surgery still suggest a very gradual rewarming. Regional sympathectomy improves the healing process at least in less severe cases.

CRYOTHERAPY

Cryotherapy is a new brand of therapeutics that relies on the local tissue changes induced by rapid freezing.

Gastric Freezing for Gastric Ulcers

Many attempts have been made in the past to develop an effective treatment for peptic ulcers without resorting to operations. Freezing, as a tool for this purpose, was pioneered by Wangensteen and co-workers in 1962.[399] They chose for this new technique an attractive name—"physiological gastrectomy."[400] Later the name was changed to "gastric freezing."[131,132,297,298,401] Wagensteen and his associates observed that in dogs,[130,321] as well as in human patients,[47] there was a profound decrease of HCl gastric secretion after gastric freezing, a decrease that lasted for 2 to 6 months.[401,402] Furthermore, development of experimental ulcers in rats was also prevented by gastric freezing.[250] A number of investigators agree that there is a decrease in gastric secretion after gastric freezing but that this decrease is a temporary one, lasting only 2 to 3 months.[174,295,323,340,384]

A temporary gastric secretory depression can be produced by "cryogenic vagotomy," freezing without destruction of the gastric mucosa.[175] Repeated treatments with gastric freezing in patients (30 for second time, 6 for third time) produced the same temporary secretory changes and relief as did the first gastric freezing.[178] In dogs 20 freezing treatments did not induce a prolonged or profound decrease in his-tamine-stimulated gastric acid output.[295] Most investigators agree, however, that there is an immediate relief of ulcer symptoms after freezing,[11,129,341,384] though much of it may be of a subjective nature.[153]

Though the freezing of peptic ulcers has already been performed on thousands of patients, reports on the results are still conflicting.[54] This especially concerns the complications after freezing, such as mucosal ulceration, necrosis, and bleeding.[46,238,239,247,248,251,341,415] Some investigators question the degree of the effectiveness of freezing in ulcer disease,[322] whereas others do not find any significant decrease in acid secretion after gastric freezing.[44,45,52,118,156,191,225,252,276] Shingleton and his associates[194] suggest an extensive selective parietal cell damage in order to achieve the inhibition of gastric acidity. Some investigators compare the effects of gastric freezing on the stomach tissues to the effects of frostbite on other tissues[198] while others find additional complications that sometimes accompany gastric freezing (for instance, atrial fibrillation).[317] There are reports that vitamin B_{12} absorption is not altered after gastric freezing[158] or that it is only temporarily decreased.[32]

Melnyk and co-workers[256] developed a gastric freezing apparatus but were unable to cool the gastric walls uniformly and therefore they could not obtain predictable responses after each gastric freezing. Improved freezing devices were recently developed by Shingleton et al[352] and by Blumgart et al[55] which might solve this problem at least partially, while Sulman and Ferguson[383] suggested gastric freezing by direct alcohol perfusion.

Although these techniques appear to be promising,[12,177,197] further development is needed to decrease complications after gastric freezing. Until that time arrives, it has been suggested that gastric freezing should be limited to carefully controlled studies in selected centers because of the complicated procedures and some of the inherent dangers.[342,407]

Gastric freezing should be distinguished from gastric hypothermia, which is sometimes called "gastric cooling" or "localized gastric cooling." Gastric hypothermia is a cooling of the stomach, above the freezing point. Gastric hypothermia is beneficial (only temporarily) for massive upper gastrointestinal hemorrhage[150,176,196,249] probably because it leads to decreased volume blood flow through the splanchnic region induced by a decreased temperature of stomach tissues.[299,372] Gastric hypothermia has the same depressing effect on the gastric secretion as gastric freezing. However, the effect of gastric hypothermia is of a much shorter duration (only 2–3 weeks) than that observed after gastric freezing.[401] The term "supercooled stomach" was introduced by McSweeney et al in 1963[253] for the cooling of stomachs in dogs to a temperature of −10 to −12 C, without freezing the stomach walls. The stomachs so cooled remained soft and pliable. However, this technique did not receive as wide an application as did the stomach freezing.

Cryosurgery for Cancers

Many of the early investigators suggested that the local application of extreme cold would facilitate the destruction of some tumors. Arnot[10] used ice-cold brine to diminish the growth of cancer tissue. Bory[57–59] employed cryosurgery for small surface tumors, mostly the tumors of the face that appear in older persons. Cryogenic surgery for the treatment of tumors was pioneered in the United States by Cooper et al in 1962[83] and in 1963.[86] Earlier Hass and Taylor[146] locally froze parts of rabbit brains to stress the fact that cryosurgical techniques are essentially hemostatic. The objective of cryosurgery is to kill all of the cells in the diseased target area with a minimum injury to the surrounding healthy tissue.[244] This is done by the insertion of a freezing probe into the tumor (penetration freezing). Freezing can be induced without the insertion of a cryocannula in the tissue. Such a technique of inducing cryosurgical lesions is called contact freezing.[69] It appears that multiple freezing increases the lethality to the target area.[243] In order to produce permanent lesions the cryoprobes must be applied at least twice. Removal of the tumor as a solid frozen mass also represents an advantage.[80] During the last several years various tumors were subjected to freezing in situ.[69,81] The necrosis after freezing became so predictable that Cahan[69] proposed the term cryonecrosis for this process. The main advantage of this technique is considerable palliation of the distressing symptoms of incurable cancers. The pain and the tumor size are reduced as well as the drainage and odor. Furthermore, many investigators have observed a decreased bleeding after cryosurgery. Contrary to these observations it has been suggested that heat in electrosurgery is still the best and the most reliable technique for control of bleeding.

Cryosurgery was used for transplanted cancers[122] and for

virus-induced tumors in hamsters but without much success except for a temporary decrease in tumor size.[205]

The survival of patients after cryotherapy is not significantly increased except in a few cases.[112] Slow thawing after cryosurgery of tumors appears to be better than fast thawing.[69] However, excellent results were obtained when cryosurgery was used to eradicate cutaneous carcinomas[413] or large malignant epitheliomas[412] and other skin cancers. The technique is simple and effective, and the surgery leaves a minimal residual scarring.

Cryosurgery was successfully employed in oral cancer treatments, especially for the tumors resistant to radiation therapy and the tumors in difficult locations, particularly in the very weak or the very sick patients.[111,113] Cryotherapy was successfully used for freezing a mandible without excision.[99] Nasopharyngeal and laryngeal cancer cryosurgery also appear to be successful.[36,37,212,370] The same also applies to inoperable rectal cancers.[81,110] After cryosurgery for rectal cancer, the sensation of tenesmus and the chronic urge to defecate are alleviated. Blood loss appears to be decreased as well as mucus secretion. Old and weak patients withstand cryosurgey rather well.[81] Bone deformity and disability after cryosurgery are small when compared with other types of surgical procedures.

Cryosurgery for brain tumors is often used either to destroy the tumor tissue or to facilitate the removal of the tumor as a solid frozen mass.[80,207,397] Cryosurgery was used for treatment of malignant tumors of other parts of the head and for tumors of the neck. Some alterations of the blood–brain barrier have been described after cryosurgery of the brain. These changes give a positive scan for several days after the lesions. However, the scan is not observed after 30 days though some alteration of blood–brain barrier is still present.[397] The treatment of Parkinsonian patients to relieve tremor and rigidity has been improved recently. Cryotherapy gave surgeons the possibility to test the effects of slight cooling on unanesthetized patients, thereby inducing reversible changes before producing the permanent freezing lesions in the ventrolateral nucleus of the thalamus.[82,216,398] Stereotoxic cryosurgery of the pituitary gland was used for treatment of carcinoma of the breast.[410] Cryosurgery was successfully applied in the treatment of glomus tumors of the middle ear.[214] Rowbotham et al[325] described the experimental and clinical results obtained with cryosurgical cannulas for cerebral neoplasms. The low thermal conductivity of the brain was considered to be a favorable factor for the use of cryogenic techniques.

It appears, therefore, that cryosurgery offers a controllable, avascular, rapid, and effective procedure for a new approach to the removal of deep intracerebral gliomas and some tumors on the base of the brain. The chance of spillage and the seeding of malignant cells are probably decreased as well. Furthermore, the period the patients remain hospitalized after cryosurgery for tumors is decreased. However, the major problem in the successful use of cryotherapy for the eradication of tumors is the involvement of the adjacent normal tissues during the freezing and thawing. Furthermore, we still need "clear confirmation of complete tumor cell death in any mass of tumor tissue"[108] to verify this hypothesis.

Cryogenic Techniques in Neurosurgery

Cryogenic techniques are used with success in neurosurgery for cryothalamectomy[85,87,309,398] or for third ventriculostomy in hydrocephalus.[63] Cooper[79] finds cryothalamectomy the treatment of choice for tremor caused by multiple sclerosis, certain cerebellar diseases, and for dystonia of various etiologies.

Cryotherapy for Other Causes

More than half a century ago investigators were calling attention to the damaging effects of freezing upon tissue[204] pointing toward clinical application of freezing injury. Controlled inactivation of tissues was advocated more recently.[146] Its use in tumor treatment and in neurosurgery cryotherapy has shown encouraging results in patients with gangrene complicated by sepsis. The mortality of 46 percent was decreased to 6 percent if the limbs of the patients were frozen (Dry Ice refrigeration).[163]

Cryotherapy has been employed to destroy lesions in the head and neck without pain or bleeding and with a minimum of tissue reaction.[395] Bellows[41] used cryotherapy for the temporary control of Herpes virus.

Cryoextraction was found to be superior to the traditional methods in cataract treatment.[34,40,42,78,89,121,173,192] Cryosurgery was also employed for the treatment of glaucoma.[409]

Painless cryotherapy without anesthesia was used for successful treatment of obstructions of the prostate in human patients[343] and in experimental animals.[127] One hundred patients, mostly poor-risk cases, were submitted to successful cryoprostatectomies at the University Clinics at Copenhagen.[144]

Cryosurgery for the uterus was reported by Cahan experimentally as well as clinically.[68,70] Cahan believes that cryosurgery of the uterus provides a simple, reliable, and economical means of producing the destruction of endometrium and, consequently, organ failure. Intrauterine cryosurgery can be accomplished with no postoperative deaths and with no morbidity attributable to the procedure.[70]

Cryotherapy was also successfully used for treatment of chronic cervicitis. Healing was complete 8 weeks after freezing.[275,280]

In experimental animals cryogenic liver lesions make a reproducible and easily controlled necrosis.[84]

Pituitary cryosurgery was performed on human patients[90] with acromegaly[91] or in treatment of breast and prostate cancers.[411] The major complications after this cryosurgical treatment in some cases are diabetes insipidus and cerebrospinal rhinorrhea.

Cryotonsillectomy by the contact freezing technique was used in experimental work[71] as well as for patients.

Cryoimmunotherapy

Possibilities that cryosurgery for tumors might induce some degree of autoimmunization was suggested by Bory[58] and by Cahan[69,126] but has not been definitely proved.[3] It appears that the tumors are more sensitive to freezing by the cryoprobes than the healthy tissue,[246] a fact which may be used in cryoimmunotherapy. The significance of the possible formation of antibodies after freezing, directed toward DNA and RNA in tumor cells, remains to be determined.[50] Several papers dealing with cryoimmunotherapy presented at one of the annual meetings of the Society of Cryobiology (1969 in Buffalo) indicate an increased interest and new possibilities for use of cryotherapy. Some of these presentations dealt with the cryodestruction and the immunological reactions of cells of the coagulating gland of male rabbits,[356] and with the immunologic response as a consequence of freezing the rabbit male accessory glands and their thyroid gland.[117]

Summary

On the basis of this discussion, it appears that cryosurgery for tumor treatment is a promising new technique, especially as an excellent additional therapy bringing a fast palliation even in the case of large and incurable tumors. Cryosurgery for other nontumor causes appears to offer some new additional benefits to the already established surgical methods. It might be especially useful for the treatment of prolonged hemorrhage in patients with blood dyscrasias, for tonsillectomy, in leukemia, for hemophiliac patients, and other cases.[69] The advantages of the cryosurgical technique are that it is essentially hemostatic, it induces conical and sharply delineated destructive changes, and it usually induces uniform, consistent, and reproducible alterations.

BIBLIOGRAPHY

1. Abbot WM: The biochemistry of freezing injury in kidneys. Cryobiology 4:266, 1968
2. Abbott WM: The physiology of renal preservation injury. I. Freezing injury and its modification. Cryobiology 5:300–305, 1969
3. Ablin RJ, Soanes WA, Gonder MJ: Prospects for cryoimmunotherapy in cases of metastasizing carcinoma of the prostate. Cryobiology 8:271–279, 1971
4. Akerblom O, de Verdier CH, Erikson A, et al: Rapid freezing of erythrocytes using glycerol in low concentrations. Proc 11th Congr Int Soc Blood Transf, Sydney, No. 29, 1966, pp 814–822
5. Altland PD, Highman B, Nelson BD, et al: Effects of dimethyl sulfoxide on serum enzymes and tissues in exercised rats. Life Sci 5:375–383, 1966
6. Altland PD, Highman B, Parker M: Induction of hypothermia by dimethyl sulfoxide in rats exposed to cold: Tissue and enzyme changes. Proc Soc Exp Biol Med 123:853–859, 1966
7. Andjus RK: Suspended animation in cooled, supercooled and frozen rats. J Physiol 128:547–556, 1955
8. Andjus RK, Lovelock JE, Smith AU: Resuscitation and recovery of hypothermic, supercooled, and frozen mammals, in Dripps RD (ed): The Physiology of Induced Hypothermia. Washington, National Academy of Sciences, 1956, pp 125–129
9. Armstrong JA, Farrant J, Walter CA: Prevention of damage to organized tissue during freezing and thawing. Cryobiology 2:301–302, 1966
10. Arnot JB: On treatment of cancer by the regulated application of an anesthetic temperature. London, Churchill, 1851
11. Artz CP, McFarland JB, Barnett WO: Clinical evaluation of gastric freezing for peptic ulcer. Ann Surg 159:758–764, 1964

12. Artz CP, McFarland JB, Fitts CT: The use of gastric freezing for the treatment of peptic ulcer disease. J Miss State Med Assoc 4:427–432, 1963
13. Asahina E: Motility of some animals and an excised tissue in supercooled state. Low Temp Sci 15:45–50, 1957
14. Asahina E: Prefreezing as a method enabling animals to survive freezing at an extremely low temperature. Nature 184:1003–1004, 1959
15. Asahina E: Intracellular freezing and frost resistance in egg-cells of the sea urchin. Nature 191:1263–1265, 1961
16. Asahina E, Takehara I: Supplementary notes on the frost-resistance of the slug, caterpillar, *Monema flavescens* I. Low Temp Sci 22:79–90, 1963
17. Asahina E, Tanno K: A large amount of trehalose in a frost-resistant insect. Nature 204:1222, 1964
18. Asahina E, Tanno K: Observations of ice crystals formed in frozen larvae (sic) of European corn-borer by the use of freeze-sectioning. Low Temp Sci 25:105–111, 1967
19. Asahina E, Tanno K: A frost-resistant adult insect, *Pterocormus molitorius* (Hymenoptera, Ichneumonidae). Low Temp Sci 26:85–89, 1968
20. Asher IM: Effects of DMSO on the electrical response of Homarus nerves frozen to −20°C, −30°C and at room temperature. Cryobiology 9:153–162, 1972
21. Ashwood-Smith MJ: Preservation of mouse bone marrow at −79°C with dimethyl sulphoxide. Nature 190:1204–1205, 1961
22. Ashwood-Smith MJ: Low temperature preservation of mouse lymphocytes with dimethyl sulfoxide. USNRDL-TR-689, 6 November 1963
23. Ashwood-Smith MJ: Blood and bone marrow preservation. Fed Proc 24, Suppl 15:S-299–S-301, 1965
24. Ashwood-Smith MJ: Radioprotective and cryoprotective properties of dimethyl sulfoxide in cellular systems. Ann NY Acad Sci 141:45–62, 1967
25. Ashwood-Smith MJ, Warby C: Protective effect of low and high molecular weight compounds on the stability of catalase subjected to freezing and thawing. Cryobiology 9:137–140, 1972
26. Athreya BH, Grimes EL, Lehr HB, et al: Differential susceptibility of epithelial cells and fibroblasts of human skin to freeze injury. Report on an improved method for storage of human skin at −196°C. Cryobiology 5:262–269, 1969
27. Bailey and Love's: Short Practice of Surgery, Philadelphia, Lippincott, 1968, pp 47–48
28. Baldini MG: Discussion on the current status of platelet preservation. Cryobiology 5:49–57, 1968
29. Barchi RL, Panuska JA, Gray I: Rate loss of dimethyl sulfoxide from tissues of euthermic and hypothermic rats. Fed Proc 28:792, 1969
30. Barlyn LW, Berggren RB, Lehr HB: Frozen skin autografts protected by dimethyl sulfoxide. Surg Forum 15:475–477, 1964
31. Barner HB: The vascular lesion of freezing as modified by dimethyl sulfoxide. Cryobiology 2:55–61, 1965
32. Barner HB, Jones TI, Garlick TB: Temporary impairment of vitamin B_{12} absorption—Another side effect of therapeutic gastric freezing. JAMA 190:779–781, 1964
33. Barner HB, Rivers BJ Jr, Cady B, et al: Survival of the canine ureter after freezing. Surgery 53:344–347, 1963

34. Barraquer JI: Keratomileusis. Int Surg 48:103–117, 1967
35. Bartlett PF, Reade PC: Cryopreservation of developing teeth. Cryobiology 9:205–211, 1972
36. Barton RT: Cryosurgical treatment of nasopharyngeal neoplasms. Am Surg 32:744–747, 1966
37. Barton RT: Cryosurgery in nose and throat tumors. JAMA 204:570–573, 1968
38. Beisang AA, Dietzman RH, Mayo CH, et al: Damage during perfusion procedures used to prepare whole organs for freezing. Cryobiology 4:263–264, 1968
39. Beisang AA, Dietzman RH, Mayo CH, et al: Damage during perfusion procedures used to prepare whole organs for freezing. Cryobiology 5:273–277, 1969
40. Bellows JG: The mechanical superiority and advantages of cryoextraction. Am J Ophthalmol 61:1003–1009, 1966
41. Bellows JG: Cryotherapy of herpesvirus keratitis in 1242 cases. Int Surg 50:489–494, 1968
42. Bellows JG: Cryoextraction of cataracts in 800 consecutive cases. Cryobiology 6:259–260, 1969
43. Bendarzewski L: Hypothermia and frostbite. Pol Tyg Lek 8:1478–1480, 1953
44. Berg CD, Nanson EM: Effects of gastric freezing on gastric secretions in dogs. Surg Forum 14:352–353, 1963
45. Berg CD, Nanson EM: Effect of antral freezing on isolated denervated gastric pouch secretions. Surg Gynecol Obstet 119:583–585, 1964
46. Berg CD, Nanson EM: Gastric ulcer: A sequela to gastric freezing. Can J Surg 7:341–346, 1964
47. Bernstein EF, Goodale RL Jr., McFee AS, et al: Interim report on results of gastric freezing for peptic ulcer. JAMA 187:436–441, 1964
48. Bickis IJ, Kazaks K, Finn, JJ, et al: Permeation kinetics of glycerol and dimethyl sulfoxide in Novikoff hepatoma ascites cells. Cryobiology 4:1–10, 1967
49. Blackshaw AW: Preservation of rabbit, sheep and ox red cells. Aust J Biol Sci 7:566–572, 1954
50. Blackwood J, Moore FT, Pace WG: Cryotherapy for malignant tumors. Cryobiology 4:33–38, 1967
51. Blair JR: Follow-up study of cold injury cases from the Korean War, in Ferrer EJ (ed): Fourth Conference on Cold Injury. New York, Josiah Macy Jr Foundation 1955, pp 9–35
52. Blixenkrone-Møller N, Olsen TS, Trophøj K: Morphological gastric changes after freezing by the method of Wangensteen. Acta Chir Scand 129:631–643, 1965
53. Bloch JH, Longerbeam JK, Manax WG, et al: Preservative solutions for freezing whole organs in vitro. Trans Am Soc Artif Intern Organs 9:139–147, 1963
54. Blumgart LH: Gastric "freezing." Gastroenterology 47:677–678, 1964
55. Blumgart LH, Naylor FD, Duthie HI: Assessment of a new inlet device for use in gastric hypothermia. J Br Soc Gastroenterol 6:407–410, 1965
56. Borchgrevink CF, Havel RJ: Transport of glycerol in human blood. Proc Soc Exp Biol Med, Suppl 113:946–949, 1963

57. Bory L: L'action biostatique et immunisante de la cryotherapie (la cytocryolyse). Therapie 8:219–222, 1953
58. Bory L: Logique de la cryotherapie dans le traitement des tumeurs. Presse Med 67:45–46, 1959
59. Bory L: De L'action du froid sur les tissus normaux et cancereux. Prog Med 4:75–77, 1960
60. Bouroncle BA: Preservation of human normal and leukemic cells with dimethyl sulfoxide at −80°C. Cryobiology 3:445–455, 1967
61. Boyne PJ: Review of the literature on cryopreservation of bone. Cryobiology 4:341–357, 1968
62. Bradham GB, Sample JJ: The vascular and thermal effects of dimethyl sulfoxide. Ann NY Acad Sci 141:225–230, 1967
63. Bryan N, Coe JE: Experimental alteration in cerebrospinal fluid production following cryosurgery of the choroid plexus. J Neurosurg 30:62–64, 1969
64. Buckner CD, Storb R, Dillingham LA, et al: Low temperature preservation of monkey marrow in dimethyl sulfoxide. Cryobiology 7:136–140, 1970
65. Bunge RG, Keettel WC, Sherman JK: Clinical use of frozen semen. Report of four cases. Fertil Steril 5:520–529, 1954
66. Bush IM, Santoni E, Lieberman PH, et al: Some effects of freezing the rat kidney in situ. Cryobiology 1:163–170, 1964
67. Cady B, Barner HB, Rivers RJ Jr, et al: Glycerolization of the canine kidney. I. Fluid exchanges. Cryobiology 3:76–80, 1966
68. Cahan WG: Cryosurgery of the uterus: Description of technique and potential application. Am J Obstet Gynecol 88:410–414, 1964
69. Cahan WG: Cryosurgery of malignant and benign tumors. Fed Proc 24, Suppl 15:S-241–S-248, 1965
70. Cahan WG, Brockunier A: Cryosurgery of the uterine cavity. Am J Obstet Gynecol 99:138–153, 1967
71. Cahan WG, Montesa-Cruz AF: Cryotonsillectomy in dogs. Arch Otolaryngol 81:372–378, 1965
72. Capella JA, Kaufman HE, Robbins JE: Preservation of viable corneal tissue. Cryobiology 2:116–121, 1965
73. Carroll PM, Lin JH: The protection of frozen-thawed rat uterus by glycerol and dimethyl sulfoxide. Cryobiology 5:226–233, 1968
74. Caujolle FME, Caujolle DH, Cros SB, et al: Limits of toxic and teratogenic tolerance of dimethyl sulfoxide. Ann N Y Acad Sci 141:110–126, 1967
75. Cavins JA, Djerassi I, Aghai E, et al: Current methods for the cryopreservation of human leukocytes (granulocytes). Cryobiology 5:60–69, 1968
76. Chilson OP, Costello LA, Kaplan NO: Effects of freezing on enzymes. Fed Proc 24, Suppl 15:S-55–S-65, 1965
77. Clark WA, Klein A: The stability of bacteriophages in longterm storage at liquid nitrogen temperatures. Cryobiology 3:68–75, 1966
78. Cole OW, Dunnigan WJ: Enzymatic zonulolysis and cryoextraction of cataracts. Int Surg 50:242–244, 1968
79. Cooper IS: Cryogenic surgery. A new method of destruction or extirpation of benign or malignant tissues. N Engl J Med 268:743–749, 1963
80. Cooper IS: Application of cryogenics to brain tumor surgery. Proceedings 3rd International Congress on Neurological Surgery, Copenhagen, 1965, pp 727–733

81. Cooper IS: Cryogenic surgery for cancer. Fed Proc 24, Suppl 15:S-237–S-240, 1965
82. Cooper IS: Cryogenic neurosurgery. Gen Pract 39:96–109, 1969
83. Cooper IS, Grissman F, Gorek E, et al: Cryogenic congelation and necrosis of cancer: A preliminary report. J Am Geriatr Soc 10:289–293, 1962
84. Cooper IS, Hirose T: Cryogenic hepatic surgery. J Cryosurg 1:116–122, 1968
85. Cooper IS, Lee A St J: Cryothalamectomy-hypothermic congelation: A technical advance in basal ganglia surgery: A preliminary report. J Am Geriatr Soc 9:714–718, 1961
86. Cooper IS, Stellar S: Cryogenic freezing of brain tumors for excision or destruction in situ. J Neurosurg 20:921–930, 1963
87. Cooper IS, Waltz JM: Cryogenic applications in neurosurgery. J Cryosurg 1:15–30, 1968
88. Cowley CW, Sawdye JA, Robbins HD: An analytical approach to the determination of processing techniques for the low temperature preservation of human erythrocytes. Cryobiology 1:324–333, 1965
89. Craig PC: Ophthalmo-cryosurgery. An international panel reports (editorial). Int Surg 49:509–512, 1968
90. Dashe AM: Medical considerations in pituitary cryosurgery. Int Surg 49:110–116, 1968
91. Dashe AM, Solomon DH, Rand RW, et al: Sterotaxic hypophyseal cryosurgery in acromegaly and other disorders. JAMA 198:591–596, 1966
92. Davies DF: Quantitative recovery of selected components of serum after rapid freezing and rapid thawing. Fed Proc 24, Suppl 15:S-249–S-252, 1965
93. Davies DF: Effects of freezing and thawing serum and plasma on selected quantitative recoveries. Cryobiology 5:87–95, 1968
94. deJong P, Golding MR, Sawyer PN, et al: The role of regional sympathectomy in the early management of cold injury. Surg Gynecol Obstet 115:45–48, 1962
95. Denko CW, Goodman RM, Miller R, et al: Distribution of dimethyl sulfoxide-35 S in the rat. Ann N Y Acad Sci 141:77–84, 1967
96. Doebbler GF: Cryoprotective compounds: Review and discussion of structure and function. Cryobiology 3:2–11, 1966
97. Dolan MF: The present status of organ freezing and possible future recourses. Cryobiology 1:199–204, 1965
98. Elford BC: Functional recovery of smooth muscle after exposure to dimethyl sulfoxide and low temperatures. Cryobiology 7:148–153, 1970
99. Emmings FG, Neiders ME, Greene GW Jr: Freezing the mandible without excision. J Oral Surg 24:145–155, 1966
100. Esterman MA, Johnson RW, Sweeney MJ: Culture of L 1210 cells stored at −190°C. Cryobiology 9:144–146, 1972
101. Farrant J: Pharmacological actions and toxicity of dimethyl sulphoxide and other compounds which protect smooth muscle during freezing and thawing. J Pharm Pharmacol 16:472–483, 1964
102. Farrant J: Mechanism of cell damage during freezing and thawing and its prevention. Nature 205:1284–1287, 1965
103. Farrant J, Walter CA, Armstrong JA: Preservation of structure and function of an organized tissue after freezing and thawing. Proc R Soc Med 168:293–310, 1967

104. Farrant J, Woolgar AE: Cryoprotective additives and hypertonic hemolysis. Cryobiology 7:56–60, 1970
105. Ferrebee JW, Billen D, Urso IM, et al: Preservation of radiation recovery factor in frozen marrow. Blood 12:1096–1100, 1957
106. Fishbein WN, Stowell RE: Studies on the mechanism of freezing damage to mouse liver using a mitochondrial enzyme assay. I. Temporal localization of the injury phase during slow freezing. Cryobiology 4:283–289, 1968
107. Fox R, Burdick JF: Preservation of rabbit spermatozoa: Ethylene glycol vs glycerol for frozen semen. Proc Soc Exp Biol Med 113:853–856, 1963
108. Fraser J, Gill W: Cryosurgery. J Coll Surg Edinb 12:207–216, 1967
109. Fuhrman FA: Experimental frostbite: Oxygen consumption and anaerobic glycolysis of rat tissues after freezing and cooling in vitro. J Appl Physiol 10:224–230, 1957
110. Gage AA: Cryotherapy for inoperable rectal cancer. Dis Colon Rectum 11:36–44, 1968
111. Gage AA: Cryotherapy for oral cancer. JAMA 204:565–569, 1968
112. Gage AA: Cryosurgery for cancer. An evaluation. Cryobiology 5:241–249, 1969
113. Gage AA, Erickson RB: Cryotherapy and curettage for bone tumors. J Cryosurg 1:60–66, 1968
114. Gage AA, Fazekas G, Riley EE: Freezing injury to large blood vessels in dogs. Surgery 61:748–754, 1967
115. Gage AA, Ishikawa H, Winter PM: Experimental frostbite—The effect of hyperbaric oxygenation on tissue survival. Cryobiology 7:1–8, 1970
116. Geisler PH, Iossifides IA, Eichman MF: Preservation of the lactic dehydrogenase activity of platelets by freezing in dimethyl sulfoxide and plasma. Blood 24:761–764, 1964
117. Ghayasuddin M, Zappi E, Shulman S: Cryo-immunization: Antibody response after sequential tissue freezing and injection of rabbit thyroid gland. Cryobiology 6:262, 1969
118. Gilat T, Clapp P, Sherlock P, et al: Effects of freezing on the gastric mucosa of dogs. Gastroenterology 46:680–690, 1964
119. Githens JH, Tschetter PN, Moscovici MG, et al: Studies of the irradiation protection effect of fetal liver in mice. II. Storage by freezing. Blood 18:344–348, 1961
120. Glazier JB, Hughes JMB, Maloney JE, et al: Measurements of capillary dimensions and blood volume in rapidly frozen lungs. J Appl Physiol 26:65–76, 1969
121. Goldberg HK: Cataract surgery by cryoextraction. Int Surg 50:109–111, 1968
122. Goldenberg DM, Sigel A, Schrott, KM, et al: Cryotherapy of heterotransplanted human cancer: Preliminary experimental findings in the Syrian hamster. Urol Int 24:166–176, 1969
123. Golding MR, Martinez A, deJong P, et al: The role of sympathectomy in frostbite with a review of 68 cases. Surgery 57:774–777, 1965
124. Golding MR, Mendoza MF, Hennigar GR, et al: On settling the controversy on the benefit of sympathectomy for frostbite. Surgery 56:221–231, 1964
125. Gollan F: Effect of DMSO and THAM on ionizing radiation in mice. Ann N Y Acad Sci 141:63–64, 1967

126. Gonder MJ, Pfeiffer L, Soanes WA, et al: Prospects for cryoimmunotherapy in cases of metastasizing carcinoma of the prostate. Cryobiology 6:262–263, 1969
127. Gonder MJ, Soanes WA, Smith V: Experimental prostate cryosurgery. Invest Urol 1:610–619, 1964
128. Gonzales F, Luyet BJ: Resumption of heart-beat in chick embryo frozen in liquid nitrogen. Biodynamica 7:1–5, 1950
129. Goodale RL Jr: Progress in gastric freezing. Arch Surg 89:1060–1062, 1964
130. Goodale RL Jr, Bernstein EF, Soucheray J, et al: Effect of duodenal freezing on the secretin mechanism. Proc Soc Exp Biol Med 112:738–740, 1963
131. Goodale RL Jr, Delaney JP, Engle JC, et al: The duration of achlorhydria attending freezing of the isolated canine gastric pouch. J Surg Res 5:370–376, 1965
132. Goodale RL Jr, Eyal Z, Largiader FA, et al: Protection afforded by low molecular weight dextran against the post-freeze gastric ulcer in the dog. J Surg Res 4:403–407, 1964
133. Greaves RIN: Serum-plasma preservation. Historical review. Cryobiology 5:76–86, 1968
134. Grieff D, Mackey S: Cryobiology of platelets. II. Effects of freezing and storage at low temperatures on the survival of isolated human blood platelets as measured by assays for aminopeptidases. Cryobiology 7:9–13, 1970
135. Grossi G, Artusi T: Sulla sopravvivenza delle cellule del midollo osseo conservate in glicerolo a −79°C. Boll Soc Ital Biol Sper 40:1090–1093, 1964
136. Guttman FM, Khalessi A: Studies on the technique of freezing canine bowel segments with cold intraarterial helium and cold ambient nitrogen after perfusion with glycerol and dimethyl sulfoxide. Cryobiology 4:258, 1968
137. Guttmann RD, Perry VP: Acquired tolerance to homografts induced with dimethyl sulfoxide protected and frozen splenic cells. Cryobiology 1:212–216, 1965
138. Hagen JH, Hagen PB: An enzymic method for the estimation of glycerol in blood and its use to determine the effect of noradrenaline on the concentration of glycerol in blood. Can J Biochem Physiol 40:1129–1139, 1962
139. Halasz NA, Orloff MJ: New freeze-protecting compounds and their screening. Surg Forum 15:214–215, 1964
140. Halasz NA, Rosenfield HA, Orloff MJ, et al: Whole organ preservation. II. Freezing studies. Surgery 61:417–421, 1967
141. Halasz NA, Seifert LN, Orloff, MJ: Whole organ preservation. I. Organ perfusion studies. Surgery 60:368–372, 1966
142. Hamilton R, Ketterer FD, Holst HI, et al: Rapid thawing of frozen canine kidneys by microwaves. Cryobiology 4:265–266, 1968
143. Hamilton R, Lehr HB: Survival of small intestine after storage for seven days at −196°C. Cryobiology 3:375, 1967
144. Hansen RI, Lund F, Backer OG: Cryosurgery of the prostate. Urol Int 24:160–165, 1969
145. Hardenbergh E, Ramsbottom R: Experimental frostbite. The effect of "double freeze" on tissue survival in the mouse foot. Cryobiology 5:336–339, 1969
146. Hass GM, Taylor CB: A quantitative hypothermal method for the production of local injury of tissue. Arch Pathol 45:563–580, 1948

147. Hauschka TS, Mitchell JT, Niederpruem DJ: A reliable frozen tissue bank: Viability and stability of 82 neoplastic and normal cell types after prolonged storage at −78°C. Cancer Res 19:643–653, 1959
148. Haynes LL, Tullis JL, Pyle HM, et al: Clinical use of glycerolized frozen blood. JAMA 173:1657–1663, 1960
149. Heber U: Freezing injury in relation to loss of enzyme activities and protection against freezing. Cryobiology 5:188–201, 1968
150. Hermann G, Karsh HB, Kauvar AJ: Gastric cooling in the management of massive upper gastrointestinal hemorrhage. Gastroenterology 47:513–516, 1964
151. Hershey FB, Trump JG, Solomon HJ, et al: Electron-irradiated and freeze-dried arterial homographs; experiences at the St. Louis City Hospital Artery Bank. Ann Surg 147:562–570, 1958
152. Highman B, Altland PD: Effect of dimethyl sulfoxide, exercise, and training on rat serum enzymes and tissues. Am J Physiol 213:779–782, 1967
153. Hitchcock CR, Ruiz E, Sutherland RD, et al: Eighteen-month follow-up of gastric freezing in 173 patients with duodenal ulcer. JAMA 195:71–75, 1966
154. Hobbs KEF, Huggins CE: Investigation of the effects of cryophylactic agents on the isolated rat heart at 37°C. Cryobiology 6:239–245, 1969
155. Holst H, Feigl P, Brown A, et al: Temperature of additive as a factor in contracture of rat skin autografts. Cryobiology 2:315, 1966
156. Horrell WR, Rose H, Fordtran JS, et al: Gastric hypothermia for duodenal ulcer. JAMA 200:290–294, 1967
157. Horwitz NH, Gokalp H, Randall J: In situ freezing of the common carotid artery and sagittal sinus of the dog. Cryobiology 2:223–228, 1966
158. Hubel KA, Faber L, Kent TH, et al: The effects of gastric freezing on vitamin B_{12} absorption, acid secretion, tissue morphology, and serum enzymes. Am J Dig Dis 9:328–336, 1964
159. Huggins CE: Prevention of hemolysis of large volumes of red blood cells slowly frozen and thawed in the presence of dimethyl sulfoxide. Transfusion 3:483–493, 1963
160. Huggins CE: Frozen blood. Ann Surg 160:643–649, 1964
161. Huggins CE: Preservation of organized tissue by freezing. Fed Proc 24, Suppl 15:S-190–S-195, 1965
162. Huggins CE, Yuasa S: Preservation of lymphocytes at −196°C in ethylene glycol. Cryobiology 4:256–257, 1968
163. Hussain SA, Gorman JF, Rosenberg JC: Preoperative freezing for sepsis complicating gangrene. Int Surg 48:515–518, 1967
164. Iossifides I, Geisler P, Eichman MF, et al: Preservation of the clot-retracting actvity of platelets by freezing in dimethyl sulfoxide and plasma. Transfusion 3:167–172, 1963
165. Iossifides IA, Gutzait L, Brand M, et al: Erythropoietic recovery in mice protected with fresh and frozen bone marrow. Proceedings, 9th Congress of the International Society for Blood Transfusions, Mexico, 1962, pp 281–286 (1964)
166. Jacob SW: Studies in organ preservation by actual freezing and reduction of the freezing point. Cryobiology 1:176–180, 1964

167. Jacob SW, Bischel M, Herschler RJ: Dimethyl sulfoxide (DMSO): A new concept in pharmacotherapy. Curr Ther Res 6:134–135, 1964
168. Jacob SW, Webb RL: An experimental approach to the supercooling of canine hearts. Surg Forum 11:200–202, 1960
169. Jacob SW, Wood DC: Notes on dimethyl sulfoxide symposium: Vienna, Austria, November 8 and 9, 1966. Curr Ther Res 9:229–233, 1967
170. Joshi RA, Blumenthal HT: Alteration of homotransplantability of rat adrenal and aorta by dehydration freezing. Lab Invest 7:19–29, 1958
171. Kalabuchov N: "Anabiosis" in vertebrates and insects at a temperature below zero on undercooling and freezing of animals. Dokl Acad Sci SSSR 7:1–8, 1934
172. Kamegai T, Sumida S: Clinical experience of frozen blood. Cryobiology 4:253–254, 1968
173. Kaplan JA, Freilich DB: Effect of cryosurgery on vitreous hemorrhage. Int Surg 50:5–9, 1968
174. Karacadag S, Klotz AP: A physiologic interpretation of gastric freezing in the human. Am J Dig Dis 9:319–327, 1964
175. Karacadag S, Klotz AP: Gastric "freezing" in peptic ulcer, an evaluation of 100 cases. Ann Intern Med 61, Suppl 6:645–649, 1964
176. Karacadag S, Klotz AP: Gastric hypothermia in the management of massive upper gastrointestinal bleeding. Am J Gastroenterol 42:505–510, 1964
177. Karacadag S, Klotz AP: Secretory comparison of gastric freezing and radiation therapy. Am J Gastroenterol 42:604–610, 1964
178. Karacadag S, Klotz AP: Multiple gastric freezing. Am J Dig Dis 10:116–121, 1965
179. Karow AM Jr: Effects of cryoprotectants on the heart. Cryobiology 4:268, 1968
180. Karow AM Jr: Biological effects of cryoprotectants as related to cardiac cryopreservation. Cryobiology 5:429–443, 1969
181. Karow AM Jr: Cryoprotectants: A new class of drugs. J Pharm Pharmacol 21:209–223, 1969
182. Karow AM, Carrier O Jr: Effects of cryoprotectant compounds on mammalian heart muscle. Surg Gynecol Obstet 128:571–583, 1969
183. Karow AM Jr., Carrier O Jr, Clower BR: Toxicity of cryoprotectrive agents at 30°C. J Pharm Pharmacol 20:297–301, 1968
184. Karow AM Jr, Carrier O Jr, Holland WC: Toxicity of high dimethyl sulfoxide concentrations in rat heart freezing. Cryobiology 3:464–468, 1967
185. Karow AM Jr, Unal MO, Carrier O Jr, et al: The comparative cryoprotective effect of Mg^{++} as assayed by pharmacological method. Cryobiology 2:299, 1966
186. Karow AM Jr, Unal MO, Carrier O Jr, et al: Preliminary observations on drug responses in viably frozen mammalian hearts. Cryobiology 3:335–340, 1967
187. Karow AM Jr, Webb WR: Effects of glycerol and freezing on skin homografts. Surgery 49:641–643, 1961
188. Karow AM Jr, Webb WR: Toxicity of various solute moderators used in hypothermia. Cryobiology 1:270–273, 1965
189. Karow AM Jr, Webb WR: Tissue Freezing A theory for injury and survival. Cryobiology 2:99–108, 1965

190. Karow AM Jr, Webb WR, Stapp JE: Preservation of hearts by freezing. Arch Surg 91:572–574, 1965
191. Kauvar AJ, Karsh HB, Hermann G: Gastric freezing, a clinical evaluation. Arch Surg 89:985–988, 1964
192. Kelman CD: Cryosurgery for cataract extraction and the treatment of other eye diseases. Boyd's Highlights Ophthalmol 7:181–209, 1964
193. Kenney J, Ketterer FD: Kidney thawing by conduction heating. Cryobiology 4:248, 1968
194. Klavins JV, Shingleton WW, Fuson RL: Alterations during the repair of injury induced by gastric freezing. Cryobiology 4:309–316, 1968
195. Kolb KH, Jaenicke G, Kramer M, et al: Absorption, distribution and elimination of labelled dimethyl sulfoxide in man and animals. Ann N Y Acad Sci 141:85–95, 1967
196. Klotz AP: Gastric "freezing" and cooling in review. Rev Surg 21:381–392, 1964
197. Klotz AP, Christodoulopoulos JB: The secretory physiology of gastric freezing. Am J Dig Dis 10:31–34, 1965
198. Kolig G, Marx FW Jr: Gastric freezing or gastric frostbite? Arch Surg 90:182–187, 1965
199. Kollarits CR, Lessler MA, Berggren RB, et al: Oxygen utilization by rat skin exposed to several cryoprotective solutions during liquid nitrogen storage. Cryobiology 7:94–99, 1970
200. Komarov LV: Revival of rabbit ear after freezing in liquid oxygen. Dokl Acad Sci SSSR 64:747–749, 1949
201. Krijnen HW, DeWit JJ, Kuivenhoven ACJ, et al: Glycerol treated human red cells frozen with liquid nitrogen. Vox Sang 9:559–572, 1964
202. Krijnen HW, Kuivenhoven ACJ, DeWit JJ: The preservation of blood cells in the frozen state. Cryobiology 5:136–143, 1968
203. Kruhøffer P, Nissen OI: Handling of glycerol in the kidney. Acta Physiol Scand 59:284–294, 1963
204. Lake NC: An investigation into the effects of cold upon the body. Lancet 2:557–562, 1917
205. Larson VM, Clark WR, Hilleman MR: Cryosurgical treatment of primary SV_{40} viral and adenovirus 7 transplant tumors in hamsters. Proc Soc Exp Med Biol 128:983–988, 1968
206. Lavrik SS: Conservation of bone marrow with polyvinylpyrrolidone by freezing in liquid nitrogen. Fed Proc Transl Suppl 25:T978–T980, 1966
207. LeBeau J, Hanau J: Etude histologique des lesions produites par l'application de grand froid en chirugie cerebrale chez l'homme. Ann Chir 18:554, 1964
208. Lehmann H: Long-term preservation of blood. Proc R Soc Med 57:625–628, 1964
209. Lehmann H: Changes in enzymes at low temperatures, long-term preservation of blood. Fed Proc 24, Suppl 15:S-66–S-69, 1965
210. Lehr HB, Berggren RB, Summers AL, et al: Freezing and thawing of large organs. Cryobiology 1:194–197, 1964
211. Leibo SP, Mazur P: The role of cooling rates in low-temperature preservation. Cryobiology 8:447–452, 1971

212. Lemariey A, Muler H: Essai d'application de la cryotherapie au traitment de la papillomatose laryngee infantile. Ann Otolaryngol (Paris), 77:279–285, 1960
213. Leunissen RLA, Piatnek-Leunissen DA: A device facilitating in situ freezing of rat heart with modified Wollenberger tongs. J Appl Physiol 25:769–771, 1968
214. Lewis JS, Cahan WG: Cryosurgical management of glomus jugular tumors. Laryngoscope 77:912–917, 1967
215. Lin JH, Carroll PM: The effect of calcium and magnesium on frozen rat uteri, and the calcium content of uteri frozen by various procedures. Cryobiology 5:105–108, 1968
216. Lin TH, Matsumoto K, Cooper IS: Electroencephalographic changes in Parkinsonian patients following cryogenic lesions in the ventrolateral nucleus of the thalamus. J Int Coll Surg 42:281–286, 1964
217. Losina-Losinsky LK: The resistance of insects to deep cooling and to intracellular freezing, in Troshin AS (ed): The Cell and Environmental Temperature. New York, Pergamon Press, 1967
218. Lotke PA, Dolan MF: Thermoelectric cooler for preservation of canine kidneys. Refrigeration Science and Technology, Supplement, Bulletin of the International Institutes of Refrigeration. Paris, 1965, p 497
219. Lovelock JE: The haemolysis of human red blood cells by freezing and thawing. Biochim Biophys Acta 10:414–426, 1953
220. Lovelock JE: The mechanism of the protective action of glycerol against haemolysis by freezing and thawing. Biochim Biophys Acta 11:28–36, 1953
221. Lovelock JE: The denaturation of lipid-protein complexes as a cause of damage by freezing. Proc R Soc B 147:427–433, 1957
222. Lovelock JE: Diathermy apparatus for the rapid rewarming of whole animals from 0°C and below. Proc R Soc B 147:545, 1957
223. Lovelock JE, Bishop MWH: Prevention of freezing damage to living cells by dimethyl sulfoxide. Nature 183:1394–1395, 1959
224. Lovelock JE, Smith AU: Studies on golden hamsters during cooling to and rewarming from body temperatures below 0°C. III. Biophysical aspects and general discussion. Proc R Soc B 145:427–442, 1956
225. Lubos MC, Viril LC, Klotz AP: A controlled study of outpatient gastric freezing. Am J Dig Dis 11:266–271, 1966
226. Luyet B: A review of research on the preservation of hearts in the frozen state. Cryobiology 8:190–207, 1971
227. Luyet BJ, Kroener C, Williams R: Determination of the amounts of ice formed in the feet of mice frozen at various temperatures. Technical Documentary Report AAL-TDR-63-29, 1964
228. Luyet BJ, Schmidt P: Determination of amount of ice formed in blood at various freezing temperatures. Fed Proc 9:81–82, 1950
229. Luyet BJ, Williams RJ: Comparative study of freezing injury in a hibernator and a nonhibernator. Technical Documentary Report AAL-TDR-63-30, 1964
230. Makin GS, Howard JM: Dimethyl sulfoxide and supercooling for storage of canine kidneys. Arch Surg 91:564–567, 1965
231. Malinin GI, Fontana DJ, Braungart DC: Distribution of C^{14}-labeled dimethyl sulfoxide in tissues of intact animals. Cryobiology 4:249, 1968
232. Malinin GI, Fontana DJ, Braungart DC: Distribution of C^{14}-labeled dimethyl sulfoxide in tissues of intact animals. Cryobiology 5:328–335, 1969

233. Malinin TI: Injury of human polymorphonuclear granulocytes frozen in the presence of cryoprotective agents. Cryobiology 9:123–130, 1972
234. Malinin TI, Pegg DE, Perry VP, et al: Long-term storage of bone marrow cells at liquid nitrogen and Dry Ice temperatures. Cryobiology 7:65–69, 1970
235. Malinin TI, Perry VP: Toxicity of dimethyl sulfoxide on Hela cells. Cryobiology 4:90–96, 1967
236. Manax WG, Bloch JH, Longerbeam JK, et al: In vitro freezing of whole organs. Cryobiology 1:157–162, 1964
237. Martinez A, Golding M, Sawyer PN, et al: The specific arterial lesions in mild and severe frostbite: Effect of sympathectomy. J Cardiovasc Surg 7:495–503, 1966
238. Marx FW Jr, Kolig G: Hemorrhagic necrosis following gastric freezing. Surg Gynecol Obstet 119:1276–1284, 1964
239. Marx FW Jr, Kolig G: The hazards of gastric freezing. Am J Dig Dis 11:272–278, 1966
240. Mazur P: Studies on the effects of subzero temperatures on the viability of spores of *Aspergillus flavus*. I. The effect of rate of warming. J Gen Physiol 39:869–888, 1956
241. Mazur P: Kinetics of water loss from cells at subzero temperatures and the likelihood of intracellular freezing. J Gen Physiol 47:347–369, 1963
242. Mazur P: Physical and chemical changes during freezing and thawing of cells with special reference to blood cells. Proc 11th Congr Int Soc Blood Transf, Sydney, No. 29, 1966, pp 764–777
243. Mazur P: Factors affecting cell injury in cryosurgical freezing. Bull Millard Fillmore Hosp 14:123–128, 1967
244. Mazur P: Physical-chemical factors underlying cell injury in cryosurgical freezing, in Thomas CC (ed): Cryosurgery. Springfield, Thomas, 1968, pp 32–51
245. Mazur P, Schmidt JJ: Interactions of cooling velocity, temperature, and warming velocity on the survival of frozen and thawed yeast. Cryobiology 5:1–17, 1968
246. McDonald DF, Mobley TL, Rudolph JH: Cryotherapy of a heterografted human bladder tumor—Long-term observations. Cryobiology 2:280–284, 1966
247. McFarland JB, Artz CP, Fitts CT: Gastric freezing for duodenal ulcer. Am Surg 30:53–55, 1964
248. McFarland JB, Fitts CT, Artz CP: Mucosal damage following gastric freezing. A warning. (Direct inspection and biopsy in conjunction with photoendoscopy using the Hirschowitz fiberscope.) Surg Forum 14:354–355, 1963
249. McFarland JB, Gow JG: Trial of gastric cooling for haematemesis. Br Med J 3:831–834, 1967
250. McFee AS, Stone NH, Goodale RL Jr, et al: Prevention of stress-induced ulcer in the rat by gastric freezing. JAMA 186:917–919, 1963
251. McIlrath DC, Hallenbeck GA, Allen HA, et al: Gastric freezing: An experimental study. Gastroenterology 45:374–383, 1963
252. McSweeney ED Jr: The effect of hypothermia on gastric secretion. Seminar, Dept. of Exp Surgery, Montreal, McGill Univ, 1963
253. McSweeney ED Jr, Melnyk CS, Deshpande PJ, et al: The supercooled stomach. Surg Forum 14:347–349, 1963

254. Melnick JL: Preservation of viruses by freezing. Fed Proc 24, Suppl 15:S-280–S-283, 1965
255. Melnick PJ: Effect of freezing rates on the histochemical identification of enzyme activity. Fed Proc 24, Suppl 15:S-259–S-267, 1965
256. Melnyk CS, Jacob SW, Benson JA Jr: Gastric freezing in dogs. Ann Surg 162:135–144, 1965
257. Meryman HT: Tissue freezing and local cold injury. Physiol Rev 37:233–251, 1957
258. Meryman HT: Review of biological freezing, in Cryobiology. London, Academic Press, 1966
259. Meryman HT: Physical limitations of the rapid freezing method. Proc R Soc B 147:452–459, 1957
260. Miller LK: Activity in mammalian peripheral nerves during supercooling. Science 149:74–75, 1965
261. Minor TM, Shumacker HB: An evaluation of tissue loss following single and repeated frostbite injuries. Surgery 61:562–563, 1967
262. Mollison PL, Sloviter HA: Successful transfusion of previously frozen human red cells. Lancet 2:862–864, 1951
263. Mollison PL, Sloviter HA, Chaplin H Jr: Survival of transfused red cells previously stored for long periods in the frozen state. Lancet 2:501–505, 1952
264. Morris GJ, Farrant J: Interactions of cooling rate and protective additive on the survival of washed human erythrocytes frozen to −196°C. Cryobiology 9:173–181, 1972
265. Moss GS, Reed PC, Riddell AG: Observations on the effects of glycerol on the cold storage of the canine liver. J Surg Res 6:147–151, 1966
266. Mueller FO, Casey TA, Trevor-Roper PD: Use of deep-frozen human cornea the full-thickness grafts. Br Med J 2(1):473–475, 1964
267. Mueller FO, Smith AU: Some experiments on grafting frozen corneal tissue in rabbits. Exp Eye Res 2:237–246, 1963
268. Mundth ED, DeFalco AJ, Jacobson YG: Functional survival of kidneys subjected to extracorporeal freezing and reimplantation. Cryobiology 2:62–67, 1965
269. Mundth ED, Long DM, Brown RB: Treatment of experimental frostbite with low molecular weight dextran. J Trauma 4:246–257, 1964
270. Narula PN, Jacob SW: The cryoprotective effect of dimethyl sulfoxide and glycerol on cell cultures at various temperatures. Cryobiology 2:32, 1965
271. Nei T: Low-temperature preservation of microorganisms. Fed Proc 24, Suppl 15:S-284–S-285, 1965
272. Nei T: Mechanism of hemolysis of erythrocytes by freezing at near zero temperatures. Cryobiology 4:303–308, 1968
273. O'Grady LF, Lewis JP: Stem cell renewal in frozen marrow. Cryobiology 5:250–253, 1969
274. O'Neill P, Mueller FO, Trevor-Roper PD: On the preservation of corneae at −196°C for full-thickness homografts in man and dog. Br J Opthamol 51:13–30, 1967
275. Ostergard DR, Townsend DE, Hirose FM: The treatment of chronic cervicitis by cryotherapy. Cryobiology 4:97–102, 1967
276. Owens FJ, Brown CH, Sullivan BH Jr: Gastric "freezing" for peptic ulcer.

Evaluation by gastroscopic, cinefluoroscopic, gastric secretory, and gastric biopsy studies. Am J Dig Dis 10:514–521, 1965
277. Panuska JA: The effect of dimethyl sulfoxide on behavioral temperature regulations. Proc Soc Exp Biol Med 127:169–173, 1968
278. Panuska JA, Malinin TI, Mentz RJ: Effect of dimethyl sulfoxide on cooling rates of unrestrained rats. Cryobiology 2:345–350, 1966
279. Panuska JA, Perez-Colon J, Banka RP: The effect of dimethyl sulfoxide on heart rate and cardiac arrest in unanesthetized rats during progressive hypothermia. Cryobiology 4:157–161, 1968
280. Pappas HJ, Collins RJ, Paloucek EP: Cryosurgical treatment of chronic cervicitis. Int Surg 49:513–515, 1968
281. Parkes AS: Viability of adrenocortical tissue transplanted after freezing and thawing. Proc. R. Soc B 144:314–328, 1955
282. Parkes AS, Smith AU: Recent Research in Freezing and Drying. Oxford, Blackwell, 1960, p 320
283. Pascoe JE: The survival of the rat's superior cervical ganglion after cooling to −76°C. Proc R Soc B 147:510–519, 1957
284. Pegg DE: In vitro assessment of cell viability in human bone marrow preserved at −79°C. J Appl Physiol 19:123–126, 1964
285. Pegg DE: Storage of human bone marrow at low temperatures and its clinical applicataions. Int Surg 48:214–220, 1967
286. Pegg DE: An apparatus for the simultaneous programmed control of dimethyl sulfoxide concentration and temperature in an organ perfusion system. Cryobiology 4:249–250, 1968
287. Pegg DE, Farrant J: Some effects of colloids and dimethyl sulfoxide on the perfusion of isolated rabbit kidneys. Cryobiology 4:264, 1968
288. Pegg DE, Kemp NH: Collection, storage, and administration of autologous human bone-marrow. Lancet 2:1426–1429, 1960
289. Pennell RB: Low-temperature preservation of proteins. Fed Proc 24, Suppl 15:S-269–S-274, 1965
290. Persidsky MD, Richards V: Mode of protection with polyvinylpyrrolidone in freezing of bone marrow. Nature 196:585–586, 1962
291. Persidsky MD, Richards V: Optimal conditions and comparative effectiveness of dimethyl sulfoxide and polyvinylpyrrolidone in preservation of bone marrow. Nature 197:1010–1012, 1963
292. Persidsky MD, Richards V: Radiation protection of mice with bone marrow and spleen preserved at low temperature using polyvinylpyrrolidone. Blood 23:337–340, 1964
293. Persidsky MD, Richards V, Leef J: Cryopreservation of bone marrow with low molecular weight polyvinylpyrrolidone. Cryobiology 2:74–78, 1965
294. Persidsky MD, Richards V, Leef J: Volume changes in bone marrow and Ehrlich ascites cells after freezing as an index of preservation efficiency. Cryobiology 3:59–67, 1966
295. Perry GT, Dunphy JV, Fruin RC, et al: Gastric freezing for duodenal ulcer. Gastroenterology 47:6–9, 1964
296. Perry VP, Malinin TI, Kerby CC, et al: Protection of lethally irradiated guinea pigs with fresh and frozen homologus peripheral blood leukocytes. Cryobiology 1:233–239, 1965

297. Peter ET, Bernstein EF, Sosin H, et al: Technique of gastric freezing in the treatment of duodenal ulcer. JAMA 181:760–764, 1962
298. Peter ET, Bernstein EF, Walder AI, et al: Effect of prolonged gastric hypothermia (gastric freezing) upon various phases of gastric secretion. Surg Forum 13:269–271, 1962
299. Peter ET, Nicoloff DN, Bernstein EF, et al: The effect of gastric hypothermia on splanchnic hemodynamics in the dog. J Surg Res 3:32–35, 1963
300. Polge C: Low-temperature storage of mammalian spermatozoa. Proc R Soc B 147:498–508, 1957
301. Polge C, Smith AU, Parkes AS: Revival of spermatozoa after vitrification and dehydration at low temperature. Nature 164:666, 1949
302. Ponten U, Siesjo BK: A method for the determination of the total CO_2 content of frozen tissues. Acta Physiol Scand 60:297–308, 1964
303. Ponten U, Siesjo BK: Acid labile carbon dioxide of rat brain after freezing the tissue in situ. Acta Physiol Scand 60:309–317, 1964
304. Popovic P, Popovic V: Survival of newborn ground squirrels after supercooling or freezing. Am J Physiol 204:949–952, 1963
305. Popovic P, Popovic V: Survival of young rats after supercooling to −3°C. Cryobiology 2:23, 1965
306. Porterfield JS, Ashwood-Smith MJ: Preservation of cells in tissue culture by glycerol and dimethyl sulfoxide. Nature 193:548–550, 1962
307. Pribor DB, Nara A: Toxicity and cryoprotection by dimethyl sulfoxide and by glycerol in isolated frog sciatic nerves. Cryobiology 5:355–365, 1969
308. Pursel VG, Johnson LA, Gerrits RJ: Distribution of glutamic oxalacetic transaminase and lactic dehydrogenase activities in boar semen after cold shock and freezing. Cryobiology 7:141–144, 1970
309. Rand RW: Cryogenic techniques in sterotaxic neurosurgery. Cryohypophysectomy and cryothalamectomy. Int Surg 49:212–216, 1968
310. Rapatz G: Cellular structural and ultrastructural modifications associated with cooling, in Musacchia SJ, Saunders JF (eds): Depressed Metabolism. New York, Am Elsevier, 1969, pp 3–38
311. Rapatz G: Some problems associated with the freezing of hearts. Cryobiology 7:157–162, 1970
312. Rapatz G, Luyet B: Effects of cooling rates on the preservation of erythrocytes in frozen blood containing various protective agents. Biodynamica 9:333–350, 1965
313. Rapatz G, Luyet B: Combined effects of freezing rates and of various protective agents on the preservation of human erythrocytes. Cryobiology 4:215–222, 1968
314. Rapatz G, Sullivan JJ, Luyet B: Preservation of erythrocytes in blood containing various cryoprotective agents, frozen at various rates and brought to a given final temperature. Cryobiology 5:18–25, 1968
315. Reaumur RAF: Memoires pour servir a l'histoire des insects. Paris, Imprimerie Royale, 1736, pp 141–147
316. Reite OB: Functional qualities of small blood vessels in tissue injured by freezing and thawing. Acta Physiol Scand 63:111–120, 1965
317. Reynolds BM, Scherl ND: Paroxysmal atrial fibrillation after gastric freezing. N Engl J Med 270:1301–1302, 1964

318. Richards V, Braverman M, Floridia R, et al: Initial clinical experiences with liquid nitrogen preserved blood, employing PVP as a protective additive. Am J Surg 108:313–322, 1964
319. Richards V, Persidsky MD, Braverman M, et al: Preservation of bone marrow and blood at cryogenic temperatures. J Cardiovasc Surg 5:313–326, 1964
320. Rinfret AP: Factors affecting the erythrocyte during rapid freezing and thawing. Ann N Y Acad Sci 85:576–594, 1960
321. Ritchie WP Jr, Breen JJ, Wangensteen OH: Freezing of the intact rat stomach: An indication of the biologic potential of the technic. Am J Dig Dis 12:379–388, 1967
322. Root HD, Barata JR: Influence of gastric pressure on effects of gastric freezing. Surg Forum 15:330–332, 1964
323. Rose H, Fordtran JS, Harrell R, et al: A controlled study of gastric freezing for the treatment of duodenal ulcer. Gastroenterology 47:10–17, 1964
324. Rostand J: Glycerine et resistance du sperme aux basses temperatures. C R Acad Sci (Paris) 222:1524–1525, 1946
325. Rowbotham GF, Haigh AL, Leslie WG: Cooling cannula for use in treatment of cerebral neoplasms. Lancet 1:12–15, 1959
326. Rowe AW, Allen FH Jr: Freezing of blood droplets to liquid nitrogen for use in blood group studies. Transfusion 5:379–380, 1965
327. Rowe AW, Cohen E: Low temperature preservation of leukocytes: Freezing technique and in vitro viability criteria. Proc 11th Congr Int Soc Blood Transf, Sydney, No. 29, 1966, pp 779–787
328. Rowe AW, Eyster E, Kellner A: Liquid nitrogen preservation of red blood cells for transfusion; a low glycerol-rapid freeze procedure. Cryobiology 5:119–128, 1968
329. Rudolph LE, Mandel S: Supercooling, intermittent perfusion, and high pressure oxygen in whole organ preservation. Transplantation 5:1159–1166, 1967
330. Ruffie J, Colombies P, Ducos J: L'optitude a la transformation blastique en culture et l'analyse chromosomique utilisee comme moyen de controle de la survive de leucocytes congeles. Proc 11th Congr Int Soc Blood Transf, Sydney, No. 29, 1966, pp 727–730
331. Russell PS, Gittes RF, Sparrow EM: Storage of parathyroid tissue in the frozen state. Surg Forum 11:21–23, 1960
332. Russell PS, Wood ML, Gittes RF: Preservation of living tissue in the frozen state. A study using parathyroid tissue. J Surg Res 1:23–31, 1961
333. Salt RW: Natural occurrence of glycerol in insects and its relation to their ability to survive freezing. Can Entomol 89:491–494, 1957
334. Sams WM Jr: The effects of dimethyl sulfoxide on nerve conduction. Ann N Y Acad Sci 141:242–247, 1967
335. Scherer WF, Hoogasian AC: Preservation at subzero temperatures of mouse fibroblasts (strain L) and human epithelial cells (strain Hela). Proc Soc Exp Biol Med 87:480–487, 1954
336. Schimmel H, Wajcner G, Chatelain C, et al: Freezing of whole rat and dog kidney by perfusion of liquid nitrogen through the renal artery. Cryobiology 1:171–175, 1964
337. Scholander PF, Flagg W, Hock RJ, et al: Studies on the physiology of frozen plants and animals in the arctic. J Cell Comp Physiol 42, Suppl 1:1–56, 1953

338. Scholander PF, Van Dam L, Kanwisher JW, et al: Supercooling and osmoregulation in arctic fish. J Cell Physiol 49:5–24, 1957
339. Schopf-Ebner E, Gross WO, Bucher OM: Pulsatile activity of isolated heart muscle cells after freezing storage. Cryobiology 4:200–203, 1968
340. Scott HW Jr, O'Neill JA Jr, Snyder HE, et al: An evaluation on the long term results of gastric freezing for duodenal ulcer. Surg Gynecol Obstet 121:723–727, 1965
341. Scott HW Jr, Shull HJ, O'Neill JA Jr, et al: Experimental and clinical appraisal of gastric freezing for duodenal ulcer. Ann Surg 159:769–786, 1964
342. Scott HW Jr, Shull HJ, O'Neill JA Jr, et al: A clinical appraisal of gastric freezing for duodenal ulcer. J Tenn Med Assoc 57:131–135, 1964
343. Sesia G, Ferrando U, Riggi G: A new apparatus for use in cryotherapy of prostate obstruction. Int Surg 49:330–338, 1968
344. Sharp DG, Sadhukhan P, Galasso GJ: The slow decline in quality of vaccinia virus at low temperatures (37°C to −62°C). Proc Soc Exp Biol Med 115:811–814, 1964
345. Sherman JK: Survival of higher animal cells after the formation and dissolution of intracellular ice. Anat Rec 144:171–190, 1962
346. Sherman JK: Dimethyl sulfoxide as a protective agent during freezing and thawing of human spermatozoa. Proc Soc Exp Biol Med 117:261–264, 1964
347. Sherman JK: Practical applications and technical problems of preserving spermatozoa by freezing. Fed Proc 24, Suppl 15:S-288–S-296, 1965
348. Sherman JK, Bunge RG: Observations on preservation of human spermatozoa at low temperatures. Proc Soc Exp Biol Med 82:686–688, 1953
349. Sherman JK, Lin TP: Effect of glycerol and low temperature on survival of unfertilized mouse eggs. Nature 181:785–786, 1958
350. Shikama K: Effect of freezing and thawing on the stability of double helix of DNA. Nature 207:529–530, 1965
351. Shikata J, Shumacker HB, Nash FD: Studies in experimental frostbite. The effect of cold acclimatization upon resistance to local cold injury. Arch Surg 81:817–823, 1960
352. Shingleton WW, Fuson RL, Roufail WM, et al: Comparison of instrumentation for experimental and clinical gastric freezing. Ann Surg 162:1053–1056, 1965
353. Shlafer M, Karow AM Jr: Ultrastructure—Function correlative studies for cardiac cryopreservation. II. Hearts frozen to various temperatures without a cryoprotectant. Cryobiology 8:350–360, 1971
354. Shlafer M, Karow AM Jr: Ultrastructure—Function correlative studies for cardiac cryopreservation. III. Hearts frozen to −10° and −17°C with and without dimethyl sulfoxide (DMSO). Cryobiology 9:38–50, 1972
355. Shorter RG, Titus JL, Kerr FWL, et al: Effects of freezing and storage on survival of thyroid autografts. Proc Soc Exp Biol Med Suppl 113:73–75, 1963
356. Shulman S, Zappi E, Ghayasuddin M, et al: Cryoimmunization: Tissue temperature gradients and tissue antigenicity. Cryobiology 6:284, 1969
357. Shumacker HB, Abramson DI: Sympathectomy in trench foot. Ann Surg 125:203–215, 1947
358. Shumacker HB, Kilman JW: Sympathectomy in the treatment of frostbite. Arch Surg 89:575–584, 1964

359. Sloviter HA: Mechanism of hemolysis caused by freezing and its prevention. Nature 193:884–885, 1962
360. Smith AU: Prevention of haemolysis during freezing and thawing of red blood-cells. Lancet 2:910–911, 1950
361. Smith AU: Frostbite in golden hamsters revived from body temperatures below 0°C. Lancet 2:1255–1259, 1954
362. Smith AU: Studies on golden hamsters during cooling to and rewarming from body temperatures below 0°C. I. Observations during chilling, freezing and supercooling. Proc R Soc B 145:391–407, 1956
363. Smith AU: Studies on golden hamsters during cooling to and rewarming from body temperatures below 0°C. II. Observations during and after resuscitation. Proc R Soc B 145:407–426, 1956
364. Smith AU: Problems in the resuscitation of mammals from body temperatures below 0°C. Proc R Soc B 147:533–544, 1957
365. Smith AU: Life at low temperatures. Nature 182:911–913, 1958
366. Smith AU: Viability of supercooled and frozen mammals. Ann N Y Acad Sci 80:291–300, 1959
367. Smith AU: Biological effects of freezing and supercooling, Baltimore, Williams & Wilkins, 1961, p 217
368. Smith AU, Lovelock JE, Parkes AS: Resuscitation of hamsters after supercooling or partial crystallization at body temperatures below 0°C. Nature 173:1136–1137, 1954
369. Smith ER, Hadidian Z, Mason MM: The single- and repeated-dose toxicity of dimethyl sulfoxide. Ann N Y Acad Sci 141:96–109, 1967
370. Smith MFW, Boles R, Work WP: Cryosurgical techniques in removal of angiofibromas. Laryngoscope 74:1071–1080, 1964
371. Solovieva NA, Lozinsky LKL: Some aspects of the metabolism of phosphorus during the diapause of the *Pyrausta nubilalis* caterpillars, in Lozinsky LKL (ed): Reaction of Cells and Their Proteins after Exposure to Extreme External Conditions. Nauka, Moscow, 1966, pp 73–81
372. Sosin H, Bernstein EF, Madsen A, et al: Mechanism of control of hemorrhage from duodenal ulcer by gastric hypothermia. JAMA 186:219–223, 1963
373. Staub NC, Storey WF: Relation between morphological and physiological events in lung studied by rapid freezing. J Appl Physiol 17:381–390, 1962
374. Steponkus PL: Effect of freezing on dehydrogenase activity and reduction of triphenyl tetrazolium chloride. Cryobiology 8:570–573, 1971
375. Stickel DC, Flemma RJ, Morgan CV Jr, et al: Temperature control in glycerolized kidneys during freezing and thawing. Surg Forum 14:178–179, 1963
376. Stowell RE, Young DE, Arnold EA, et al: Structural, chemical, physical, and functional alterations in mammalian nucleus following different conditions of freezing, storage and thawing. Fed Proc 24, Suppl 15:S-115–S-141, 1965
377. Strumia MM: Freezing of whole blood. Science 110:398–400, 1949
378. Strumia MM, Colwell LS, Strumia PV: Preservation of whole blood in frozen state for transfusion. Science 128:1002–1003, 1958
379. Strumia MM, Colwell LS, Strumia PV: The preservation of blood for transfusion. IV. In vitro recovery after freezing and thawing of red cells modified with sugars. J Lab Clin Med 56:576–586, 1960

380. St Whitelock O, Furness FN, Sturgeon PA, et al: Freezing and drying of biological materials. Ann NY Acad Sci 85:501–734, 1960
381. Suda I, Kito K, Adachi C: The viability of long-term frozen cat brain in vitro. Nature 212:268–270, 1966
382. Sugiura K, Tortolani AJ, Sargent MG: Viability of various solid and ascites tumors after prolonged storage at −78°C. Cryobiology 4:177–183, 1968
383. Sulman D, Ferguson DJ: Gastric freezing by alcohol perfusion. Surg Forum 15:325–327, 1964
384. Sutherland RD, Bitter JE, Hitchcock CR: Rebound hyperacidity after gastric freezing, clinical study of treatment for duodenal ulcer. Arch Surg 89:208–214, 1964
385. Thomas GD, Gresham RB: Comparative tensile strength—Study of fresh, frozen and freeze-dried fascia lata. Surg Forum 14:442–443, 1963
386. Thurston RJ, Harris GC Jr: Calcium-45 uptake as a measurement of freeze-thaw injury to chicken spermatozoa in the presence or absence of cryopreservatives. Cryobiology 7:100–106, 1970
387. Torney H, Bordt DE: Viability quantitation of leptospires after rapid and controlled rate freezing. Cryobiology 5:352–354, 1969
388. Tran PT, Bender MA: Factors affecting survival of mouse bone marrow cells during freezing and thawing in glycerol. J Appl Physiol 15:939–942, 1960
389. Trump BF, Young DE, Arnold EA, et al: Effects of freezing and thawing on the structure, chemical constitution, and function of cytoplasmic structures. Fed Proc 24, Suppl 15:S-144–S-168, 1965
390. Turner MD, Pitts HR, Turner AC: Respiratory changes in isolated perfused rat kidneys after freeze-thaw and hypothermic storage. Cryobiology 4:140–146, 1967
391. Umminger BL: Physiological studies on supercooled killifish (*Fundulus heteroclitus*). III. Carbohydrate metabolism and survival at subzero temperatures. J Exp Zool 173:169–174, 1970
392. Valeri CR: Effect of resuspension medium on in vivo survival and supernatant hemoglobin of erythrocytes preserved with glycerol. Transfusion 5:25–35, 1965
393. Valeri CR, Brodine CE: Current methods for processing frozen red cells. Cryobiology 5:129–135, 1968
394. Valeri CR, Brodine CE, Moss GE: Use of frozen blood in Vietnam. Proc 11th Congr Int Soc Blood Transf, Sydney, No. 29, 1966, pp 735–738
395. Von Leden H, Rand RW: Cryosurgical technics in head and neck surgery. Am Surg 33:36–39, 1967
396. Walker TM, Albrigo JL, Panuska JA: The effect of dimethyl sulfoxide on oxygen consumption in cold-exposed rats and hamsters. Cryobiology 3:265–268, 1966
397. Waltz JM, Cooper IS: Temperature gradients, the blood-brain barrier and the brain tumor. Bull Millard Fillmore Hosp 14:96–102, 1967
398. Waltz JM, Riklan M, Stellar S, et al: Cryothalamectomy for Parkinson's disease: A statistical analysis. Neurology 16:994–1003, 1966
399. Wangensteen OH, Peter ET, Bernstein, EF, et al: Can physiological gastrectomy be achieved by gastric freezing? Ann Surg 156:579–591, 1962
400. Wangensteen OH, Peter ET, Nicoloff DM, et al: Achieving "physiological gastrectomy" by gastric freezing. JAMA 180:439–444, 1962

401. Wangensteen SL, Barker HG, Smith RB III, et al: Gastric "freezing": A double blind study. Am J Dig Dis 10:420–435, 1965
402. Wangensteen SL, Magill T, Reber R, et al: Gastric "freezing," temperatures and morphologic changes. Arch Surg 90:286–289, 1965
403. Way MJ: Glycerol-containing insects. Proc R Soc B 147:551, 1957
404. Webb WR, Dodds RP, Unal MO, et al: Suspended animation of the heart with metabolic inhibitors. Ann Surg 164:343–351, 1966
405. Webb WR, Karow AM Jr: Hypothermic organ preservation—Comparison of cooling and warming methods. JAMA 191:1012–1014, 1965
406. Weyer E, Hutchins H, Krauss M, et al: Conference on biological actions of dimethyl sulfoxide. Ann NY Acad Sci 141:1–671, 1967
407. White RR, Hightower NC Jr, Adalid R: Problems and complications of gastric freezing. Ann Surg 159:765–768, 1964
408. Whittingham DB, Leibo SP, Mazur P: Survival of mouse embryos frozen to −196° and −269°C. Science 178:411–414, 1972
409. Wiesinger H: Experiences with a modified technic for cyclocryotherapy. Int Surg 48:425–429, 1967
410. Wilson CB, Winternitz WW, Bertan V, et al: Stereotaxic cryosurgery of the pituitary gland in carcinoma of the breast and other disorders. JAMA 198:587–590, 1966
411. Wilson CB, Winternitz WW, Rush BF, et al: Cryohypophysectomy: Indications, technic, and results. Int Surg 48:28–40, 1967
412. Zacarian SA: Cryosurgery in dermatology. Int Surg 47:528–534, 1967
413. Zacarian SA, Adham MI: Cryotherapy of cutaneous malignancy. Cryobiology 2:212–218, 1966
414. Zacarian SA, Stone D, Clater M: Effects of cryogenic temperatures on microcirculation in the golden hamster cheek pouch. Cryobiology 7:27–39, 1970
415. Zikria BA, DeJesus RS, Cunnick WR, et al: Gastric "freezing"—A clinical double-blind study. Am J Gastroenterol 47:208–214, 1967

2

Body Fluids

INTRODUCTION

Some changes in body fluids and electrolytes are to be expected in hypothermic animals and patients. Claude Bernard's concept of the maintenance of a constant milieu interieur ("internal environment") includes the stability of temperature for all tissues and organs in the body. This stability of temperature, however, does not exist in hypothermia. Therefore, it is not surprising that, concomitant with changes in the temperature, other elements of the internal environment are also changed.

In order to understand the physiology of body fluids in cooled organisms better, it is important to remember that the various types of cooling rarely induce the same changes in water or electrolyte distribution in animals or in man. Accidental hypothermia in cases of alcoholic stupor, clinical hypothermia under anesthesia, or experimental hypothermia induces different and sometimes even opposite changes. Additional physiological alterations are brought about by the state of the organism before cooling as well as by the depth and length of hypothermia. Therefore, it is not surprising that the inconsistencies of many findings on blood constituents, blood electrolytes, and water metabolism in hypothermia have recently led to a lessening of interest for investigations in this field. Some researchers, for instance Reed and Gavrilescu,[127] argue that serum potassium and serum bicarbonate determinations are the only meaningful measurements that one can undertake while studying the blood chemistry in hypothermic patients. At present it is difficult to interpret the scanty information concerning body fluids which varies with the hypothermic state and with type of organism. Therefore, one can only draw a spotty sketch of the physiological changes induced by a decrease in body temperature. Further research will help to round this sketch into a composite picture to permit a better understanding of the basic physiological processes that regulate water and electrolyte balance in hypothermia.

VOLUME AND COMPOSITION OF BODY FLUIDS

Water represents 70 percent of body weight and is the universal solvent in a normothermic body. This applies to the hypothermic state, also, where any water shift plays an extremely important role.

Blood Volume

The blood volume of patients and of experimental animals cooled to a low body temperature is decreased.[13,38,82,92] The longer animals stay at a low body temperature, the more profound is the observed decrease in circulating blood volume (Fig. 2-1). This blood volume is decreased to 60 percent of the normal volume after 6 to 8 hours at a body temperature of 15 C.

The circulating blood volume increases during rewarming. This increase is rather large, up to 130 percent of the normothermic value as seen in dogs after surface cooling to a body temperature of 23 C.[82] This fact was applied to dogs cooled to a body temperature of 4 C with 1 or 2 hours of circulatory arrest and led to successful resuscitation of the animals.[123] However, when hypervolemia was not induced during rewarming, all of the dogs succumbed during the last part of rewarming or immediately afterward. Since the plasma protein concentration is actually reduced during rewarming, the observed hypervolemia suggests an inflow of a low-protein or protein-free fluid into the blood compartment.[45,82]

The decreased blood volume is accompanied by a pronounced hemoconcentration, particularly in profound hypothermia.[91,106,120,122,157,165]

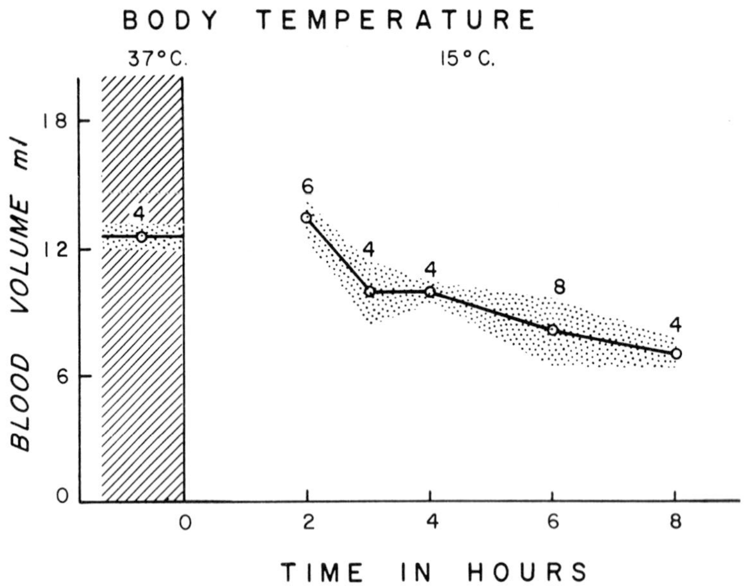

Fig. 2-1. Circulating blood volume of white rats in normothermia (37 C) and during sustained hypothermia (15 C). Number above the open circle shows number of animals.

Hemoconcentration occurs in artificially cooled animals, in hypothermic patients,[8] and even during normothermic cold exposures.[9] In rats cooled to a body temperature of 15 C and maintained at this temperature for hours, the hematocrit ratio increases continuously from a value of 42 to 70 percent or more.[120,122] The same is observed in artificially cooled hibernators (*not* in hibernation) except that in this case the large increase in hematocrit ratio is seen after several days in hypothermia,[120] not several hours. It appears that after splenectomy, cooling induces smaller changes of the hematocrit ratio.[82]

The mechanism of hemoconcentration induced during cooling is not well understood. Hemoconcentration might be induced by a decrease in pO_2 of the arterial blood in the early phase of hypothermia. Lowering of the pO_2 brings forth an adrenergic discharge and splenic concentration of the formed elements in the blood.[74] The cause of hemoconcentration might also be an adherence of the formed elements in the venules of the splenic region of cooled organisms. Sludging of red blood cells,[46] intravascular aggregation,[24,93,148] and "sequestering" of blood[76] have also been observed in hypothermia, though some investigators dispute these findings. Glucose, saline, or low-molecular-weight dextran decreases sludging,[57] but high-molecular-weight dextran seems to be less effective. Johansson[71] believes that there is little or no sludging of the red blood cells when cooling is well controlled. Thus, Johansson's work supports the idea that tissue oxygenation is adequate in hypothermia. The answer to the often-asked question, should the blood of patients during profound cooling be diluted, has still not been completely answered though it appears that hemodilution will be accepted eventually as the best solution.[33,79,121,123]

The increased hematocrit ratio induced in hypothermia can be returned to the normal level by dextran saline or glucose administration or by rewarming.[41,95,98]

It is important to note that profound hemodilution naturally occurs in hibernators,[79,121] and that these animals can decrease their body temperature to a level close to the freezing point, and live at this body temperature for days or weeks.

Therefore, it appears that hemodilution, or some blood replacement therapy, might be beneficial whenever a decreased circulating blood volume is observed, especially when the cooling is profound. For these reasons determination of the circulating blood volume has an important prognostic value during the rewarming of cooled organisms.

The water content of the heart or the brain is unaffected by moderate hypothermia,[104] but profound or extended hypothermia leads to water swelling in almost all hypothermic tissues. This swelling may be caused by a decrease or a cessation of the ionic active transport. Brendel[26] believes that in the higher mammals cold-induced swelling of the brain is one of the limiting factors for survival at low body temperatures. Cold swelling of the brain appears to be similar to the changes witnessed during intracellularly developing edema of the brain.[128] This brain swelling is greatly decreased when the circulation of hypothermic animals is extracorporeally supported, especially when the extracorporeal volume blood flow is high[99] and when an increased pCO_2 of the blood is induced. Cold swelling is observed in artificially cooled hibernators during the summer, but not during the winter months.

In Summary

In hypothermia one observes intracellular hydration and extracellular dehydration. These changes disappear after rewarming. An increased circulating blood volume is observed during the final phases of rewarming and indicates a successful recovery from hypothermia.

Electrolytes

Cationic changes induced by cooling have been studied many times.[26,27] Most investigators agree that these changes are not striking and that their trend is sometimes controversial. However, one must keep in mind that even a small increase or decrease in the concentration of some ions, especially hydrogen and potassium, can induce profound changes in normothermia as well as in hypothermia.

Cationic changes induced by hypothermia are as follows: Serum potassium in hypothermia is increased,[145] unchanged,[20,25] or decreased.[53,58,73,166,169] If the potassium concentration in hypothermia is really increased, this alteration might help to explain the hyperexcitability of the heart and its increased tendency toward the ventricular fibrillation sometimes observed in hypothermia.[146]

This potassium cation concentration during hypothermia can be compensated by glucose administration which tends to return the excitability of the hypothermic heart to normal levels.[128] Serum potassium is increased in hibernation as well.

Distribution of the potassium ions in various parts of the hypothermic heart is quite uneven.[97] This is especially observed during total cardiac bypass, when the major portion of potassium ions become concentrated in the ventricular septum.[75] An isolated perfused rat heart loses intracellular potassium and the perfusion fluid becomes acidic due to an accumulation of lactic acid. This phenomenon develops only when the perfusion fluid is deeply cooled.[153] After hypothermic cardiac arrest the concentration of potassium ions in tissues is decreased greatly. A decrease in the potassium level and an increase in the sodium content of the brain, heart, lung, and liver were reported in profound hypothermia. But even in shallow hypothermia there is a shift in the equilibrium of the cell potassium ions. This shift is from an easily exchangeable to a nonexchangeable fraction of potassium ions, leading toward a loss of potassium from the cell.[81]

It appears that one of the main causes of fluctuation in the potassium ion concentration in hypothermia is the change in cell membrane permeability induced by cooling.[84] Decreased effectiveness of the sodium–potassium pump and of the active ionic transport is another important factor that induces the observed changes in potassium ion concentration during hypothermia.[68] A decrease in the effectiveness of the sodium pump was observed even in poikilothermic animals cooled to a body temperature of 3 C.[100] The potassium exchange rate is independent of the heart rate, whether the heart is beating spontaneously or whether it is driven electrically.[153,154]

In moderate hypothermia there is no change in serum sodium concentration, but the plasma sodium level falls when the body temperature of an experimental animal is decreased below 25 C.

Hypothermia induces hyperphosphatemia as well, in the plasma[36,67] and in the muscles.[159] The calcium level appears to be unchanged during hypothermia,[59,110,151] though earlier reports mention an increase and sometimes even a decrease in calcium level.

During induced hypothermia in air-cooled patients, hyperphosphatemia has been observed also. Curiously, an important early finding that profound electrolytic changes induced by traumatic shock are much reduced in hypothermia[49] has not yet brought either confirmation or rejection.

Hypothermia increases the magnesium ion level in the plasma[71,105,110,117,135] This increase might be induced by cessation of kidney function, or it may be a direct consequence of the unloading of magnesium by the cold cells themselves. This increase might be of physiological importance for the proper maintenance of a profoundly decreased metabolism. Surface-cooled dogs with a high plasma magnesium ion concentration withstand deep cooling better than dogs with a low plasma magnesium ion concentration. However, a large infusion of magnesium ions leads to death of the animals at a somewhat higher body temperature. When cooled during the winter months, rats showed a small serum magnesium increase.

Summary

Hypothermia induces some changes in the electrolyte metabolism, but the overall picture is still quite obscure. It appears that potassium and magnesium levels of plasma are changed in hypothermia, cellular potassium being decreased and magnesium being increased. Different techniques of cooling, different species of animals, and the precooling state of experimental animals or patients greatly affect the results obtained during cooling.

Carbohydrate Metabolism

The most frequent observation is that hypothermia leads to hyperglycemia.[48,80,119] The rise in blood sugar level is probably elicited by an increased epinephrine release and a decreased utilization of glucose in the cold tissues.[1] During prolonged hypothermia in rats kept at a body temperature of 15 C, glycemia of the blood decreases continuously, initially being very high, however. After 9 hours at this low body temperature, just before death, glycemia has a very low level of only 35 mg percent.[120] The same happens with artificially cooled hibernators. They also start with a pronounced hyperglycemia which diminishes continuously. Just before death, which in their case occurs after spending several days in hypothermia, the artificially cooled hibernators have a very low blood glycemia.[120] Intravenous injection of glucose does not prolong the survival of hypoglycemic animals in extended hypothermia. This suggests that the blood sugar level is not the limiting factor for survival of animals during prolonged hypothermia. Contrary to this, in some animal species (chickens, rabbits, etc.) cooling induces hypoglycemia from the beginning.[129,130] A profound hypoglycemia is also witnessed in hibernators entering hibernation.[1] It is also known that hypoglycemia is induced after a long-term exposure to a very cold environment. In this case hypoglycemia and hypothermia appear together.[134]

In hypothermic patients the blood glucose changes depend mostly on the nutritional status of patients, the rate of cooling, and the depth of anesthesia.[137] When the body temperature is decreased to 25 C or lower, administration of epinephrine no longer leads to hyperglycemia.[37] In moderate hypothermia glucose continues to enter active cells from the extracellular spaces.[19] The same probably happens in profound hypothermia though it is less obvious (inhibition of the enzymes responsible for glucose transfer, reduced insulin activity, depressed liver function, or a combination of these factors).

Hyperlactacidemia is present in hypothermic patients,[10] especially during occlusin of the circulation when the lactate–pyruvate ratio increases. Hyperlactacidemia is probably caused by a decreased liver function. The myocardial lactate concentration in hypothermic guinea pigs is slightly elevated[61] but the concentration of cardiac lactic acid returns to the "normal" level when the animals are cooled more profoundly or when they are kept in hypothermia for several hours. It appears, therefore, that hypothermia is not the cause of the increased lactate in the blood occasionally observed in cooled organisms, again indicating that the cooled tissues of a hypothermic animal or patient do not suffer from hypoxia.

Cardiac glycogen was studied in cooled guinea pigs[101] and in other animals. Survival of hypothermic rats kept in pure nitrogen depends on the cardiac glycogen reserves.[101]

Proteins and Enzymes of Blood

The plasma protein level is decreased in hypothermic chickens,[147] goats,[158] and in other animals.[114] But other investigators found that the concentration of proteins in the blood is increased.[15] Thauer[156] believes that the plasma protein concentration is unchanged in hypothermia and deduces from this that the reduction in plasma and blood volume during cooling is caused by trapping of part of the blood in the peripheral tissues.

Free amino acid concentration in the blood is unchanged in hypothermia, except for taurine, which appears to be elevated.[83] It does not seem, however, that hypoproteinemia and inadequate nutritive levels of proteins in the blood are the cause of the decreased wound healing often seen after cooling.[94] Furthermore, changes in the serum protein fractions, observed during intracranial surgical interventions in hypothermic patients, do not appear to be induced by the lowering of the body temperature only. In artificially cooled hibernators the level of free amino acids in the blood is decreased.[83]

In profound hypothermia serum histamine is increased.[70,150] Thus the well-known effect of hypothermia on slowing down the symptoms of shock cannot be explained on the basis of histamine levels only or depletion of histamine depots. The level of blood ammonia is decreased in hypothermia.[162]

It is well known that the concentration of enzymes in the plasma is rather small, much smaller than in the cells. But after the cells are damaged, the enzymes are liberated and eventually enter the blood. The transaminase concentration of the glutamic oxalacetic acid increases after a cardiac infarct, first in the heart tissue and later in blood as well. The same applies to the increased amount of plasma lipase which indicates destructive processes in the pancreas. In hypothermic animals or patients an increased concentration of these plasma enzymes probably indicates an increase in membrane permeability of all cells, or at least cells that are more sensitive to cooling than others.[102] Some of the enzymatic changes induced by hypothermia are specific for certain animals.[158] Glutamic oxalacetic transaminase is increased in the serum of anesthetized dogs kept hypothermic for 12 hours, but after rewarming, this increase does not lead to necroses[23] or to damage of the liver cells.[103] After rewarming, the glutamic oxalacetic transaminase activity of serum does not return to normal level immediately but remains elevated for several hours.[163] The elevated transaminase values in deeply cooled patients is further increased (to 2 or 3 times the normal level) during cardiac arrest.[125]

In hypothermia one does not see the release of lysosomal enzymes[88] always observed in anoxia. This finding also points toward a normal oxygen supply to the heart and the other vital tissues in hypothermia. Furthermore, the acid hydrolase activity, a test often used to evaluate possible hypoxic conditions of tissues, remains unchanged in hypothermia.[88] Hypothermia does not change the binding status of lysosomal enzymes.[89]

Summary

Cooling usually leads to hyperglycemia. The passage of glucose into the hypothermic cell is somewhat decreased. This probably is caused by inhibition of the enzymes responsible for glucose transfer, by a reduced insulin activity, by a depressed liver function, or by a combination of any of these factors. Glucose utilization in the cooled cell is decreased too. The plasma protein level is decreased in hypothermia while the level of glutamic oxalacetic transaminase is increased, indicating an increased cell membrane permeability.

BLOOD GASES

Several years ago it was believed that an increased CO_2 tension is needed in profound hypothermia for the facilitation of oxygen dissociation from oxyhemoglobin and thus for a better supply of oxygen to the cooled tissues.[30] However, this idea had to be abandoned when it was discovered that changes in the O_2 dissociation curve induced by hypothermia are much smaller than expected[50,118] and that the release of oxygen from the cold red blood cells is almost as easy as from normothermic ones. Furthermore, a decrease in the blood pH helps the hemoglobin dissociation curve to return toward normal.[113]

The oxygen tension in the blood leaving the ventilated lungs of anesthetized dogs is the same whether or not the blood is cooled. Furthermore, an increased solubility of gases in cold plasma permits a greater amount of oxygen (per unit of volume of plasma) to be delivered to the tissues at the same oxygen tension of the blood.[132] The amount of physically dissolved oxygen in plasma of dogs core cooled to a body temperature of 10 to 15 C is increased by a factor of 2 and in plasma cooled to a temperature of 5 C by a factor of 7 (from 0.6 to 4.0 volume percent).

Until early 1960 it was thought that a drastic temperature increase might cause bubble formation in blood[140,142] which might be harmful especially during extracorporeal circulation. However, even during fast blood rewarming, bubbles were not observed. Microwaves are used for extra rapid rewarming of blood in the extracorporeal circuit without any detrimental effect.

The arteriovenous (AV) oxygen difference (volume percent) in hypothermia is the same as in normothermia.[2,111,122,132] This also applies to the AV oxygen difference of the coronary blood and to the blood in other organs. However, the presence of a normal AV oxygen difference in moderate or even more in profound hypothermia does not necessarily mean that the volume blood flow through every tissue in the body is normal. It is possible that during surface cooling the blood in the capillaries and in the venules of some tissues stagnates and that these tissues are hypoxic. If this should be the case, the AV oxygen difference of the whole organ would still appear normal.

A very profound cooling decreases AV oxygen difference. At a body temperature of 10 to 14 C, the AV oxygen difference often becomes negligible. However, the normal or near-normal oxygen saturation in hypothermic animals and in cooled patients is greatly reduced in special situations, for example after long-lasting circulatory arrest in experimental animals or patients cooled to a body temperature of 10 to 20 C. In this case the oxygen saturation of arterial blood is decreased to 40 to 50 percent. An increased pCO_2 of blood sometimes widens the AV oxygen difference of blood,[3] indicating a better tissue perfusion in surface-cooled animals. In prolonged hypothermia the AV oxygen difference increases continuously. In rats kept at a body temperature of 15 C for 9 hours, the AV oxygen difference increases from 5 to 15 volume percent.[122] Hibernating animals have a normal oxygen AV difference.[121]

A nomogram is now available showing the O_2 tensions of fully saturated blood at different temperatures.[64] When blood is cooled from a temperature of 37 to 20 C the amount of oxygen dissolved is increased by 30 percent.[63] Deoxygenation (half-complete) is greatly decreased (from 0.04 to 0.8 seconds) when human blood is cooled to a temperature of 7 C.[86] However, it is important to recognize that the transit time of red blood cells in cooled tissues is longer than in normothermia.[32] Thus the rate of release of oxygen from red blood cells does not appear to be a limiting factor for peripheral utilization of oxygen.[85]

The temperature coefficients for pCO_2 and for pH of whole blood have also been established[56,77] and the CO_2 dissociation curves in hypothermic animals and in hypothermic patients have been studied.[62] The CO_2 binding properties of cooled blood appear to be the same in nonhibernating and in hibernating animals.[116] A temperature-dependent nomogram for pCO_2 of blood has been found to be helpful for the estimation of values of the acid–base balance in hypothermia.[90] The CO_2 and O_2 binding ability of sheep erythrocytes is increased after cooling by 50 percent.[144] It appears that the values of pCO_2 and pH remain unchanged during hibernation.[79]

Summary

In hypothermia oxygen solubility in plasma is increased. Furthermore, the arteriovenous oxygen difference of the blood does not change in cooled patients or in cooled animals. This is so in the whole body as well as in the various organs, indicating a normal oxygen supply to cold cells. But whether this finding applies to all tissues, especially every part of the brain tissue, still remains an unanswered question.

VISCOSITY OF COOLED BLOOD

The relative viscosity of a suspension solution is not affected by temperature itself, unless the volume fraction or the shape of the suspended particles is changed. Due to the hemoconcentration and a change in the shear rate of blood induced by low temperature, hypothermia leads to an increased blood viscosity.[57,126] This increase might be very important for the performance of the cooled heart, especially in patients or animals kept hypothermic for hours, when the hematocrit rate increases to values of 70 volume percent or more.[120,122] In this case the hypothermic heart must perform additional work in order to pump the increasingly viscous blood.

The viscosity of cold blood is often compared to the viscosity of blood at normal body temperature or to the viscosity of water. The calculated viscosity values seldom correspond to the measured ones.[14] Earlier literature describes appreciable changes of blood viscosity induced by cooling, as for instance an increase of 2 percent in relative viscosity of blood for each temperature decrease of 1 C.[42] However, recent data show that the relative viscosity of blood is increased by only 10 percent when blood is cooled from a normal temperature to a temperature of 17 C.[14] It is likely that this increase in viscosity is induced mostly by an increase in the volume of each red blood cell. In experiments with rats a decrease in body temperature to 20 C did not change the viscosity of blood whatsoever.[143] Further decreases in body or blood temperatures to 2 to 10 C increase the blood viscosity by 50 to 100 percent. The critical body temperature at which the viscosity of blood suddenly becomes augmented for rats and other small laboratory animals appears to be a temperature of 14 to 16 C. This critical body temperature probably varies from species to species. For man it appears to be at a somewhat higher level. The precipitous increase in blood viscosity at this critical temperature is physiologically very important. This is the body temperature at which the adequate functioning of the heart of cooled animals and patients is impaired. Thus, before this critical temperature is reached, one should consider employing extracorporeal circulatory support combined with some blood dilution.

Summary

Viscosity of blood is increased in hypothermia but probably to a smaller degree than was thought a few years ago. However, a very profound surface cooling of human patients and of experimental animals might decrease the temperature of the blood below a critical level and thus suddenly increase the viscosity of blood.

FORMED ELEMENTS OF THE BLOOD

It is known that the velocity of the blood determines the leukocyte count. Thus, it is not surprising that hypothermia often leads to leukocytopenia (often with relative lymphocytosis), which is observed in hypothermic patients and in cooled animals as well.[15,124,139] The same has been seen in hibernators entering hibernation. Sarajas[138] believes that leukopenia is induced by a decreased tissue perfusion. After cooling, the eosinophil count of dogs decreases to 80 percent of the normothermic value.[66] In hypothermic patients a change in the shape of erythrocytes was also described.[43]

COAGULATION IN HYPOTHERMIA

Blood clotting in hypothermia has been the object of study in many papers.[107,160] Most authors agree that the clotting time increases as the body temperature decreases.[4,60,155]

Clinical experience also points toward an increase in bleeding tendency, though there are some reports about unchanged coagulation time in cooled human patients[28] and hypothermic dogs.[34] It appears that clotting factors are changed less when proper cooling techniques are used.[28] Hypothermia of long duration seems to prolong the coagulation time even more. This increased coagulation time is probably the consequence of a decreased number of platelets.[65,152,164] The increased coagulation time is observed in hibernators during hibernation[21,87] and in hibernators during estivation (hibernation during the summer season).[149]

Heparin activity is modified little in hypothermia.[31] Therefore, small amounts of administered heparin increase the platelet count in normothermic as well as in hypothermic patients[72,164] and have proved to be useful in decreasing the bleeding tendency in posthypothermic patients. Heparin prevents the hypothermic decrease of fibrinogen.[72,161] The fibrinogen content in hypothermic dogs is slightly decreased or remains unchanged. During hypothermic open-heart surgery some investigators observed an increased fibrinolytic activity which increases the danger of posthypothermic hemorrhage.[136] This increased fibrinolytic activity in hypothermia is prevented by the administration of epsilon aminocaproic acid, although some investigators believe that clinical use of epsilon aminocaproic acid is contraindicated except for a very prolonged bleeding combined with high fibrinolytic activity.

Prothrombin time is unchanged in hypothermic animals[155] and in hypothermic human patients. Consumption of prothrombin is decreased in hypothermia.[28] The production of plasma thromboplastin appears to be unaffected by a low temperature, while the action of thromboplastin on prothrombin or thrombin–fibrinogen interaction appears to be inhibited.[109]

Summary

Some changes in the formed elements of blood and profound changes of the clotting mechanisms are observed during cooling. After rewarming, all these changes disappear except for a temporary reduction in the number of platelets and a temporary prolongation of the coagulation time. Prophylactic use of epsilon aminocaproic acid or the administration of fresh blood after rewarming are recommended for the correction of clotting problems.

ACID–BASE BALANCE IN HYPOTHERMIA

Proper evaluation of the acid–base balance in hypothermia is a rather complicated procedure because of an increased CO_2 solubility, a small p*K* factor in the Henderson-Hasselbach equation, and some other problems. Still most investigators agree that in hypothermic animals and patients one observes both respiratory and metabolic acidosis. While the pH value of the blood at a normal body temperature is 7.4, the pH of blood in men or experimental animals cooled to a body temperature of 18 to 20 C is around 7.1 to 7.2. This phenomenon has been called "cold acidosis."[7,35,112] Sometimes even lower values than 7.1 to 7.2 have been reported.[18,120] During the cooling of human patients the values of the arterial pH vary more than the values of the venous pH[18] indicating changes in respiratory activity. Striking changes in the arterial pH have been associated with a high mortality of hypothermic patients.[112] Hyperventilation prevents respiratory acidosis.

During profound surface cooling, metabolic acidosis probably appears before respiratory acidosis, but during fast cooling this may be reversed. Acidosis might lead to the opening of the arteriovenous shunts and some tissue hypoxia.[141] This would lead further to the production of excessive amounts of lactic acid both during the cooling and during the rewarming process.[17,108] The metabolic acidosis is reinforced by a decreased utilization of lactic acid in the cold liver and in the cold heart.[131] It has been suggested that the low blood pressure observed, especially during the final stages of cooling, might be the consequence of hypothermic acidosis, slight hypoxia, or an inadequate blood flow.[44,47,113,167] It is likely that the increased tissue perfusion during core cooling decreases the amount of metabolic acidosis.

During hypothermic circulatory occlusion this acidosis is even more pronounced,[16,52,54,55] probably due to changes in the liver function.[52] The profound acidosis observed during hypothermic circulatory arrest might be elicited by changes induced in cell membranes.[84]

During rewarming, metabolic acidosis occurs even if it were not observed during the cooling process. However, the acidosis disappears after rewarming is completed.[40]

The degree of metabolic acidosis also depends on the species of the animal cooled[78] and on the precooling status of the patient, as well as on the cooling technique. The depth of anesthesia, the temperature at which hypothermia is maintained, the length of hypothermia, and perhaps the existence of large temperature gradients within the cooled organism also regulate the degree of acidosis.

Metabolic acidosis depresses the tissue metabolism and the activity of the respiratory center, thereby inducing a respiratory acidosis, also.

The metabolic acidosis and the respiratory acidosis in hypothermic patients and in cooled experimental animals are easily compensated by administration of sodium bicarbonate.[96] Furthermore, it appears that hyperventilation (with additional carbon dioxide) restores a normal pH and a normal pCO_2 of the blood as well as a normal buffer base.

Renal function is depressed in profound hypothermia. This leads to derangements in the acid–base balance. When marked differential hypothermia is observed during fast core or fast surface cooling, hypoxic acidosis can easily develop.[12] This hypoxic acidosis disappears, or at least it is much decreased, during the stabilization period, when the temperature of the body becomes more uniform.[11] A few investigators think that an induced alkalosis has a certain protective effect upon the heart in hypothermic animals.

When the coronary blood vessels of cooled dogs (body temperature 26 C) are perfused with warm heparinized blood, no acidosis develops even during occlusion of the inflow tract. Acidosis and the loss of potassium from the myocardium seen during hypothermic ventricular fibrillation, are ameliorated by a warm cardiac lavage.[39]

It is interesting to note that hypothermia does not increase the tolerance toward respiratory acidosis.[69]

For hypothermic patients the pH of the blood should be maintained at normal or, even better, at somewhat lower than normal values.[5] The correction factor (adjusted to a temperature of 37 C) for the measurement of the pH of blood with Astrup electrodes is 0.0147 for each degree centigrade below the normal body temperature.[6,22,133] Furthermore, pH meters could be calibrated or preset to the theoretical values of the buffer solutions at a lowered body temperature, the temperature which is under observation.[51,168] In order to assess the acid–base metabolism in human hypothermic patients new methods for the study of arterial blood samples have been developed.[115]

In hypothermia, the pCO_2 is maintained in a range close to 40 mg Hg, which helps to correct any metabolic imbalance easily.[29]

Summary

During cooling and rewarming the pH value of the blood of experimental animals or of patients decreases (“cold acidosis”), sometimes even when bicarbonate is administered. Both respiratory and metabolic acidosis develop during cooling. This acidosis is very pronounced but does not appear to be harmful. However, during surface cooling, a much decreased pH of the blood might be associated with an increased tendency toward ventricular fibrillation.

BIBLIOGRAPHY

1. Agid R, Ambid L: Effects of corporeal temperature on glucose metabolism in a homeotherm, the rat, and a hibernator, the garden dormouse, in Musacchia XJ, Saunders JF (eds): Depressed Metabolism. New York, Am Elsevier, 1969, pp 119–157
2. Albers C, Brendel W, Hardewig A: Blutgase in Hypothermie. Pfluegers Arch Ges Physiol 266:373–393, 1958
3. Aleksic A, Mitrovic M: The influence of partial CO_2 tension on arterio-venous oxygen difference in deep hypothermia. J Cardiovasc Surg 8:81–83, 1967
4. Anstall HB, Huntsman RG: Influence of temperature upon blood coagulation in a cold- and a warm-blooded animal. Nature 186:726, 1960
5. Astrup P, Engel K: Acid-base problems in hypothermia. Arch Intern Med 116:739–742, 1965
6. Austin WH, Lacombe EH, Rand PW: pH-temperature conversion factors and pCO_2 factors for hypothermia. J Appl Physiol 19:893–896, 1964
7. Axelrod DR, Bass DE: Electrolytes and acid-base balance in hypothermia. Am J Physiol 186:31–34, 1956
8. Axelrod DR, Bass DE: Electrolytes and acid-base balance in hypothermia. Surv Anesthesiol 1:117–118, 1957
9. Baker DG: Influence of cold exposure on electrolyte metabolism. Fed Proc 19, Suppl 5:125–130, 1960
10. Ballinger WF II, Templeton JY III, Vollenweider H, et al: Acidosis in patients during hypothermia and biventricular bypass. J Cardiovasc Surg 3:323–326, 1962
11. Ballinger WF II, Vollenweider H, Pierucci L Jr, et al: The accumulation and removal of excess lactate in arterial blood during hypothermia and biventricular bypass. Surgery 51:738–745, 1962
12. Ballinger WF II, Vollenweider H, Templeton JY III, et al: Acidosis of hypothermia. Ann Surg, Suppl 154:517–523, 1961
13. Barlow G, Spurr GB, Bowe RL: Circulating levels of 17-hydroxycorticosteroids in prolonged hypothermia. J Appl Physiol 14:777–780, 1959
14. Bayliss LE: The rheology of blood, in Hamilton WF (ed): Handbook of Physiology, Circulation I. Washington, American Physiology Society, 1962, pp 137–150
15. Beaton JR: Haematologic and serum protein alterations in the hypothermic rat. Proc Soc Exp Biol Med 107:426–428, 1961
16. Bernhard WF, Carroll SE, Schwarz HF, et al: Metabolic alterations associated with profound hypothermia and extracorporeal circulation in the dog and man. J Thorac Cardiovasc Surg 42:793–803, 1961
17. Bernhard WF, McMurrey JD, Ganong WF, et al: The effect of hypothermia on the peripheral serum levels of free 17-hyroxycorticoids in the dog and man. Ann Surg 143:210–215, 1956
18. Bessman SP, Cowley RA: Biochemical changes in human beings during refrigeration anesthesia. Ann NY Acad Sci 80:540–546, 1959
19. Bickford AF, Mottram RF: Glucose metabolism during periods of induced hypothermia. J Physiol 143:37P–38P, 1958
20. Bigelow WG, Lindsay WK, Greenwood WF: Hypothermia: Its possible role

in cardiac surgery. An investigation of factors governing survival in dogs at low body temperatures. Ann Surg 132:849–866, 1950

21. Biorck G, Johansson BW, Nilsson IM: Blood coagulation studies in hedgehogs, in a hibernating and a non-hibernating state, and in dogs, hypothermic and normothermic. Acta Physiol Scand 56:334–348, 1962
22. Bjork VO, Aletras H, Intonti F: The use of hypothermia in open heart surgery. J Cardiovasc Surg 3:182–194, 1962
23. Blair E, Hook R, Tolley H, et al: Serum glutamic oxalacetic transaminase content in hypothermia. Science 133:105–106, 1961
24. Bond TP, Derrick JR, Guest MM: Microcirculation during hypothermia. Arch Surg 89:887–890, 1964
25. Boyd JW, Webb WR: Serum and tissue electrolyte changes during profound hypothermia. Am Surg 27:186–192, 1961
26. Brendel W, Muller C, Reulen HJ, et al: Elektrolytveranderungen in tiefer Hypothermie. II. Beziehungen zur klinischen und biologischen Uberlebenszeit. Pfluegers Arch Ges Physiol 288:220–239, 1966
27. Brendel W, Reulen HJ, Aigner P, et al: Elektrolytveranderungen in tiefer Hypothermie. IV. Die Kalteschwellung des Gehirns beim Winterschlafer. Pfluegers Arch Ges Physiol 292:83–89, 1966
28. Bunker JP, Goldstein R: Coagulation during hypothermia in man. Proc Soc Exp Biol Med 97:199–202, 1958
29. Burton GW: Metabolic acidosis during profound hypothermia. Anaesthesia 19:365–375, 1964
30. Callaghan PB, Lister J, Paton BC, et al: Effect of varying carbon dioxide tensions on the oxyhemoglobin dissociation curves under hypothermic conditions. Ann Surg, Suppl 154:903–910, 1961
31. Calogera E: The behavior of heparin activity in heat shock and in freezing. Folia Med 34:461–471, 1951
32. Chang CB, Shoemaker WC: Effect of hypothermia on red cell volumes. J Thorac Cardiovasc Surg 46:117–124, 1963
33. Connolly JE, Roy A, Guernsey JM, et al: Bloodless surgery by means of profound hypothermia and circulatory arrest. Effect on brain and heart. Ann Surg 162:724–737, 1965
34. Couves CM, Overton RC Jr, Eaton WL: Hematologic changes in hypothermic dogs. Surg Forum 6:102–106, 1956
35. Cranston WI, Pepper MC, Ross DN: Blood reaction during hypothermia. J Physiol 125:20P–21P, 1954
36. Crawford AL, Haist RE: Some effects of insulin on the blood sugar and inorganic phosphorus levels of normothermic and hypothermic rats. Can J Physiol Pharmacol 43:137–146, 1965
37. Crawford AL, Henderson MJ, Hawkins RD, et al: The effect of glucagon on blood sugar and inorganic phosphorus levels in normothermic and hypothermic rats. Can J Physiol Pharmacol 43:601–610, 1965
38. D'Amato HE, Hegnauer AH: Blood volume in the hypothermic dog. Am J Physiol 173:100–102, 1953
39. DeWeese JA, Jones TI, Mahoney EP: Myocardial metabolism during hypothermia with caval occlusion and low flow coronary perfusion. Surg Forum 8:298–302, 1957

40. Donatelli R, Pellegrini A: Modificazioni fisiopathologichi da circolazione extracorporea in normothermia ed ipotermia profonda. Chir Patol Sper 9:1131, 1960
41. Drake CT, Lewis FJ: The plasma volume expanding effect of low molecular weight dextran in the hypothermic dog. Surg Forum 12:182–184, 1961
42. Eckstein RW, Book D, Gregg DE: Blood viscosity under different experimental conditions and its effect on blood flow. Am J Physiol 135:772–775, 1942
43. Eiseman B, Spencer FC: Effect of hypothermia on the flow characteristics of blood. Surgery 52:532–544, 1962
44. Ellis FH, Kirklin JW: The use of extracorporeal circulation in cardiac surgery. Dis Chest 36:173–178, 1959
45. Fedor EJ, Fisher B: Simultaneous determination of blood volume with Cr-51 and T-1824 during hypothermia and rewarming. Am J Physiol 196:703–705, 1959
46. Gelin LE, Lofstrom B: A preliminary study on peripheral circulation during deep hypothermia. Observations on decreased suspension stability of the blood and its prevention. Acta Chir Scand 108:402–404, 1954/1955
47. Gerbode F, Osborn JJ, Johnston JB: Experience with perfusion hypothermia using an improved rotating disc oxygenator. Thorax 15:185–192, 1960
48. Giaja J, Stefanovic M: Relation between hypothermia and glycemia in asphyxia. C R Acad Sci (Paris) 232:751–753, 1951
49. Gibertini G, Malaguti G, Porro A, et al: Alcuni aspetti della reazione dell'organismo al trauma in corso di ibernazione. II. Comportamento della kalemia e della natremia. Att Soc Lomb Sci Med Biol 9:17–19, 1954
50. Gleichmann U, Lohr B, Lubbers DW, et al: Untersuchungen zur Diagnostik und Therapie der metabolischen Azidose sowie uber Blutgase bei Herzoperationen mit extrakorporaler Zirkulation und Hypothermie. Thoraxchirurgie 11:251–269, 1963-64
51. Gleichmann U, Lohr B, Roskenbleck H: Verhalten der O_2 Dissoziationkurve des Blutes wahrend der extrakorporalen Zirkulation, kombiniert mit Hypothermie. Zentralbl Chir 88:509–516, 1963
52. Gleichmann U, Lubbers DW, Ringler W: Vergleichende Untersuchungen des Kohlensauredruckes mit der Mikro-pH-Methode (Astrup) under der stabilisierten Ganzglas-pCO_2-Elektrode in Normo- und Hypothermie. Pfluegers Arch Ges Physiol 273:190–198, 1961
53. Gollan F, Rudolph GG, Olsen NS: Electrolyte transfer during hypothermia and anoxia in dogs. Am J Physiol 189:277–280, 1957
54. Gordon AS, Jones JC, Luddington LG, et al: Deep hypothermia for intracardiac surgery: Experimental and clinical use without an oxygenator. Am J Surg 100:332–337, 1960
55. Gordon AS, Meyer BW, Jones JC: Open heart surgery using deep hypothermia without an oxygenator. J Thorac Cardiovasc Surg 40:787–812, 1960
56. Greenburg AG, Moulder PV: Temperature coefficients for pCO_2 and pH in whole blood: Finding pCO_2 and pH at low temperatures. Arch Surg 91:867–871, 1965
57. Grossman R, Lewis FJ: The effect of cooling and low molecular weight dextran on blood sludging. J Surg Res 4:360–362, 1964
58. Grote W, Schweikhardt F: Electrolytes in serum, and lactic and pyruvic acid

in blood under normothermia and hypothermic conditions in rabbits. Pfluegers Arch Ges Physiol 305:351–360, 1969

59. Gutherie JR, Nayler WG: Effect of hypothermia on radiocalcium movement in cardiac muscle. Comp Biochem Physiol 20:657–665, 1967
60. Halinen MO, Suhonen RE, Sarajas HS: Characteristics of blood clotting in hypothermia. Scand J Clin Lab Invest 21, Suppl 101:65, 1968
61. Hanson A, Johansson BW: Myocardial lactate concentration in guinea pigs, normothermic and hypothermic, and hedgehogs, in a hibernating and a non-hibernating state. Acta Physiol Scand 53:137–141, 1961
62. Harms H, Bartels H: CO_2-Dissoziationskurven des menschlichen Blutes bei Temperaturen von 5–37°C und unterschiedlicher O_2-Sattigung. Pfluegers Arch Ges Physiol 272:384–392, 1961
63. Hedley-Whyte J, Laver MB: O_2 solubility in blood and temperature correction factors for pO_2. J Appl Physiol 19:901–906, 1964
64. Hedley-Whyte J, Radford EP Jr, Laver MB: Nomogram for temperature correction or electrode calibration during pO_2 measurements. J Appl Physiol 20:785–786, 1965
65. Helmsworth JA, Stiles WJ, Elstun W: Changes in blood cellular elements in dogs during hypothermia. Surgery 38:843–846, 1955
66. Helmsworth JA, Stiles WJ, Elstun W: Leukopenic and thrombocytopenic effect of hypothermia in dogs. Proc Soc Exp Biol Med 90:474–476, 1955
67. Herak M, Timet P: The activity of serum alkaline and acid phosphotase in thc rat during hypothermia and posthypothermia. Yugosl Physiol Pharmacol Acta 3:282–285, 1967
68. Hercus V, Bowman S: Cation studies during experimental hypothermia. Aust Ann Med 8:123–128, 1959
69. Holmdahl MH: The tolerance of the dog under hypothermia to respiratory acidosis. Proceedings, 1st World Congress on Anesthesia, 1955, pp 109–112
70. Holobut W, Modrzejewski E: Changes of histamine content in peripheral blood during hypothermia. Arch Int Pharmacodyn Ther 163:28–31, 1966
71. Johansson BW: Electrocardiographic changes in depressed metabolism, in Musacchia XJ, Saunders JF (eds): Depressed Metabolism. New York, Am Elsevier, 1969, pp 313–374
72. Johansson BW, Nilsson IM: The effect of heparin and epsilon aminocaproic acid on coagulation in hypothermic dogs. Acta Physiol Scand 60:267–277, 1964
73. Kanter GS: Regulation of extracellular potassium in hypothermia. Am J Physiol 205:1285–1289, 1963
74. Kanter GS: Hypothermic hemoconcentration. Am J Physiol 214:856–859, 1968
75. Kaplan A, Fisher B: Potassium ion as a cardioplegic agent in total cardiac bypass and during hypothermia with coronary perfusion. J Thorac Cardiovasc Surg 39:468–477, 1960
76. Keen G, Gerbode F: Observations on microcirculation during profound hypothermia. J Thorac Cardiovasc Surg 45:252–260, 1963
77. Kelman GR, Nunn JF: Nomograms for correction of blood pO_2, pCO_2, pH, and base excess for time and temperature. J Appl Physiol 21:1484–1490, 1966
78. Kent KM, Peirce CE II: Acid-base characteristics of hibernating animals. J Appl Physiol 23:336–340, 1967

79. Kent KM, Popovic V: Cardiovascular responses in hypothermia and hibernation. Physiologist 8:318, 1965
80. Kilburn KH: Effect of adrenergic blockage with Hydergine on hyperglycemia accompanying hypothermia in dogs. Am J Physiol 199:955–958, 1960
81. Klein RL: Effects of active transport inhibitors on K movements in Acanthamoeba sp. Exp Cell Res 34:231–238, 1964
82. Klussmann FW, Lutcke A, Koenig W: Uber das Verhalten der Korperflussigkeiten wahrend kunstlicher Hypothermie. Pfluegers Arch Ges Physiol 268:515–529, 1959
83. Kristofferson R, Broberg S: Free amino acids in blood serum of hedgehogs in deep hypothermia and after spontaneous arousal. Experientia 24:148–150, 1968
84. Langdon L, Kingsley DPE: Changes in serum and urinary potassium levels during profound hypothermia in man. J Clin Pathol 17:257–259, 1964
85. Lawson WH Jr, Forster RF: Oxygen tension gradients in peripheral capillary blood. J Appl Physiol 22:970–973, 1967
86. Lawson WH Jr, Holland RAB, Forster RE: Effect of temperature on deoxygenation rate of human red cells. J Appl Physiol 20:912–918, 1965
87. Lechler E, Penick GD: Blood clotting defect in hibernating ground squirrels (*Citellus tridecemlineatus*). Am J Physiol 205:985–988, 1963
88. Leighty EG, Ressallat MM, Passananti GT, et al: Effects of hypoxia and hypothermia on the release of lysosomal enzymes in the dog heart. Surg Forum 17:181–183, 1966
89. Leighty EG, Stoner CD, Ressallat MM, et al: Effects of acute asphyxia and deep hypothermia on the state of binding of lysosomal acid hydrolases in canine cardiac muscle. Circ Res 21:59–64, 1967
90. Lenfant C: Nomogram for rapid determination of pCO_2 when in vivo temperature of blood is different from 37°C. J Appl Physiol 16:909–910, 1961
91. Lewis RA, Satoskar RS, Gaitonde BB, et al: Biochemical changes during hypothermia. Surv Anesthesiol 1:120, 1957
92. Lofstrom B: Changes in blood volume in induced hypothermia. Acta Anaesthesiol Scand 1:1–13, 1957
93. Lofstrom B: Induced hypothermia and intravascular aggregation. Acta Anaesthesiol Scand 3:Suppl III:1–19, 1959
94. Lofstrom B, Zederfeldt B: Wound healing after induced hypothermia. IV. Importance of the rewarming phase. Acta Chir Scand 129:341–344, 1965
95. Marshall R, Gunning AJ: The measurement of blood gas tensions during profound hypothermia. J Surg Res 2:351–356, 1962
96. Maurath J: Blutgase und Saure-Basen-Gleichgewicht bei Langzeithypothermie. Klin Wochenschr 39:1149–1150, 1961
97. Mavor GE, Harder RA, McEvoy RK, et al: Potassium and the hypothermic heart. Am J Physiol 185:515–520, 1956
98. Meiselman HJ, Merrill EW, Salzman EW, et al: Effect of dextran on rheology of human blood: Low shear viscometry. J Appl Physiol 22:480–486, 1967
99. Messemer K, Brendel W, Reulen HJ, et al: Die Uberlebenszeit von Hunden in tiefer Hypothermie bei extrakorporalem Kreislauf. Pfluegers Arch Ges Physiol 281:60–61, 1964
100. Miller DA, Standish ML, Thurman AE Jr: Effects of temperature on water and electrolyte balance in the frog. Physiol Zool 41:500–506, 1968

101. Miller JA Jr, Zakhary R, Miller FS: Hypothermia, asphyxia, and cardiac glycogen in guinea pigs. Science 144:1226–1227, 1964
102. Mitin V, Timet D, Biscan J: The activity of transaminases in rats blood plasma during hypothermia and post-hypothermia. Biol Glas (Yugosl) 18:1–7, 1965
103. Mitin V, Timet D, Biscan J: The activity of the transaminases in the blood plasma of the rat following carbon tetrachloride poisoning and compared with the same activity in hypothermia. Vet Arch (Yugosl) 39:1–5, 1969
104. Moulder PV, Eichelberger L, Roma M, et al: Biochemistry of blood, heart, and skeletal muscle under induced, controlled hypothermia. Arch Surg 78:37–44, 1959
105. Moussa SL, Boba A: Exogenous plasma magnesium increases during hypothermia in dogs. Am J Physiol 199:1090–1092, 1960
106. Munday KA, Blane GF, Chin EF, et al: Plasma electrolyte changes in hypothermia. Thorax 13:334–342, 1958
107. Negre E, Izarm P, du Cailak J, et al: Modification des facteur de l'homostase au cours de l'hypothermie profonde. Ann Chir Thorac Cardiovasc 1:646–651, 1962
108. Neville WE, White RJ, Verdura J: Relationship of flow rate, "excess lactate," and buffer base during closed chest profound hypothermic perfusion with a pump oxygenator. Surgery 55:281–290, 1964
109. Nour-Eldin F: Hypothermia and blood coagulation. Acta Haematol 29:218–225, 1963
110. Nowell NW, White DC: Season variation of magnesium and calcium in serum of the hypothermic rat. J Appl Physiol 18:967–969, 1963
111. Orihata H, Nakayama K, Ichii K: Studies in extension of interruption period for blood circulation in heart, particularly on head cooling method. Bull Heart Inst Jap 2:77–101, 1958
112. Osborn JJ: Experimental hypothermia: Respiratory and blood pH changes in relation to cardiac function. Am J Physiol 175:389–398, 1953
113. Osborn JJ, Gerbode F, Johnston JB, et al: Blood chemical changes in perfusion hypothermia for cardiac surgery. J Thorac Cardiovasc Surg 42:462–476, 1961
114. Ostashkov KV: Blood serum proteins under conditions of artificial hypothermia. Biokhimiia (Moskva) 26:966–969, 1961
115. Patterson RH Jr, Sondheimer HM: Assessing acid-base metabolism with samples of arterial blood obtained from hypothermic subjects. J Surg Res 6:19–23, 1966
116. Person RS: Effect of the temperature upon the binding of CO_2 by the blood of some mammals. C R Acad Sci USSR 70:339–342, 1950
117. Platner WS, Hosko MJ Jr: Mobility of serum magnesium in hypothermia. Am J Physiol 174:273–276, 1953
118. Popovic V: Mecanisme de la mort de l'homeotherme refroidi. Acta Med Yugosl 7:40–62, 1953
119. Popovic V: De L'hypothermie lethargique prolongee. Arch Sci Physiol (Paris) 9:219–229, 1955
120. Popovic V: Physiological characteristics of rats and ground squirrels during prolonged lethargic hypothermia. Am J Physiol 199:467–471, 1960

121. Popovic V: Cardiac output in hibernating ground squirrels. Am J Physiol 207:1345–1348, 1964
122. Popovic V, Kent KM: Cardiovascular responses in prolonged hypothermia. Am J Physiol 209:1069–1074, 1965
123. Popovic V, Kostolny I, Pass KA, et al: Survival of extracorporeally cooled dogs after one hour circulatory arrest. Cryobiology 8:330, 1971
124. Puchkov NV: On the influence of cooling upon the organism. Zentralbl Allg Pathol 81:289, 1943
125. Quinn JW, Sirak HD, Shabanah EH, et al: Transaminase values following open heart surgery. Ann Surg 152:45–50, 1960
126. Rand PW, Lacombe E, Hunt HE, et al: Viscosity of normal human blood under normothermic and hypothermic conditions. J Appl Physiol 19:117–122, 1964
127. Reed PI, Gavrilescu KE: The value of laboratory tests in hypothermia. J Clin Pathol 11:220–223, 1958
128. Reulen HJ, Aigner P, Brendel W, et al: Elektrolytveranderungen in tiefer Hypothermie. I. Die Wirkung akuter Auskuhlung bis 0°C und Wiedererwarming. Pfluegers Arch Ges Physiol 288:197–219, 1966
129. Rodbard S: Relationship between body temperature and blood sugar in chicken. Am J Physiol 150:67–69, 1947
130. Rodbard S, Goldstein MS: Neurogenic control of the blood sugar elicited by induced variations in the body temperature of the chick. Am J Physiol 162:175–181, 1950
131. Rosenfeld JB: Acid-base and electrolyte disturbances in hypothermia. Am J Cardiol 12:678–682, 1963
132. Rosenhain FR, Penrod KE: Blood gas studies in the hypothermic dog. Am J Physiol 166:55–61, 1951
133. Rossing RG, Cain SM: A nomogram relating pO_2, pH, temperature, and hemoglobin saturation in the dog. J Appl Physiol 21:195–201, 1966
134. Sahovic K, Orescanin B: Contribution to the physiopathology of the hypothermia of homeotherms; effect of deep hypothermia on glycemia; effect of adrenalin, insulin, and adrenalectomy. Glas Srp Akad Nauka (Med) 204(4):87–97, 1951
135. Sahovic K, Orescanin B, Milhailovic L: Les modifications biochimiques et les variations des elements sanguins chez les animaux en hypothermie. Glas Acad Serbe Sci 208:153–182, 1954
136. Samama M, Yver J, Weiss M: Mecanisme de l'activation du systeme fibrinolytique en chirurgie cardiaque avec C.E.C. et hypothermie profonde. Hemostase 2:335–336, 1962
137. Sarajas HSS: The appearance of immature myeloid cells and allied changes in the peripheral blood of dogs rendered hypothermic, with or without subsequent rewarming. Ann Chir Gynaecol Fenn 51:146–158, 1962
138. Sarajas HSS: Blood glucose and plasma potassium levels in hypothermic dogs. Ann Chir Gynaecol Fenn 51:253–263, 1962
139. Sarajas HSS: The circulating leukocyte pool versus the circulatory status in hypothermic dogs. Ann Acad Sci Fenn 106:3–11, 1964
140. Sealy WC, Brown IW, Young WG, et al: Hypothermia and extracorporeal circulation for open-heart surgery. Ann Surg 150:627–639, 1959

141. Sealy WC, Lesage MA, Young WG Jr: Vascular responses during hypothermia. J Thorac Cardiovasc Surg 46:795–810, 1963
142. Shields TW, Lewis FJ: Rapid cooling and surgery at temperatures below 20°C. Surgery 46:164–174, 1959
143. Shorrock JET, Hillman H: The viscosity of rat blood between the temperatures of 2 and 35°C. Cryobiology 5:324–327, 1969
144. Sirs JA: Uptake of O_2 and CO by hemoglobin sheep erthrocytes at various temperatures. J Appl Physiol 18:166–170, 1963
145. Smith RT: Electrolyte studies in experimental animals during hypothermia. Am J Surg 92:228–232, 1956
146. Spurr GB, Barlow G, Lambert H: Influence of prolonged hypothermia and hyperthermia on cardiac response to inject potassium. Am J Physiol 196:696–702, 1959
147. Sturkie PD: Effects of hypothermia upon specific gravity and proteins of blood of chickens. Am J Physiol 148:610–613, 1947
148. Svanes K: Studies in hypothermia: VI. Intravascular aggregation in hypothermic mice. Acta Anaesthesiol Scand 10:123–131, 1966
149. Svihla A, Bowman HR, Ritenour R: Prolongation of clotting time in dormant estivating mammals. Science 114:298–299, 1951
150. Szilagyi T, Csaba B, Damjanovich S, et al: Effect of hypothermia on the histamine level of blood plasma. Acta Physiol Sci Hung (Budapest) 20:141–144, 1961
151. Szorady I, Koltay M, Dombradi G, et al: Investigation of the electrolyte distribution in artificial hibernation. Kiserl Orvostud 13:335–344, 1961
152. Tadzer IS: Fibrinolysis and platelet adhesiveness in hypothermic rats. Physiol Pharmacol Acta 3:436–439, 1967
153. Taylor IM: Factors contributing to the damaging effect of cold upon mammalian tissues. Final Technical Report DA-49-007-MD-999, 1964
154. Taylor IM, Huffines WD, Young DT: Tissue water and electrolytes in an isolated perfused rat's heart preparation. J Appl Physiol 16:95–102, 1961
155. Terzioglu M, Ozer F: Blood heparin level and the status of blood coagulation in cats during hypothermia. Arch Int Physiol Biochem 64:1–19, 1956
156. Thauer R: The circulation in hypothermia of nonhibernating animals and men, in Hamilton WF (ed): Handbook of Physiology, Circulation III. Washington, American Physiology Society, 1965, pp 1899–1920
157. Timet D: Red and white blood picture of the goat in hypothermia and posthypothermia. Rad JAZU 329:121–159, 1962
158. Timet D, Mitin V: Serum protein concentration in the goat during hypothermia and posthypothermia. Rad JAZU 345:225–236, 1967
159. Timet D, Mitin V, Tranger M, et al: Study of the phosphorus metabolism in the liver and in the muscles during hypothermia and posthypothermia carried out by means of isotope P-32. Physiol Pharacol Acta 3:439–442, 1967
160. Von Kaulla KN: Is 37°C the optimal clotting temperature for human blood? Acta Haematol 25:56–61, 1961
161. Weiss M, Guery J, DuBost C; Hemorrhagie, coagulation, hemostase des operes a "coeur ouvert." II. Influence favorable sur 6 saignement postoperatoire de l'injection d'acide epsilon-amino-caproique. Ann Chir Thorac Cardiovasc 3:366–381, 1964

162. Welch HF, Affifi R, Rosano CL: Effect of hypothermia on blood ammonia formation. Surgery 50:390–394, 1961
163. Wendel OW: Serum glutamic oxalacetic transaminase activity following hypothermia. Anaesthesia 16:24–31, 1961
164. Wensel RH, Bigelow WG: Use of heparin to minimize thrombocytopenia and bleeding tendency during hypothermia. Surgery 45:223–228, 1959
165. Willson JT, Miller WR, Eliot TS: Blood studies in the hypothermic dog. Surgery 43:979–989, 1958
166. Yonce LR, Dykers JR Jr, McGee JW: Vascular resistance and venous blood K^+ during hypothermia in skeletal muscle. Am J Physiol 202:277–280, 1962
167. Young WG, Sealy WC, Brown IW, et al: Metabolic and physiologic observations on patients undergoing extracorporeal circulation in conjunction with hypothermia. Surgery 46:175–184, 1959
168. Zingg W: The calibration of a pH meter for pH determinations at varying temperatures. Can Med Assoc J 90:490, 1964
169. Zotti EF, Lesage MA, Wallace AG, et al: Conduction and excitability of the intact hypothermic heart. Studies using chronically implanted electrodes and controlled deep hypothermia. Trans Am Soc Artif Intern Organs 11:139–142, 1965.

3

Circulation

"And this distilling liquor drink thou of,
When presently through all thy veins shall run
A cold and drowsy humor—for no pulse
Shall keep his native progress, but surcease;
No warmth, no breath shall testify thou livest."

". . . and cold appear like death,
And in this borrow'd likeness of shrunk death
Thou shalt continue two and forty hours
And then awake as from pleasant sleep."

Romeo and Juliet (IV, 1), W. Shakespeare

Hypothermia decreases the metabolism of all living tissues: the deeper the cooling of an organism, the more profound is the depression of the metabolism. The circulation in hypothermia, as in normothermia, closely follows the metabolic needs of an organism. However, during a very profound cooling, the circulation is considerably decreased and might even be failing. The profound and extended cooling eventually leads to circulation failure and it is probably the main factor limiting the safe survival ("biological survival") of cooled organisms. However, in profound hypothermia one observes the "protective role of hypothermia." The organism is much less sensitive to the detrimental effects of the external or the internal environment than at normal body temperature. The circulation of a cooled homeotherm can be interrupted for 1 or even 2 hours without harmful effects. This striking difference, between 4 and 5 minutes (in normothermia) and 2 hours in profound hypothermia, has been the major factor that has attracted so many investigators, experimental as well as clinical, to this field.

Circulatory changes induced by cooling have been the subject of many investigations. These changes have been discussed in detail.[59,60,62,108,195,360,491,515]

HYPOTHERMIC HEART

Introduction

In the many animal species studied, the heart activity during cooling undergoes changes similar to those in human patients. Cooling of the heart can be accomplished either by cooling the whole body or by selective cooling of the heart only. Selective cooling of the heart can be induced either by coronary perfusion with cold blood or saline[368] or by surface cooling of the heart. It appears that the physiological changes observed during the cooling are directly produced by a decreased temperature. This applies to the slowing of the heart rate, prolongation of the systole, prolongation of the isovolumetric relaxation phase,[28] and prolongation of the conduction velocity.[99,116] Johansson,[271] who studied the ECG changes induced by hypothermia in detail, believes that alterations in the ventricular conduction (determined mostly by S-T segments and the T-wave) are brought about by these effects of cooling.

Electrocardiographic Changes

A number of specific ECG changes are seen in cooled animals[13,67,271,272,450,539,556] as well as in hypothermic patients.[48,530] Hypothermia prolongs some parts of the ECG, for instance the PR and S-T intervals and the QRS complex itself.[67,160,428]

Hypothermic animals and hypothermic patients have altered patterns of deflection in their ECG which are not observed in normothermia. The specific deflection which appears between the QRS and S-T segments was called a J-wave[166] or O-wave.[70,136] It should be mentioned that some time ago (but not any more) this "hypothermic wave" was considered to be caused by a current of injury.[114,236]

Blood dilution with dextran decreases the "sludging" of blood corpuscles in hypothermia, but it does not change the modifications of the ECG brought on by cold, indicating that the changes in the ECG are not induced by hypothermic sequestration of the red blood cells, as was once believed. The fact that the lactate content of the hearts of animals in hibernation is the same as in hypothermic nonhibernators indicates that the hearts of hypothermic animals or of cooled patients do not suffer from hypoxia and that the ECG changes induced by cooling should not be considered the result of hypoxia.[238] Furthermore, the somewhat elevated lactate content of the hearts in guinea pigs cooled to a body temperature of 30 C remains unchanged when the body temperature of the animals is lowered further.[238] These observations also indicate an absence of tissue hypoxia brought on by hypothermia.

The ECG changes induced by the cooling of patients and experimental animals are not always identical. One must keep in mind that such comparisons are often made between the healthy animals and sick, often poor-risk patients.

All ECG changes induced by the cooling disappear after rewarming.[194,241]

The ECG in hypothermia is profoundly influenced by the central nervous system, as it is in normothermia. During a shallow surface cooling of patients who already have pronounced ECG irregularities, additional anesthesia restores the ECG pattern to a normal configuration. It appears that centrally induced cardiac irregularites are also potentiated by hypothermia.[438]

SUMMARY

Many ECG changes are induced during the cooling of experimental animals and of patients. Some of these changes are caused by the direct effects of cold per se upon the heart, while others are induced by changes in the blood chemistry, changes in the nervous tone, or abnormal activities in the central nervous system. The hypothermic ECG changes do not appear to be the consequence of induced hypoxia of the cold myocardium. After rewarming all ECG changes disappear quickly.

Excitability and the Conductive System

In hypothermia the excitability and the function of the conductive system are relatively well preserved.[86] The responsiveness of a heart to electrical stimuli is unchanged until a temperature of 20 to 25 C is reached. Below this temperature the diastolic ventricular excitability appears to be depressed.

The resting potential of the heart is unchanged during cooling, at least until a body temperature of 20 C.[120,189] The action potentials eventually disappear at a low body temperature of 10 and 15 C and occasionally even at temperatures lower than that.[346] This might be caused either by a less efficient sodium pump or by a differential effect of the low temperature on the active transport of sodium versus potassium ions. During cooling the sino-atrial node and the atrium lose the ability for rhythmic excitation earlier than do the ventricles. This happens at a body temperature of 20 to 25 C when the sino-atrial pacemaker becomes inactive, whereas the AV node is still sending out impulses and the ventricles are still conducting. The Purkinje fibers conduct even at a temperature of 10 C. Action potentials of any part of a cooled heart are prolonged.

The amplitude of the action potentials of the heart remains constant during cooling except when the body temperature is decreased below 20 C.[515] The speed of depolarization is affected little by the cooling, whereas repolarization is considerably slowed.

The relative and especially the absolute refractory periods of the cooled heart are prolonged in hypothermia. At a body temperature of 22 C the prolongation is twofold.[12,520] During the rewarming from profound hypothermia the recovery of excitability of the ventricular muscle is not uniform.[236] Ventricular vulnerability appears to be increased during cooling.[415,526]

SUMMARY

Even in profound hypothermia the excitability of the whole myocardium is well preserved. Further cooling will abolish the performance of the sino-atrial pacemaker but the ventricles will continue to beat. The refractory period of the heart is prolonged in hypothermia.

Cardiac Metabolism

The energy sources for the heart are glucose and in somewhat lesser degrees lactic acid, pyruvic acid, free fatty acids, and proteins. The relative consumption of these nutrients in hearts cooled to a temperature of 25 C appears to be practically unchanged as compared to the consumption under normothermic conditions.[35]

Surface hypothermia induces a marked depletion of glycogen in the rat heart. After rewarming, the glycogen is rapidly restored.[311] There is an increased conversion of ATP to ADP in animals cooled to a low body temperature.[555] After several hours spent at a low body temperature the inadequate amount of ATP, caused by a decreased metabolism or by an inefficient coupling, might become the basis for myocardial failure and thus the beginning of the vicious cycle which leads to death in prolonged hypothermia.

During the cooling of dogs to a body temperature of 25 C the potassium concentration of their hearts increases but the water content does not change.[490]

Oxygen Consumption and Mechanical Efficiency

The myocardial oxygen consumption is decreased during cooling but probably to a smaller degree than in other organs.[61,521] During the selective cooling of the dog's heart to a temperature of 10 C, the decrease in O_2 consumption is smaller than expected.[143] The oxygen consumption of isolated hearts cooled to a temperature of 15 C is still relatively high (1.6 ml/100 gm/min, as compared to 2.2 ml/100 gm at a normal body temperature).[36] This observation has led some investigators to believe that a hypothermic perfusion of the coronaries does not offer much advantage over a normothermic one.[143]

The oxygen supply to an animal heart cooled to 20 to 25 C appears to be adequate. There is no lactate increase in the perfused blood. But when the heart ceases to beat during surface-induced hypothermia, the oxygen supply becomes insufficient. Blair[60] estimates that at a body temperature of 3 C, the oxygen dissolved in the plasma might be adequate to supply the needs of the cooled heart. Thus, hemoglobin is not required at a very low body temperature.[195]

A hypothermic heart utilizes less oxygen than a normothermic heart while performing the same stroke work against the same pressure.[1]

A positive correlation exists between the mechanical efficiency and the increased output load of healthy hypothermic hearts. Very deep cooling, to a temperature of 20 C or lower, reverses this trend and decreases mechanical efficiency of the left ventricle.[123] The increased mechanical efficiency of hypothermic hearts[252] has been attributed to either a metabolic effect of the cold per se or a profound slowing and better filling of the hypothermic heart. It is important to note that most of the observations about the increased efficiency of hypothermic hearts were obtained in heart–lung preparations. It is not quite clear whether the same phenomenon fully applies to the heart in the organism.

The profound decrease in the total oxygen consumption during cooling permits long periods of cardiac arrest. Hypothermic hearts survive anoxia or other detrimental effects longer than normothermic ones. Metabolic changes of the hypothermic myocardium after circulatory arrest are smaller in hypothermia than in normothermia.[443]

SUMMARY

Cooling decreases the oxygen consumption of the heart less than that of any of the other organs. It appears that the heart does not suffer from hypoxia during the initial stages of cooling. The hypothermic heart is a mechanically more efficient pump than the normothermic heart.

Cardiac Cycle

Prolongation of the ventricular systole and especially prolongation of the isovolumetric relaxation phase are always observed in hypothermia.[28,410] The duration of the isovolumetric relaxation period can be increased as much as 12-fold as compared to normothermic conditions.[175] The duration of diastole is extended more than that of systole.[204] However, the heart still spends much time in systole.[239] During more profound cooling one observes a twofold increase in duration of systole. Probably because of these changes the use of electrical pacemakers does not seem to be recommended in hypothermia.

SUMMARY

The duration of both systole and diastole is prolonged in hypothermia. The extended diastole permits adequate filling of the heart and an increased stroke volume. Use of electrical pacemakers, with a high discharge rate, decreases the filling of the heart as well as the cardiac output.

Contractile Force of the Ventricles

Hypothermia improves myocardial contractility.[17,466] However, some investigators find a decreased isovolumetric peak in hypothermia.[11,18,252] This decrease might be the consequence of anesthesia and of drugs. A very profound cooling always decreases the contractile force of the heart[266,364,440] and decreases the velocity of contraction.[246,499] The duration of the ejection part of systole is also lengthened and the mean velocity of the blood ejected in systole is decreased during hypothermia.[175]

In profound hypothermia the end-diastolic pressure is either unchanged or slightly decreased while left atrial pressure is decreased.[28,192,388,508] The peak systolic pressure is increased during cooling to 27 C.[18] Deeper cooling decreases the peak systolic pressure. Ouabain augments the left ventricular contractile capacity at a normal body temperature but appears less effective in hypothermia.[212] The acute pressure load leads to temporary changes of the left ventricular end-diastolic pressure of the cooled hearts as it does in normothermic hearts. However, the adaptation time is much longer in cooled animals.[177]

SUMMARY

Cardiac contractility appears to be improved in hypothermia though the velocity is decreased. In hypothermia the end-diastolic pressure is unchanged. The peak systolic pressure is increased in the initial phases of cooling and then during further cooling is decreased.

Heart Rate

During progressive cooling of experimental animals or patients, the heart rate decreases. Some investigators think this decrease is exponential[82] while others believe it is linear.[3,10,47,92,170,414] The presence or absence of thermoregulatory reflexes (abolished by deep anesthesia) determines the relationship between the heart rate decline and body temperature. The heart rate of curarized animals, isolated hearts, or hearts in heart–lung preparations decreases exponentially during cooling.[2] Isolated hearts of hibernators also follow the Arrhenius equation but with an unexpectedly high Q_{10} of 3.5.[353]

The main cause of the decreased heart rate observed during cooling is the slowing of the depolarization of the sino-atrial pacemaker. Abnormal rhythms and abnormal excitability patterns (brought forth by a decrease in conductivity) further increase the refractory period in hypothermia and decrease the heart rate even more.

The heart rate in dogs remains unchanged when the whole body is cooled but the temperature of the heart remains normal.[157] Cold adaptation does not change cardiac responses to hypothermia.[539]

The heart rate of rats cooled to a body temperature of 15 C is 55 to 75 beats per minute (Fig. 3-1) and remains unchanged during the 8 hours of survival at this low body temperature.[424,431] This also applies to artificially cooled hibernators who have the same heart rate for 3 to 4 days when kept at 10 C.[424]

SUMMARY

During cooling the heart rate of experimental animals or patients decreases exponentially or linearly, probably depending on the amount of anesthesia that is used. Prolongation of the repolarization phase of the sino-atrial pacemaker is the cause of the bradycardia.

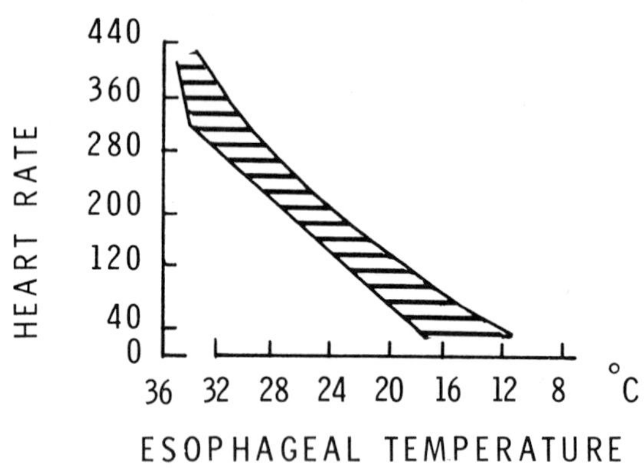

Fig. 3-1. The heart rate of rats progressively cooled to a body temperature of 12 to 15 C. Similar temperature-dependent curves were obtained for other animals and men.

Control of Excitation

Although moderate hypothermia appreciably decreases the heart rate of experimental animals and human patients, the effect of cold on the reflex regulation of cardiac activity is rather small.[156,348] Cutting the vagus nerve or the administration of atropine does not ameliorate hypothermically induced bradycardia. However, a positive chronotrope effect of the cardioaccelerating nerves is present in dogs even at a body temperature of 19 C.[511] Baroreceptor reflexes from the carotid sinus are not reduced[286,297] and may even be augmented[296] during cooling to a body temperature of 20 C. Vagal inhibition of the heart disappears only when the rats are cooled to below 10 C.[4,480] In rats, vagal inhibition is still present at a body temperature only a few degrees higher than the temperature at which the heart itself ceases to beat.[4] The nervous control of circulation is abolished when the cerebral ventricles are cooled by perfusion to a temperature of 10 C. In hypothermia chemoreceptors respond to hypoxia.[165] Unanesthetized rats have different cardiovascular characteristics during cooling to a body temperature of 18 C than during rewarming.[17] It seems likely that a decrease of baroreceptor reflexes is observed in human patients at a higher body temperature than in the experimental animals.[64] The reflex changes of the heart rate evoked by thermal stimulation of the skin observed in normothermic dogs are also observed in dogs cooled to a body temperature of 20 C.[82] In hamsters and in ground squirrels (hibernators) artificially cooled to a body temperature of 2 C, one still observes the effect of stimulation of the vagus nerves.[327] Hibernating ground squirrels have a very active vasomotor system even at a body temperature of 2 C.

Acetylcholine is more effective in rats at a body temperature of 20 C than in normothermia.[302] However, the positive inotropic action of isoproterenol and of epinephrine upon the cold heart vanishes in rats cooled to a temperature of 12 C. At this same body temperature norepinephrine is still capable of increasing the systemic arterial pressure of rats, which indicates that vasoconstriction persists.[371] Therefore, it appears that at a body temperature of 12 C alpha-adrenergic receptors of the peripheral vasculature respond to stimulation, whereas beta receptors of the cardiac muscle fail to do so. This is another example of the possibilities hypothermia offers as an effective physiological tool for separating many intertwined processes that cannot be studied easily in normothermic conditions.

SUMMARY

The reflex regulation of cardiac action is well preserved in hypothermia. Even at a low body temperature of only a few degrees above the temperature at which cold induces cardiac arrest, one observes sympathetic and parasympathetic effects upon the heart.

Cardiac Arrhythmias

Different kinds of arrhythmias—supraventricular or ventricular extrasystole, atrial flutter, atrial fibrillation, and especially various types of atrioventricular blocks—are often described in hypothermic patients[484] and in cooled animals.[347] One type of ventricular arrhythmia known as ventricular bigemini is sometimes observed in hypothermic patients. This arrhythmia is probably induced more by artificial respiration than by hypothermia.[396] Five or even 10 percent carbon dioxide in a breathing mixture reduces the incidence of arrhythmic irregularities of cooled animals. Ouabain increases the incidence of arrhythmias of cooled isolated atria in nonhibernators and even to a higher degree in artificially cooled hibernators. The occurrence of arrhythmias is increased after a hypothermia of long duration, particularly during the last hour of survival at a low body temperature.[424,431,490] After restoration of circulation, the arrhythmias disappear.[398]

SUMMARY

Profound cooling induces arrhythmias in experimental animals and in human patients. After rewarming, the arrhythmias disappear.

Ventricular Fibrillation

Ventricular fibrillation is often observed during the surface cooling of human patients or of large experimental animals[164,504] but much less frequently during core cooling. A pathologically changed normothermic or hypothermic heart fibrillates more easily than a healthy heart. Ventricular fibrillation appears below a body temperature of 28 C,[337] but sometimes it is not seen even at 18 C.[334] Irregular electrical activity of the phrenic nerve in the form of short bursts of high amplitudes frequently precedes ventricular fibrillation.[22] In dogs surface cooled to a body temperature of 22 C the ventricular fibrillatory threshold is lowered by a factor of 5, thus indicating a hypersensitive heart. It has been suggested that treatment of ventricular fibrillation in surface-induced hypothermia presents a more difficult problem than the treatment of ventricular fibrillation at a normal body temperature.[386] But Blair[60] stresses that in hypothermia "terror of ventricular fibrillation is entirely manmade."

To avoid problems associated with ventricular fibrillation, many surgical operations in human patients were performed, until recently, at body temperatures above 28 C. However, once extracorporeal circulatory support was combined with hypothermia, ventricular fibrillation ceased to be a major problem.

The mechanisms of ventricular fibrillation are unknown.[367] The administration of 100 percent pure oxygen to hypothermic animals or to cooled human patients does not decrease the critical temperature at which ventricular fibrillation appears. Studies on heart–lung preparations in dogs and on coronary blood flow during ventricular fibrillation indicate that hypoxemia is neither the cause of ventricular fibrillation nor the cause of hypothermic cardiac arrest. The high degree of myocardial hyperexcitability observed during cooling might be an important factor for the increased tendency toward ventricular fibrillation. Prolongation of the refractory period due to cold per se might be another factor in precipitating fibrillation in hypothermia.[16] Decreased conductivity of the heart muscle could also lead to ventricular fibrillation. Some investigators believe that ventricular fibrillation in hypothermia may be related to a discrepancy between the work output and energy output of the heart.

As in normothermic conditions, the ventricular fibrillation in hypothermia has been explained either by the "circus movement" concept or by the occurrence of ectopic foci. The circus movement theory appears to be more widely accepted[113] due to the fact that the heart of cooled small laboratory animals always stops in asystole but never fibrillates during cooling. The hearts of hibernators do not fibrillate either. It has been suggested that the absence of sympathetic innervation of their ventricles is the cause of the inability of hibernator hearts to fibrillate.[385,386] However, all hibernators are animals of rather small size and the circus movement theory would probably not apply to them anyhow. During the cooling of bears, ventricular fibrillation appears at a body temperature of 15 C. Bears are not hibernators and their body temperature stays relatively high (30–34 C) throughout the entire winter season.

Several factors increase the incidence of ventricular fibrillation in hypothermia. These factors are hypoxia (even in a mild form), profound acidosis, profound electrolyte changes of blood, mechanical stimuli[333] (but not according to Castberg[98]), presence of catheters, increased work load, high central venous pressure, and possibly differential cooling[366] or differential warming of the heart and congenital pathologic abnormalities. Anesthesia can often precipitate hypothermic ventricular fibrillation, therefore deep anesthesia should be avoided in hypothermia. While some anesthetics (thiopental) seldom induce ventricular fibrillation in hypothermia, others do this more often (pentobarbital,[446] halothane[481,489]). However, total epidural anesthesia permits animals to be cooled to a lower body temperature before their hearts start to fibrillate.[180–183]

Sympathetic discharge increases the tendency for ventricular fibrillation.[384,385] The concentration of epinephrine in cooled hearts is decreased.[386] Though some investigators believe that administration of physiological amounts of epinephrine is beneficial to coronary circulation in hypothermia,[340] epinephrine administration combined with trishydroxymethylaminomethane does not prevent ventricular fibrillation during cooling.[25]

Isolated normothermic rabbit atria lose potassium during fibrillation. In profound hypothermia the potassium outflow from fibrillating atria is decreased. Though it has been suggested that there is no correlation between the plasma potassium level and ventricular fibrillation, it is known that sometimes the large ionic imbalance brought on by hypothermia increases the incidence of arrhythmias and that the correction of these changes, especially of those associated with potassium, reduces the danger of fibrillation.[24] Thus, for instance, a very high potassium level (7–9 mEq/liter) brings forth an obvious deterioration of the heart action, especially during recovery periods, leading to rising venous pressures, and sometimes to cardiac arrest. A decrease in the postassium concentration during rewarming from hypothermia diminishes the danger of ventricular fibrillation.

In surface-cooled patients or experimental animals, the temperature differences between various parts of the heart are rather small.

However, cooling of a very restricted zone of the myocardium appreciably slows the conduction through this zone and, if continued long enough, may cause a reversible diastolic depolarization of the cooled area,[250] eventually leading to ventricular fibrillation. Differential warming of the heart by pericardial space perfusion with warm saline appears to be successful in preventing fibrillation during hypothermia.[280]

Any danger of ventricular fibrillation in surface hypothermia of dogs and cats can be prevented by the destruction of the sympathetic nerves innervating the heart.[385,479] The innervation can be achieved by cardiac autotransplantation of the heart or by the technique of complete bilateral sympathetic denervation of the heart. After such an operation, cats can be cooled to a colonic temperature of 15 C without ventricular fibrillation. Sympathetic ganglion blocking agents, blockade of the sino-atrial node,[444] and vagal stimultion tend to decrease ventricular fibrillation. Buffers, such as THAM (trishydroxymethylaminomethane), Tris (trihydroxymethylaminomethane), or bretylium tosylate greatly decrease the hypothermic acidosis in surface-cooled dogs and decrease the tendency toward ventricular fibrillation.[25] The same applies for hyperventilation.[117] Ten percent carbon dioxide used in a breathing mixture has a beneficial effect during the cooling of dogs and monkeys.

Some drugs have beneficial effects in preventing the onset of hypothermic ventricular fibrillation. Prenylanine and reserpine decrease the norepinephrine content of the mammalian heart and thereby might lower the critical temperature at which ventricular fibrillation appears. Procaine amide and quinidine[75,273] appear to be effective also. Although levophed increases coronary volume blood flow,[400] this drug appears to increase the tendency toward ventricular fibrillation. Blair[60] states that many drugs which were used to "protect the heart from fibrillation proved to be executor drugs in hypothermia." He urges that all drugs should be avoided, as much as possible, especially for patients with cardiac problems.

In normothermic conditions defibrillation can be accomplished by the administration of electrical countershocks. Defibrillation of hypothermic hearts (after a short-lasting cardiac arrest but still much longer than in normothermia) can be achieved by the same means or by the administration of potassium. Defibrillation of the hypothermic heart always works if it is undertaken early enough. A kind of defibrillation can always be induced by further cooling the heart to cause a cardiac arrest. Electrical defibrillation of the cooled heart is more effective when it is applied to a strongly fibrillating heart.[314] Defibrillation of the hypothermic heart can be induced by "myocardial lavage."[339] Cardiac massage is also effective in the reversal of hypothermic ventricular fibrillation. After ventricular fibrillation or after induced cardiac arrest (by more profound cooling or by drugs), a normal sinus rhythm is usually observed.

Hypertonic glucose has a beneficial effect on hearts during rewarming.

Although it is recognized that ventricular fibrillation is a reversible condition and that it can be managed satisfactorily[60,372] many investigators, especially those involved in clinical work, try to correct it as soon as it appears. But while ventricular fibrillation can be withstood in normothermia for only 5 to 7 minutes, ventricular fibrillation can be reversed in moderate hypothermia even after 50 minutes.[339] In profound hypothermia dogs can be fully resuscitated after 60 or more minutes of ventricular fibrillation.[463] A more prolonged ventricular fibrillation in profound hypothermia (lasting 1.5 or 2 hours) may, however, induce irreversible brain damage, unless the circulation is supported extracorporeally.

During rewarming from cardiac arrest one often observes first a superficial and then later a more vigorous ventricular fibrillation. During the rewarming of deeply cooled (surface) exanguinated dogs and after a "clinical death" that lasted 15 to 80 minutes, Negovskii[372] always observed fibrillation of the animals' hearts.

During surface rewarming one observes a reversion of the hypothermic heart to a normal sino-atrial rhythm. This occurs spontaneously at a body temperature ranging from 33 to 36 C, and sometimes even at lower body temperatures. In some cases electric countershocks or temporary potassium arrests are needed to induce defibrillation.

Left ventricular pumping efficiency is decreased to 50 percent of the normal value after normothermic ventricular fibrillation of a short duration. On the other hand, ventricular fibrillation of the same duration preserves normal ventricular function in animals cooled to a body temperature of 29 C.[496]

SUMMARY

During profound surface cooling the hearts of large experimental animals and of human patients have a tendency toward ventricular fibrillation. This tendency is increased in the case of damaged hearts or of hearts that are mechanically disturbed. Hypoxia or deep anesthesia has a similar effect. Certain drugs and certain sympathetic blockage agents decrease the tendency for ventricular fibrillation. In hypothermia, defibrillation is easily accomplished by countershocks, cardiac massage, and a temporary cardiac arrest. The sino-atrial rhythm returns, however, during rewarming. This happens at a somewhat higher temperature than the one at which it disappeared during cooling.

Mechanisms of Cardiac Arrest

The hearts of various species of animals stop beating at different depths of hypothermia.[153,492,529] The critical temperature that permits the last heartbeat, called the "biological zero for the heartbeat," depends on the level of anesthesia, the technique of cooling (appreciably lower during perfusion cooling,[208]) the animal species, and condition of the animal or of the patient before cooling.[267,538] In most nonhibernators the heart stops beating at a temperature of 8 to 20 C. In rhesus monkeys, other animals, and man, arrhythmias usually precede cardiac arrest.[159] Strong electrical stimulation can elicit cardiac contractions even at a temperature of 5 C.[283] In rats cooled with carbon dioxide or after administration of acetazolamide[265] the pumping action of the heart is maintained even at a body temperature of 0 to 3 C. Rats and dogs whose circulation is extracorporeally supported sometimes have organized beats even at a body temperature of 2 to 4 C. The hearts of artificially cooled hibernators cease beating at a temperature close to the freezing point.[421,556] The same applies for newborn or very young rats and other animals.[418,419]

A normothermic cardiac arrest lasting 4 to 5 minutes permanently damages the cells of the brain by decreasing the volume blood flow in the arterioles and the capillaries to a very low value.[344] Textbooks on surgery suggest in this case a prompt generalized cooling to a body temperature of 30 C. However, the induction of generalized hypothermia is an inefficiently slow process, especially when surface cooling is used.

The means for a safe and extended cardiac arrest permitting open-heart surgery and other surgical operations have been discussed at several symposia.[79] Cardiac arrest can be imposed by several different methods. Cardiac arrest brought by hypothermia is superior (longer lasting and with less damage) to cardiac arrest caused by potassium, hypoxia, acetylcholine, or other means.[30,154,169,243,335,374,442,465] Cessation of the heartbeat can be achieved in hypothermia even before the biological zero for cardiac action is attained. This can be done by the administration of potassium, magnesium, atropine, acetylcholine, or anoxia.[350] However, only profound hypothermia fully protects the heart during cardiac arrest. A shallow cooling to a temperature of 30 C does not protect the heart in the case of occlusion of the circumflex coronary artery.[171] Hence, in order to protect the heart better, to permit cardiac arrest and open-heart surgery, deep selective cooling of the heart alone was used during generalized shallow hypothermia.[480] Intermittent[36] or continuous perfusion of cold blood maintains an extended (20 minutes or longer) cardiac arrest. Coronary occlusion of hearts cooled to a temperature of 10 C neither decreases the myocardial glycogen reserve nor the coronary pO_2 or pCO_2.

Profound localized myocardial cooling, with coronary perfusion[301] (in the form of cold slush application or pericardial cavity perfusion) or without,[460] is used to induce cardiac arrest or to stop the heart from bleeding. The principal advantage of local cardiac cooling is that the cooling and rewarming of the myocardium is more swiftly accomplished than the cooling and rewarming of the entire body.[480]

Protection is greater when the perfusion is performed at a heart temperature of 4 C than at a temperature of 20 C.[554] An electrolyte solution cooled to a temperature of 0 C and injected into the clamped ascending aorta will also induce a prompt cardiac arrest. In such a case temperature is kept below 30 C with a safe cardiac arrest of much longer duration than in normothermia.[41]

In some instances cardiac arrest in hypothermia is combined with hyperbaric oxygenation which is supposed to increase hypothermic tolerance toward cardiac arrest.[281,519]

The detection of glycolysis during cardiac arrest seems to indicate that the maximum safe period of arrest is at least 1 hour or even longer.[37]

After a short cold-induced cardiac standstill, the contractile force of the left ventricle is not appreciably changed. After a cardiac arrest of 30 minutes (induced by generalized cooling to a body temperature of 15 C) the ventricular function is relatively unimpaired. After a selective, hypothermic, cardiac arrest of 14 minutes myocardial contractility recovers promptly.[31] While after a cardiac arrest induced by cooling, the contractile force of the heart is decreased by only 20 percent, a normothermic potassium arrest of the same duration leaves the contractile force of the heart decreased by a full 75 percent.[153] At a body temperature of 37 C, a 5-minute-long myocardial ischemia (due to occlusion) results in a significant depression of cardiac function. A similar depression of cardiac function is observed after 10 minutes at a body temperature of 30 C, after 20 minutes at a temperature of 20 C, and after 30 minutes at a body temperature of 12 C.[451] In general, one can say that ventricular work capacity is greater after an arrest induced by cooling than after a normothermic cardiac arrest by the use of chemicals.[221]

SUMMARY

The biological zero for the spontaneous beating of the heart is found at different temperatures for various animal species. Although there are wide variations, anesthesia and drugs increase the critical temperature at which cardiac arrest occurs. Combination of an increased pCO_2 in the breathing mixture decreases the temperature of the biological zero for the heartbeat. A decreased metabolism brought about by cooling extends safe cardiac arrest. The deeper the hypothermia, the more prolonged is the safe period of cardiac arrest, except that a very profound cooling might bring inadequate pumping of the heart. In this case, core cooling is recommended. Hypoxia, potassium, and some other drugs that induce normothermic cardiac arrest can induce cardiac arrest in hypothermia also. However, the safest arrest of the heart is induced by action of cold on the myocardium. After resuscitation by rewarming, the myocardial contractile force and oxygen consumption of a deeply cooled heart are little changed.

Metabolism in Cardiac Arrest

During cardiac arrest in profound hypothermia the myocardial oxygen consumption is 1.0 to 1.6 ml/min/100 gm[221] and depends on the depth of cooling.[38] Cooling of the heart to 25 C reduces the myocardial oxygen consumption of the cold-arrested heart to 7 percent of that observed in the beating normothermic heart. Intermittent coronary perfusion with cold oxygenated blood permits open-heart surgery for extended intervals.[38] But when the temperature of the myocardium is decreased to 10 C, one observes signs of enzymatic depression and some enzymatic impairment. It is important to note that the depression is not equal for all enzyme systems that were studied, indicating that while some processes of the heart may be temporarily interrupted others might be only decreased.

Metabolic processes of the arrested hearts become altered less after 1 hour in hypothermia than after ½ hour in normothermia.[163] Although slight lactacidemia is witnessed after 30 minutes of cold cardiac arrest, the elevated lactic acid returns to a normal level after cardiac resuscitation.[162] During normothermic ischemic cardiac arrest, the heart loses potassium but in a much lesser degree than during the hypothermic arrest. Acidosis of the coronary blood is observed during the occlusion of the heart in hypothermia. In this connection it should be noted that the arrested hearts in normothermia utilize 4 times more glycogen and produce 3 times more lactic acid than hearts at a temperature of 17 C.[219,220]

The ATP, phosphocreatine, and glycogen levels of the heart fall much more rapidly during a potassium citrate arrest in normothermia than during a selective hypothermic arrest.[219] During a hypothermic arrest of the dog hearts cooled to a temperature of 17 C, the ATP level of the heart decreases 3 times slower than during potassium citrate arrest at a normal body temperature.[220] Selective cardiac hypothermia and an arrest lasting 45 minutes deplete depots of the heart's glycogen and ATP much less than does a normothermic potassium arrest with a perfusion lasting merely 10 minutes.[79] Normothermic hearts arrested by potassium consume 2 to 3 times more oxygen than hearts arrested by cold.[153] The oxygen reserves after a hypothermic cardiac arrest are 2 times larger than those after a normothermic pharmacological cardiac arrest of the same duration.

After rewarming and the resumption of normal activity, the hypothermic heart has a normal oxygen consumption, while the oxygen consumption after a chemically induced normothermic arrest is decreased by 50 percent.[153] A decrease in the plasma potassium and the plasma calcium concentration is observed after a cardiac hypothermic arrest.[523] However, after an extended cardiac arrest in hypothermia, intracellular edema is sometimes observed.[95] During a very prolonged (1–2 hours or more) cardiac arrest by generalized or selective cooling the cardiac action may be impaired.

In such cases one observes a decreased stroke volume and a decreased general circulation during the rewarming which may lead to death.

SUMMARY

The arrested heart utilizes several times more oxygen, glycogen, and other substrates in normothermia than it does in hypothermia. The changes in high-energy compounds are smaller after a hypothermic cardiac arrest than after a normothermic arrest.

Reversible or Irreversible Changes of the Hypothermic Heart

Sarajas[461,462] believes that the heart is damaged during hypothermia. According to his and other [5,281] findings, the damage occurs because of the hypoxia produced by cooling which could result in microscopic tissue changes, accumulation of extracellular fluid, formation of inflammatory cells, and necrotic foci. Although these findings were not confirmed by other investigators, it appears that a long-lasting hypothermia (for instance, cooling of dogs to a body temperature of 25 C for 24 hours) brings myocardiac glycolysis and an interruption of the pyruvate utilization.[455,456] On the other hand, the profound cooling of mice, rats, rabbits, dogs, and other animals for shorter periods does not leave any microscopic changes of their heart, lung, liver, spleen, or kidney tissues.[233,271]

Most investigators have concluded that hypoxemia does not develop in hypothermia and that the low body temperature alone does not detrimentally affect the functions of the myocardium.[291] However, an extended hypothermic circulatory arrest, especially when the body temperature is not sufficiently decreased, can induce irreversible damage to the heart muscle. A circulatory arrest of 50 minutes and the intracardiac surgical maneuvers in dogs cooled to a body temperature of 17 C induced localized pericarditis and necrobiotic myocardial changes.[461] Prolonged exposure of the heart to saline slush in the percardium may also cause myocardial and pericardial damage in man and in animals and lead to extensive congestive failure.[485]

The heart could be considered a critical organ in prolonged hypothermia. However, the results obtained on rats kept hypothermic for several hours do not support such a conclusion. The pulse rate and the ECG of the cooled rats were essentially the same during several hours of hypothermia.[422,424,431]

SUMMARY

Hypothermia does not induce any irreversible changes of the myocardium. This applies to the generalized cooling of the entire body or to the local cooling of the heart even when the cooling is very deep. However, long-lasting hypothermia, a decrease in body temperature for many hours (up to 1 or 2 days), or prolonged circulatory arrest result in irreversible changes in the myocardium.

Myocardial function in hypothermia appears to be adequate for the work required by the heart at a reduced temperature.[294]

SYSTEMIC CIRCULATION IN HYPOTHERMIA

Introduction

Although the peripheral circulation in hypothermic animals and patients has not been studied as extensively as the performance of the cooled heart, the basic alterations of the circulation during hypothermia have become well established. Hypothermia reduces the metabolism and oxygen consumption of the tissues as it reduces the blood flow proportionally. It appears that the circulatory support in hypothermia is adequate until a body temperature is reached which is only a few degrees above the critical temperature for the cessation of the heart's pumping activity. Regional distribution of the blood flow in hypothermia might be less adequate and some tissues might become hypoxic, especially during profound, long-lasting hypothermia. In such a case, "circulatory shock" is sometimes observed. In general, after short cooling and rewarming, the circulation returns promptly to normal. In profound hypothermia the biological survival time, the time after a cooled organism can be resuscitated, is limited.[421,423,425] Microcirculatory changes induced during cooling are not yet fully understood, though most tissues have a normal oxygen tension even at a body temperature of 15 C.[96] These changes appear to be the limiting factor for survival in profound hypothermia. As it appears now, the restoration of the microcirculation in hypothermia might be the clue for prolonging the survival time.

Blood Pressure

During cooling the mean arterial blood pressure always decreases as the period of cooling is extended. However, during the initial phases of surface cooling one often notices a transient elevation of the blood pressure.[63] In large anesthetized laboratory animals surface cooled to a body temperature of 16 C, the mean arterial blood pressure is about 40 to 50 mm Hg. A similar value is observed in hibernators in hibernation at the same body temperature.[426] However, in small nonanesthetized animals (such as rats) surface cooled to a body temperature of 16 C, the mean arterial pressure is somewhat higher—about 70 mm Hg.[424,431] Epinephrine increases the mean arterial blood pressure even in profound hypothermia.[100]

A low arterial blood pressure in profound hypothermia does not appear to have a detrimental effect on the survival of the organism. Norepinephrine, which elevates the blood pressure in hypothermia, does not increase the survival of hypothermic dogs but often leads to ventricular fibrillation. It has been suggested that a high arterial blood pressure in profound hypothermia might even be harmful because of an increased permeability of the cold capillaries which would lead to edema and hemoconcentration.[431] It is surmised that hibernators have a protective mechanism against an excessively high arterial blood pressure. In hibernation they may lower the "set point" for their baroreceptors. An increase of the systolic arterial blood pressure above 40 to 50 mm Hg in a hibernating ground squirrel induces an electrical and mechanical standstill of the heart that can last several minutes (Fig. 3-2).

The arterial blood pressure of artificially cooled ground squirrels kept for 70 hours at a body temperature of 10 C ranges from 65 to 85 mm Hg. If these animals are kept longer at this temperature, their blood pressure decreases gradually to 30 mm Hg.[424] This occurs during the last 24 hours of their survival.

In homeothermic animals the pulse pressure decreases continuously during cooling whereas the central venous pressure is unchanged. Sometimes a small rise of the central venous pressure can be observed around a temperature of 25 C, then a return to the normal values is observed in deeper hypothermia.[277] During the rewarming all circulatory parameters return to normal at a body temperature of 34 C.[63]

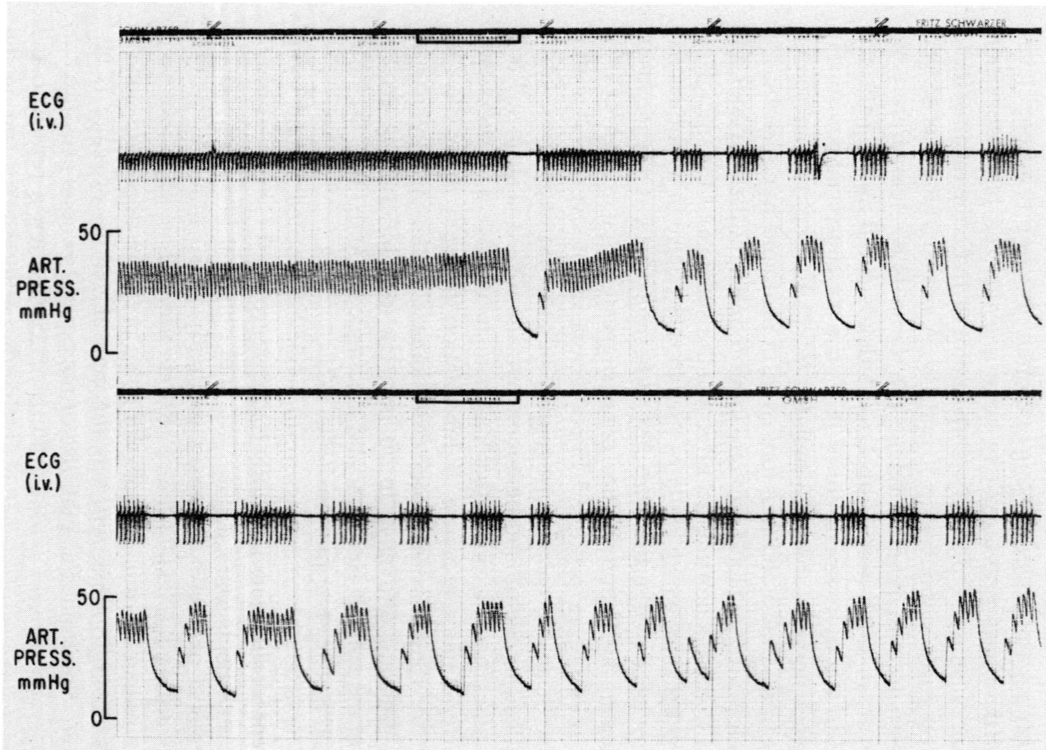

Fig. 3-2. In hibernating ground squirrels at a body temperature of 4 to 6 C, the systolic arterial pressure is kept below a value of 50 mm Hg. If the arterial pressure increases above this value, electrical and mechanical standstill of the heart is observed which can last several seconds or even minutes. Upper line represents time. Time interval of 1 minute is marked in the form of an elongated box.

SUMMARY

Arterial blood pressure decreases continuously during cooling. In profound hypothermia the arterial blood pressure is about 40 to 50 mm Hg. This low arterial blood pressure is sufficient for an adequate supply of nutrient substances to the cells. An artificially increased arterial blood pressure in deep hypothermia can lead to tissue edema which may be caused by an increased permeability of cold capillaries.

Total Peripheral Resistance

Total peripheral resistance increases during surface cooling to a body temperature of 22 C.[27,501] At this temperature the peripheral resistance is 2 to 2.5 times higher than in normothermia. The same is observed in rats cooled to a body temperature of 15 C.[277] However, the coronary resistance decreases during cooling.[74,249,494] Pulmonary vascular resistance is increased proportionally more than systemic resistance.[306] Cooling to lower temperatures decreases the peripheral resistance below the normothermic values.[326,395] This decrease may be caused by a profound vasodilation.[458] In some cases the decrease of the peripheral resistance is only temporary[192] but rises again with further cooling. This increase in peripheral resistance is probably caused by vasoconstriction, especially of some circulatory beds, and by passive effects of a decreased arterial blood pressure. Furthermore, nonuniform cooling probably has differential effects upon various tissues which have different "biological zeros." It should be mentioned that possible shunting of blood through arteriovenous anastomoses might also decrease total peripheral resistance.

In rats kept at a body temperature of 15 C for 9 hours, the already increased peripheral resistance increases still more toward the last part of survival.[431]

Stroke Volume

During moderate cooling the stroke volume remains unchanged.[91,92] Further cooling increases the stroke volume.[121,224,431] This happens even at temperatures that decrease the cardiac output considerably. When deep barbiturate anesthesia is combined with cooling the stroke volume is decreased, even at body temperatures of 26 C or lower, leading to a disproportionally steep decline of cardiac output and to an earlier cardiac arrest[82] (Fig. 3-3).[515] This can be detrimental especially during surface cooling when the circulatory arrest often occurs before the protective effects of hypothermia are present and when a further fast cooling (as in the case of perfusion cooling) is not possible.

The stroke volume decreases continuously during prolonged surface hypothermia, for instance when rats are kept for hours at a body temperature of 15 C. The cardiac output is not maintained by a "compensatory" increase of the heart rate in this case and consequently cardiac output decreases. The stroke volume reaches only 30 percent of the initial value after rats have spent 8 hours in stabilized hypothermia (Figs. 3-4, 3-5).[431] It is not clear what causes

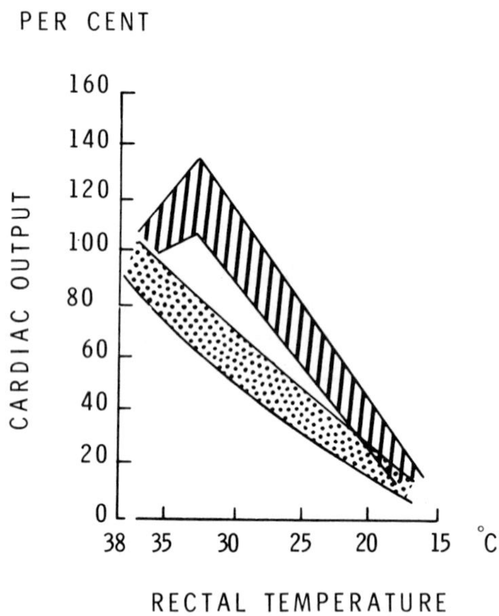

Fig. 3-3. Cardiac output of men, dogs, and rats expressed in percent of the control values at normal body temperature in relation to the rectal temperature. Stripped area: during cooling with little or no anesthesia. Dotted area: after deep anesthesia.[515]

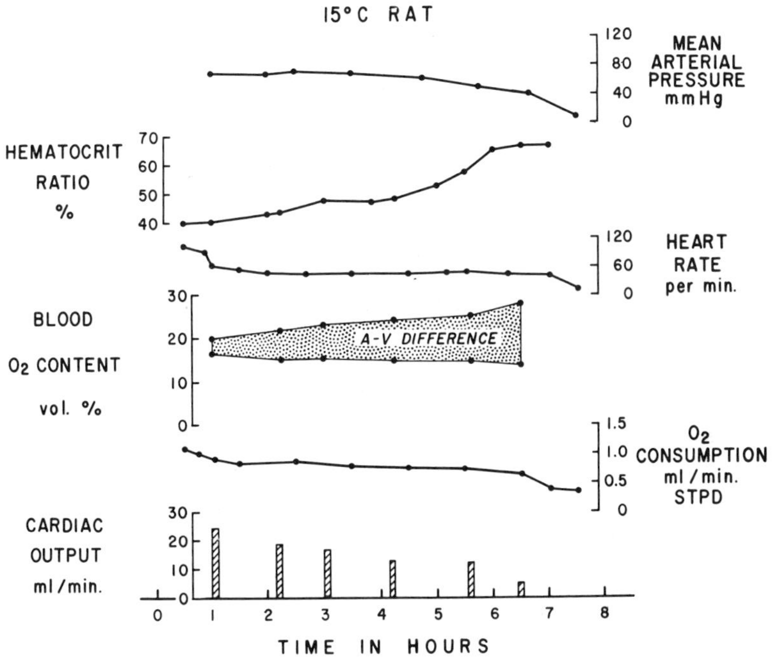

Fig. 3-4. Cardiac output and related data of a rat cooled to a body temperature of 15 C and kept in this hypothermic state as long as it lived.[431]

the continuously decreasing stroke volume in long-term hypothermia. It is possible that an increased heart work load during the phase of the initially increased stroke volume and the initially increased peripheral resistance might contribute to the circulatory failure, though this is less likely. Another possibility would be to associate the continuously increased stroke volume with a slowly failing hypothermic heart. A third possibility is that the venous return is continuously decreased, mediated by a progressively increasing hematocrit ratio and a progressively increasing viscosity (venous return is inversely proportional to viscosity of blood). Whatever the reason (hemoconcentration, hypovolemia, hyperviscosity, etc.), once the stroke volume and cardiac output are appreciably decreased the animals cannot be resuscitated by rewarming and die when their body temperature reaches 28 to 30 C.

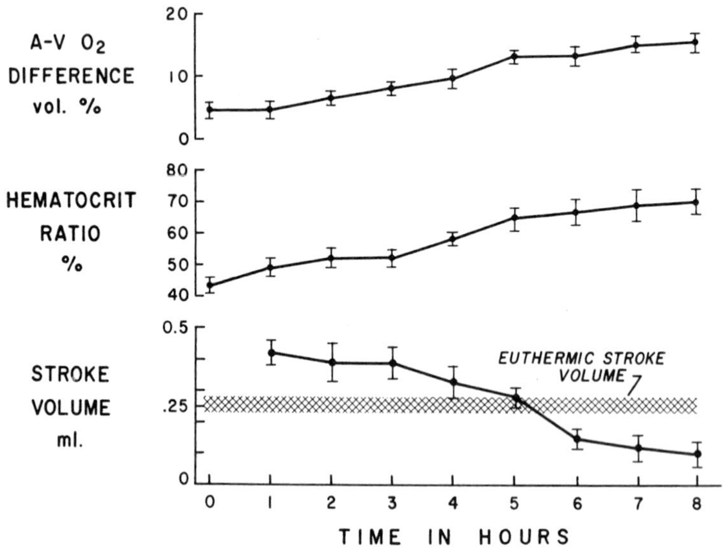

Fig. 3-5. Stroke volume, hematocrit ratio, and AV O_2 difference of rats in prolonged stabilized hypothermia.[431]

SUMMARY

The prolongation of the diastolic period in hypothermia permits a better filling of the heart and brings about an increased stroke volume. In a long-lasting stabilized hypothermia this increased stroke volume declines steadily, having a value of only 30 percent just before the death of experimental animals, as compared to the initial value of the stroke volume at the same body temperature.

Cardiac Output

In lightly anesthetized animals, the cardiac output increases initially during cooling,[534] reaching a maximal value at a body temperature of 32 to 34 C. Such a shallow cooling has no protective effects because both the metabolisms and the circulation are increased above their normothermic values. Therefore, exposure to hypoxemia or hypoxia is very damaging in shallow hypothermia, even more than in normothermia. This does not apply to deeper hypothermia. Further cooling of the body always decreases cardiac output.[293] In profound hypothermia the cardiac output is always decreased. The decrease of cardiac output during cooling appears to be exponential.[237] When dogs are cooled to a body temperature of 25 C their cardiac output declines from 130 to 40 ml/kg.[288] The cardiac output is decreased to 25 percent or even to 10 to 15 percent of the normothermic value in animals cooled to a body temperature of 20 and 17 C, respectively.[123]

In hypothermia the ultimate reduction of cardiac output is caused by a slowing of the heart as the direct action of cooling on the frequency of discharges from the pacemaker and the slower impulse conduction in the cold heart. The decrease in cardiac output during cooling is proportional to the decrease of myocardial oxygen consumption.

As in normothermia, the circulation in hypothermia closely follows the changes in tissue metabolism.[109,491,514,516,517] The temperature coefficients for cardiac output, heart rate, and oxygen consumption are very similar. During generalized cooling, the heart probably provides an adequate volume blood flow throughout the body until a body temperature of 20 to 25 C is reached. The volume blood flow appears to be adequate—until the critical body temperature is attained at which cold cardiac arrest occurs. This naturally applies to situations in which the cooling technique is adequate and in which deep barbiturate anesthesia and drugs are avoided.

In rats cooled to a body temperature of 15 C and kept at this body temperature for hours, the cardiac output decreases steadily and after 8 hours reaches only 25 percent of the value observed initially at the same body temperature.[431,432] The resulting progressive decline of tissue perfusion is brought about by a continuously diminishing stroke volume uncompensated by an increase in the heart rate.

The velocity of the blood flow is decreased in hypothermia. After the volume blood flow in hypothermic animals or patients is decreased to one-half of its initial value or even lower, the movement of blood becomes less uniform and often intermittent.

While cardiac output can be adequate even in profound hypothermia, the changes in regional distribution of blood volume flow[122] may affect some tissues adversely. Fortunately, the tissues that suffer more from hypoxia in normothermic conditions become relatively better supplied with blood in hypothermia.[9] The tissues that are proportionally less perfused during cooling are the ones which are less important for the survival of a hypothermic organism.[92] Various types of cooling techniques and especially anesthesia affect the redistribution of the volume blood flow in hypothermia. Shallow cooling and a mild anesthesia that does not entirely suppress shivering alter the cardiac output very little; however, they decrease renal and carotid volume blood flow. When deeply anesthetized dogs are cooled to low body temperature, without a shivering reaction, the cardiac output and renal and femoral blood flow are throttled, but the volume flow through the carotid artery is enhanced.[535] It appears that each vascular region responds in an individualized fashion when the cardiac output is diminished by cooling.

In prolonged stabilized hypothermia the blood flow in muscles decreases continuously. The decrease of the regional blood flow through the iliolumbar muscles is somewhat greater than that of the cardiac output observed in these conditions (Fig. 3-6).[424]

During rewarming the cardiac output increases, but the curve of the increase is less steep than during cooling. This slow increase of cardiac output during the rewarming brings an increased arteriovenous oxygen difference and a sluggish rise in the mean arterial pressure. In an extreme form this leads to a circulatory collapse ("rewarming shock"), and to death either during or shortly after the rewarming. Since the peripheral resistance during rewarming is roughly the same as during cooling, Thauer[515] concluded that the slow increase in the blood pressure during rewarming is caused mainly by a reduced cardiac output. During the last phase of rewarming, therefore, it appears very important to avoid the initiation of this vicious circle which might lead to posthypothermic circulatory collapse.[66] Overloading of the circulation should probably be avoided during the early part of rewarming, while the heart is still cold. Some circulatory beds increase their blood flow during rewarming more than others. For instance, the femoral volume blood flow increases during the rewarming above the normothermic values.[535]

SUMMARY

In hypothermia changes in circulation are closely correlated with changes in metabolism. After initial increase, cardiac output decreases during cooling. In general, circulatory support of the tissues is adequate even in a profound hypothermia of short duration, although it is possible that some of the tissues undergo hypoxia

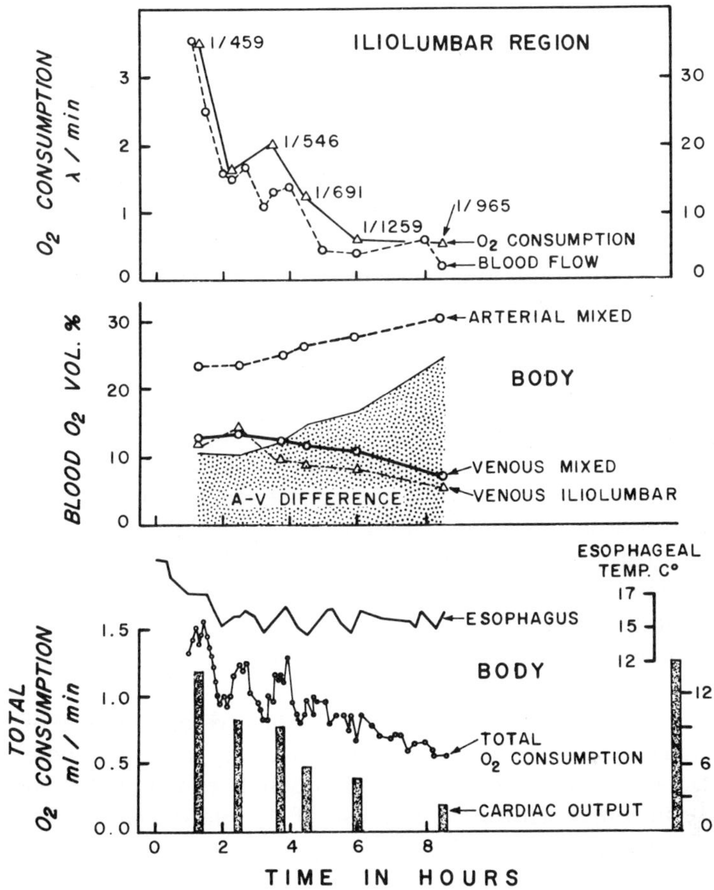

Fig. 3-6. Cardiac output and blood flow through iliolumbar region during 15C stabilized hypothermia of a rat.[424]

because of the redistribution of the cardiac output. Fortunately, this does not apply to the myocardium. During the rewarming phase the increase of cardiac output is less steep than during cooling.

Microcirculation

In vitro, blood loses normal hemostatic properties during cooling. Cold agglutinins appear when blood is cooled to a temperature of 5 C. Even less profound cooling may induce a similar change.[278]

Several investigators have observed that hypothermia induces intravascular aggregation, sludging, and subsequent capillary occlusion.[272] If this aggregation exists, it is probably induced by an inadequate volume blood flow through the peripheral bed brought forth by the combined effect of anesthesia (especially barbiturate anesthesia) and hypothermia. Anesthesia itself decreases cardiac output even in normothermia.[430] But there are many reports that hypothermia does not lead to vascular aggregation.[81] If aggregation should take place, low-molecular dextran[359] or glucose administration[435] should be effective in preventing it.

In some cases of deep hypothermia intravascular clotting was reported. This clotting was caused by sequestration of blood in the liver, spleen, and some capillaries.[50,500] Microscopic tissue destruction was also observed. The cessation of blood flow in 50 percent of the small blood vessels in the mesocecum of rats cooled to a body temperature of 20 C[328] could be the consequence either of a profound decrease in the cardiac output and its redistribution in the surface-cooled organisms or of intravascular cell agglutination. On the other hand, some investigators believe that during "adequate" cooling, intravascular sludging does not occur. Hemodilution[131,255] or extracorporeal circulatory support helps to maintain an adequate capillary support.[197,223,256,341]

The ear chambers of hypothermic rabbits were the object of a microcirculation study. Increased blood viscosity, arterial hypotension, and pooling of blood in the capillaries and venules lead to poor tissue perfusion.[500] However, because of the redistribution of the blood flow in hypothermia the ears of hypothermic animals are far from being the representative tissue for microcirculation studies.

It has been mentioned often that microcirculatory exchange might be impaired during very profound cooling due to the opening of the arteriovenus shunts permitting the blood to bypass capillaries.[377,432] If this should happen, the administration of low-molecular dextran ought to be beneficial. It effectively increases the blood flow and inhibits pool formation.[19] This problem, concerning the microcirculatory exchange, as well as many other problems associated with microcirculation, is far from being understood well. Local rewarming increases the circulation several-fold in the affected tissues.[420,427,433,434]

SUMMARY

The physiology of microcirculation in hypothermia is still not understood. Sludging, aggregation, and intravascular coagulation probably do not take place during adequate cooling and adequate rewarming. Hemodilution probably increases the capillary circulation substantially, and induces better venous drainage in cooled animals and patients.

Nervous Regulation of Circulation

The oxygen supply in hypothermia is regulated by the tissues themselves, as it is in normothermia. Lynch and Adolph[328] reported that the diameters of arterioles, capillaries, and venules are unchanged when the body temperature of the animal is decreased from 37 to 15 C. However, the vascular reactivity of the arterial and of the venous system is somewhat reduced at a body temperature of 30 C or below.[473] This change is rather slight. The baroreceptor reflexes function well at a body temperature as low as 24 C[286] or lower, but at the same temperature the thermoreceptors are rather sluggish.[397] Cooling to a body temperature of 20 C increases the activity of alpha and beta receptors. A cooling to a body temperature of 8 C depresses, but does not abolish, the activity of the vascular bed. Responses to norepinephrine and acetylcholine at these low body temperatures are still present,[473] but responses to hypoxia are absent.[395] It appears that at these very low body temperatures (10 C or lower) reflex mechanisms that regulate the level of the cardiac output according to the needs of oxygen to the tissues are temporarily lost.[515,517] Under these conditions the effects of metabolic products on the capillary circulation are very small.

One of the problems associated with the core cooling of patients or experimental animals is that during the initial phases of cooling a pronounced vasoconstriction may occur. It is brought about by a sudden decrease of temperature of centrally located organs. This vasoconstriction can lead to an inadequate perfusion of some organs and to temporary hypoxemia. Vasoconstriction is observed in some instances during surface cooling. It also occurs in mice after immersion cooling, but is not observed in mice cooled by the hypoxic-hypercapnic technique.[356] For this reason 5 or even 10 percent carbon dioxide in the oxygen breathing mixture is highly recommended for the cooling of experimental animals and patients.

When profound hypothermia is reached, vasoconstriction is replaced by a pronouned vasodilation which might lead to pooling of the blood in the splanchnic bed and in the lung. This is observed especially during core cooling[138] when the centrally placed organs have a temperature several degrees lower than the peripheral tissues. Cardiovascular reflexes cease at a body temperature of 15 C or below.

SUMMARY

Vasoconstriction is often observed during early phases of cooling, especially when the cooling is sudden as in the case of core cooling. Early vasoconstriction in this case might redistribute the volume blood flow throughout the body and induce hypoxia in some tissues. A very profound hypothermia induces vasodilation and might lead to pooling of the blood.

Coronary Blood Flow

According to the earlier literature, coronary blood flow in hypothermia was thought likely to be decreased.[342,399] For this reason, it was recommended that the administration of vasopressor agents could improve the coronary blood flow.[400] Recently it has been demonstrated that the coronary blood flow increases progressively during cooling,[341] whereas the coronary resistance decreases. At a body temperature of 18 C the coronary blood flow reaches a peak that is relatively 2 times as high as in normothermia.[341] Further cooling, to a temperature of 5 to 10 C, brings a decrease in the coronary blood flow[550] although even in profound hypothermia the heart appears to have an adequate blood flow.[237,275] This increase in the coronary blood flow during cooling is physiologically very important. It results in the additional protection of the hypothermic myocardium while its metabolic rate is decreased. The coronary blood flow of a cooled heart in a heart–lung preparation is also adequate. The cardiac arteriovenous difference of the oxygen content remains unchanged during progressive cooling, also indicating an adequate coronary blood flow in hypothermia. Cooling to a body temperature of 10 C leads to a decrease in the AV difference of oxygen content and its eventual disappearance.[550] An increased coronary blood flow in hypothermia occurs despite a falling arterial blood pressure even while the slightly increased blood viscosity indicates coronary dilation induced by the direct action of the cold.[231,341,399] This explains why there was decreased resistance to blood flow in the coronary arteries after cooling as was reported by Berne.[29]

During rewarming, the coronary blood flow follows the mirror image pattern observed during cooling. Return to normothermia brings back the normal values of the coronary blood flow.[341]

Hypoxia dilates the coronary blood vessels. However, in the case of a failing hypothermic heart, the decrease in pO_2 of the blood does not change the coronary vasomotor tone.[115] The same happens to a healthy heart in a very profound hypothermia.[341]

The technique of cooling plays an important role in determining the level of the coronary blood flow in hypothermia. Hematocrit ratio, hemoglobin concentration, acid–base balance, blood velocity, venous pressure, and hormones influence the coronary volume blood flow in hypothermia.[29,399]

The coronary blood flow of an electrically driven cold heart is decreased. This decrease might lead to coronary insufficiency.[515] Epinephrine increases the coronary circulation in deep hypothermia[336,338] but may lead concomitantly to ventricular fibrillation.

SUMMARY

During cooling the coronary blood flow is adequate for the decreased metabolic needs of a cooled heart. Hypothermic cardiac arrest occurs, however, at temperatures which appear to be higher than those at which the heart would be fully protected by the direct effect of cold during extended periods of time. Thus in the case of adult surface-cooled organisms, deeper cooling is needed to fully protect the heart from hypoxia. This can be done only with core cooling (especially when complete circulatory arrest of significant duration is contemplated). During rewarming, the heart resumes its action at higher temperatures than those at which the last beat was observed during the cooling. This is of importance for surface rewarming which is a rather slow process. After rewarming the coronary volume blood flow returns to the normal level. Pathologic changes of the heart decrease the coronary blood flow and may lead to coronary insufficiency either during cooling or during rewarming.

Hemorrhagic Shock

Hemorrhagic shock has often been studied in hypothermic experimental animals. The reason for this interest has been that the tissue perfusion in hemorrhagic shock is inadequate and that hypothermia, which lowers the tissue metabolism, was expected to decrease the deleterious consequences of hemorrhagic shock. It was observed that cooling can be beneficial in some instances but not in all situations as had been expected. Hypothermic dogs can tolerate hypovolemic hypotension induced by hemorrhagic shock for 2 hours, whereas normothermic animals die in a corresponding situation after 1 hour.[142,143] The posthemorrhagic hypotensive tolerance of cooled dogs is greater than that of normothermic animals. Hypothermia protects dogs against oligemic shock also.[468] After a hind-limb tourniquet application lasting 5 hours, normothermic dogs die, but when the tourniquet is applied to a limb cooled to 18 C or lower, the dogs survive.[235] Monkeys cooled to a body temperature of 17 C withstand an acute blood loss and the appearance of a 30-minute-long "clinical death."[373,374] Capillary atony, associated with irreversible shock, is delayed in hypothermia.[126] It is interesting to note that during experimental hemorrhagic shock in hypothermic dogs the arterial pressure is decreased but the heart rate remains unchanged.[232]

However, in some experimental situations hypothermia does not exert a protective effect during hemorrhagic shock. For example, a decreased plasma volume brought forth by hemorrhagic shock cannot be corrected by cooling.[394] Hypothermia does not change the effects of irreversible shock in animals.[394,436,437] There are also reports that severe hemorrhage is not well tolerated at a body temperature of 30 C.

The variance in results may be explained by the different levels in the depth of cooling and the different techniques of cooling used in the experiments described. The duration of hypothermia also determines the survival rate in experimental hemorrhagic shock. Rats survive hemorrhage and a profound lowering of arterial blood pressure if their body temperature is kept at 15 C for 2 to 3 hours. However, a hypothermia of longer duration (4–5 hours) combined with hemorrhage leads to death.[424] This can probably be attributed to the decreased cardiac output and the decreased circulating blood volume observed in advanced stages of prolonged hypothermia.

The protective mechanisms of hypothermia involved in hemorrhagic shock are unknown. A greatly lowered metabolism and a decreased sensitivity toward hypoxia are probably the main factors. Some investigators believe that protection of the antibacterial system might be one of the reasons for this protective role of hypothermia.[178,179]

SUMMARY

Hypothermia increases the survival in hemorrhagic shock. The deeper the cooling, the greater are the protective effects of hypothermia. However, in hemorrhage the hypothermic organism must be rewarmed relatively soon, otherwise it will die during hypothermia or during the rewarming. An adequate fluid replacement is needed in this particular case before the rewarming is completed. Long-lasting deep hypothermia increases the sensitivity toward hemorrhagic shock.

Circulatory Arrest

Some of the problems that are associated with circulatory arrest have already been discussed.

How long a cooled animal or patient will survive circulatory arrest depends mainly on two factors: the degree of hypoxia that develops and the protective effects of hypothermia.[363] The duration of a safe circulatory arrest depends on the depth and on the technique of the cooling. At higher body temperatures hypoxia develops faster and the protective role of hypothermia is rather limited; protection is good in profound hypothermia. Considering only aerobic metabolism, the time of circulatory arrest will depend on the body temperature, the age of the organism, the body weight, and the level of the basal metabolism of the organism.[527] However, due to the technical difficulties associated with measurements, the anaerobic metabolism, which plays a very important role in hypothermia, is not taken into account.

The theoretical calculation of the safe time for a circulatory arrest in a young adult based on the amount of oxygen reserve and on the oxygen consumption[527] gives the following values: The safe circulatory arrest is 6 minutes at a body temperature of 30 C; 10 minutes at a body temperature of 25 C; 18 minutes at 20 C; 30 minutes at 15 C; 56 minutes at 10 C; 100 minutes at 5 C; and 180 minutes at a body temperature of 0 C. The duration of safe circulatory arrest is appreciably longer for younger organisms.

In practice, the duration of a safe circulatory arrest appears to correspond closely to the theoretical values. The safe circulatory arrest obtained on experimental animals (dogs, rabbits, guinea pigs, and rats) can be expressed by the following equation:

$$\text{Bst} = 150 \times E^{-b\ 0.108}$$

where Bst is the biological survival time, and E is rectal temperature.[515,517] The equation was worked out by Thauer[515] on the basis of numerous data collected.

According to these measurements one may ask: what is the longest duration of safe circulatory arrest? Here are some examples of the results obtained. At a body temperature of 37 C the time for safe circulatory arrest is approximately 4.5 minutes. At a body temperature of 34 C the safe circulatory arrest is 5.5 minutes; at a body temperature of 28 C, 8.5 minutes.[465] Safe circulatory arrest of dogs cooled to a body temperature of 18 C is 60 minutes[447,449] or more.[26,215,217,359,451]

When the body temperature is decreased to 0 to 10 C, the safe circulatory arrest period ranges from 20[216,319] to 60 minutes[3,7,379–381,472,488] or even 2 hours.[6,8,295,375,382,495,531]

Surface-cooled infants and young animals tolerate circulatory arrest much better than adults. Mohri and his collaborators have shown in human patients[133,259,357–360] what Miller somewhat before him[355] and Popovic[419] have shown in experimental animals. Supercooled baby ground squirrels survive a circulatory arrest of 11 hours.[418]

After safe circulatory arrest during hypothermia, one sometimes observes metabolic acidosis during rewarming. Deep cooling with circulatory arrest and sometimes even without the arrest occasionally leads to neurological damage.[50,137,158,215,248] The causes of this damage are unknown. Extracorporeal cooling and circulatory arrest protect the brain adequately.[323]

It is likely that repeated short extracorporeal circulatory support might extend the overall duration of a safe circulatory arrest in hypothermia. In such a case the second or third inflow occlusion should be supplied only after an adequate correction of the acid–base balance.[55]

SUMMARY

The duration of safe circulatory arrest is increased from 4.5 minutes as observed in normothermia, to 60 to 120 minutes when the body temperature of experimental animals is decreased to 2 to 8 C. It appears that man is not different in this respect. Intermittent short circulatory support appears to be able to extend the safe duration of a circulatory arrest.

Cardiovascular Surgery in Surface-Cooled Patients

As in experimental situations hypothermia is also used clinically to protect tissues and organs from ischemia during a decrease or interruption of the circulation. It should be remembered, however, that clinical hypothermia is understood less well than experimental hypothermia. Anesthesia and serious pathologic conditions, especially those of the cardiovascular system, change the physiological processes in hypothermia profoundly. Various depths and lengths of cooling make it even more difficult to compare the results of the experimental with the clinical work. In the most exaggerated cases it appears that one is forced to compare the results obtained in healthy rats and other small laboratory animals with those obtained in stray dogs (that were caught by city pound catchers because of starvation and illness) or with the results obtained in very sick, often poor-risk patients. Perhaps future research will provide data that are much better controlled. Despite these difficulties, some trends of response obtained in surface-cooled patients are fairly evident. We shall concentrate our discussion primarily on these points.

The first successful clinical application of surface hypothermia to human patients (after experimental work done by Bigelow et al[43–46]) was reported by Lewis and Taufic,[321] while Swan and coworkers used hypothermia for corrections of congenital heart lesions.[505,506] In 1958, Niazi and Lewis were the first to cool a human patient to a very low body temperature.[383]

Today surface hypothermia is used in many centers as the technique of choice for the correction of atrial septal defects of the secundum type either for experimental or for clinical work.[53,101,103,322,369] Hypothermia is employed for the correction of ventricular septal defects or for other types of open-heart surgery.[23,58,106,129,130,168,226,259,260,309,310,402,448,478,495,503] Zindler reported over 1000 successful cases of hypothermic open-heart surgery; all were accomplished during a period of 6 to 8 minutes of safe cardiac exclusion.[557,558] Surface hypothermia can be safely used even for poor-risk patients.

In order to decrease the use of anesthetic agents, hypothermia was added to anesthesia and was used in patients with mitral stenosis and pulmonary valvular stenosis.[557,558] Surface cooling has been used for the correction of tetralogy of Fallot.[185]

A number of investigators chose to perfuse the coronary arteries during hypothermic correction of septal defects.[52,325]

Open-heart surgery was often performed on surface-cooled children. They can withstand deep body cooling by surface means much better than adult patients.[102,259,260] In some cases the body temperatures of the young patients were decreased to 18 to 25 C with total circulatory interruption of 15 minutes or longer.[133,258,260,357,359] Surface hypothermia was also used for surgical operations during pregnancy.[242]

Surface hypothermia has been used for the correction of coarctation of thoracic aorta or for surgery of the abdominal aorta[349] and for patch graft repair.[234] Surface cooling has been successfully used during the occlusion of the aorta.[97] Surface hypothermia permits the interruption of the circulation by a tourniquet or by placement of ligatures in the region of the abdomen.

In most instances, the body temperature of surface-cooled patients was decreased merely to 26 to 30 C or even less. In 1961 Swan suggested a more profound cooling, with the idea that a much deeper surface hypothermia would permit prolongation of a safe circulatory arrest.[502] And, indeed, deeper cooling (below 28 C) has permitted longer lasting open-heart surgery.[488]

Safe circulatory arrest of 60 minutes was reported by Mohri et al[133,359,495] but in most clinical cases, the circulatory arrest is shorter. Cerebral damage was occasionally reported after an extended circulatory arrest.[154] About 2 percent of surface-cooled children had some neurological disorders (e.g., choreoathetosis). Unfortunately, some of the physiological and neurological changes are not parallel with histological information.[357] It is still unknown why the gray matter in children and in adult patients is more sensitive to the hypothermic circulatory arrest than are the other tissues. It may be possible that the brain or some parts of the brain are cooled less than the whole body and consequently these tissues are more sensitive to hypoxia. Whatever the reason, it is clear that the neurological damage observed after rewarming (and not merely the survival) becomes the most important criterion in deciding how long a safe circulatory occlusion can last. Because of occasional neurological damage, the difficulties associated with both the slow cooling and rewarming of human patients, and with the danger of circulatory failure, profound hypothermia has been gradually abandoned except in a few clinical centers in the United States and abroad.

SUMMARY

Twenty years have passed since surface hypothermia was suggested as an adjunct to surgery. Today surface cooling is being used for surgical operations, mostly of short duration. Surface-induced hypothermia does not require the complicated procedures necessary for core cooling, but it still provides many technical advantages for the surgeon. When the cooling is more profound, surface hypothermia—as well as perfusion hypothermia—offers more protection from ischemia and from hypoxia. Unfortunately, in profound hypothermia, the survival time (biological survival time) becomes rather short. Some of the early dangers associated with surface hypothermia already have been overcome, especially the danger of ventricular fibrillation. It should be noted, however, that clinical hypothermia is always modified by drugs, and thus a study of clinical hypothermia becomes more complicated than a study of unmodified hypothermia. Clinical hypothermia is even less predictable than "pure" hypothermia. Hypothermic cardiac arrest induced by surface cooling offers many advantages for open-heart surgery: bloodless field, extended circulatory arrest, and increased resistance to hypoxia. Surface cooling is especially advantageous in the surgery of children who do not tolerate perfusion cooling because of the large priming volumes and the serious blood volume inbalances due to the mixing of large volumes of blood. Surface hypothermia for children is quite adequate when 1 hour or less of circulatory arrest is needed.

PERFUSION COOLING

Introduction

The main objective of perfusion hypothermia is to induce a fast and safe profound cooling, especially of the internal or "core" part of the body. In clinical practice the main objective of perfusion hypothermia is to permit surgery under the conditions of extremely low tissue perfusion or of complete circulatory arrest.[88] Total circulatory arrest of an appreciable duration can be achieved only in profound hypothermia.[105] It is one of the most desirable, yet rarely employed, techniques for various surgical procedures. Profound and safe hypothermia can be achieved with the help of extracorporeal circulation. Presently in surgical practice the induction of hypothermia is almost always brought about by extracorporeal circulation except when short surgical procedures are contemplated, or when the patients are babies or very young children.

Historical

The principles of extracorporeal circulation were conceived about 150 years ago.[199] Extracorporeal circulation was first used on dogs under normothermic conditions and later for developing the experimental procedures which permitted open-heart surgery.[49] Extracorporeal support of the circulation was first employed for clinical applications in 1951.[331] Initially, clinical applications of the heart–lung bypass were not wholly successful, being limited to a very low level of extracorporeal flow rates. Thus there arose the idea that the combination of heart–lung bypass with hypothermia might become a safe procedure. Pump oxygenators were used in 1952 to induce the cooling of an organism to a temperature of 28 C.[124,125,127,203,204] Gollan used extracorporeal cooling with a pump oxygenator in closed-chest dogs. Soon he was able to cool dogs to a body temperature approaching the freezing point.[210] Perfusion hypothermia was used also by Sealy for clinical purposes.[470] Somewhat later Drew[138,139] and others[217] employed autogenous oxygenation, pumps without oxygenators, to cool patients to a body temperature of 13 to 15 C, sometimes with a circulatory arrest lasting from a few minutes to a full hour. The elmination of oxygenators obliterated some of the early hazards observed in perfusion cooling. Bjork[50] used the same technique, but after observing a few cases of brain damage in the patients, he felt prompted to introduce an oxygenator and a higher rate of blood flow into his system of perfusion cooling.[56,57] Now most investigators use oxygenators in order to avoid the hypoxic damage. Several years ago cardioplegia was also introduced by the local cooling of the heart.[551] At about this same time perfusion cooling was combined with immersion cooling in order to provide a more uniform cooling of the body.

Problems of Perfusion Hypothermia

Currently perfusion hypothermia is used in numerous surgical cases. However, because of the improper use of profound perfusion cooling by inexperienced investigators and because of some of the technical difficulties arising from the combination of deep cooling and extracorporeal circulation, profound perfusion hypothermia has not been as successful as originally envisioned. Unfortunately, nonuniform techniques, the use of various species of experimental animals, and the different states of health of the patients make an evaluation or a comparison of the results obtained rather difficult. New approaches and better techniques will eventually solve these problems and permit a safe profound cooling with long-lasting circulatory arrest. The use of profound extracorporeal hypothermia has been abandoned except in a few experimental or clinical centers.

Perfusion hypothermia is radically different from surface hypothermia and from normothermic extracorporeal circulation. It represents more than the simple sum of its two components. Brown[88] pointed out that "although more information is beginning to accumulate on deep hypothermia induced by perfusion, at present little is known by which to assess its clinical possibilities and its limitations." Although there are several comprehensive books[110,184] and several review articles that cover the field of perfusion hypothermia, differences of opinion still exist. This especially refers to the limits of deep perfusion hypothermia, the duration of safe circulatory arrest, and the choice of techniques which should be used for the cooling as well as for the rewarming.

SUMMARY

After an initial successful effort, perfusion hypothermia is not being used extensively in either experimental or clinical situations. It is hoped that better techniques and new approaches will bring hypothermia back into the center of attention again and permit the full use of the appreciable physiological protective roles that hypothermia affords.

Cooling Techniques

Many perfusion-cooling techniques have been described. Most investigators suggest that the cooling should be fast and should be induced by a high-volume blood flow. This appears to be beneficial for the extended surgical procedures or for the long-term circulatory arrest (where a slow cooling extends the duration of perfusion hypothermia appreciably). It appears that during fast cooling with a high perfusion rate the myocardial oxygen tension is kept within the normal limits, whereas during slow cooling and low perfusion rates (in man, below 60 ml/kg/min) the oxygen tension falls below the normal values.[330] During slow cooling the total oxygen consumption is also decreased.[76] There are some investigators who suggest the use of slow cooling and low perfusion rates, especially for cooling the body to a temperature above 20 C.[230,324]

During rapid perfusion cooling, the temperatures of the most vital organs are decreased first, whereas the temperatures of the peripheral tissues (muscles, skin) are still high.

In some instances generalized perfusion cooling has been modified by an additional even deeper cooling of the heart (or less often by the cooling of some other organ) especially when cardioplegia is desired. Such a cooling can be achieved by using an additional small perfusion circuit[14,524] or by local external cooling. The latter can be done either with externally placed pads soaked in ice-cold saline or by irrigating the pericardial cavity with ice-cold saline.[262,480] This combination of deep body cooling and an even deeper heart cooling is presently used for long-lasting operations in cardiac surgery, for defects of the ventricular septum, tetralogy of Fallot, total anomalous pulmonary venous drainage, Senning's correction of transposition of the great vessels, correction of aneurysms involving the proximal portion of the ascending aorta, and so on. When circulatory arrest is contemplated, the perfusion cooling is usually continued for 5 to 15 minutes after the desired body temperature is reached so that the core of the body, and especially the brain, is adequately cooled. The more profound the cooling that is achieved, the better are the heart, brain, and other vital organs protected during a decrease or during an interruption of the circulatory support. Although there is probably no limit for the safe cooling of experimental animals or of patients to a freezing temperature, it is unfortunate that with the techniques presently available profound cooling always results in shorter periods of biological survival (safe duration of hypothermia).[423–425]

Anesthesia

Most investigators prefer to use an anesthesia as light as possible in hypothermia, though a few employ deep anesthesia too.

Barbiturates (such as Nembutal and other long-term anesthetic agents) were often used for perfusion cooling until it was discovered that most drugs, especially barbiturates, are very toxic in deep hypothermia. It is important to note that they decrease the cardiac output in animals by 30 to 40 percent even in normothermia.[430] The increase in toxicity is tenfold, leading to an increased mortality in profound hypothermia.[229] Chloralose and halothane[513] appear to be much less toxic and are recommended for perfusion hypothermia. Surital, a short-term anesthetic, also appears to be adequate, permitting fast cannulation procedures and the induction of the early stages of perfusion cooling.[105] Once the cooling is initiated, hypothermic physical anesthesia takes over and there is no need for additional amounts of anesthetics.[261] The administration of muscle relaxants (succinylcholine or others) is recommended during the cooling of experimental animals or of patients.

SUMMARY

The lightest possible anesthesia is recommended for perfusion cooling. During fast extracorporeal cooling the physical anesthesia of cold replaces the chemical anesthesia of drugs. The recovery after cooling is much faster if only a light anesthesia was applied.

Cannulas

In order to decrease the resistance and to avoid turbulent flow, thin-walled catheters (Teflon or stainless steel) are recommended. Herparin loss is reduced in perfusion hypothermia. For this reason reheparinization should not be administered as often as in normothermia.[549]

Body Temperature Measurements

The temperature of several vital organs (heart, brain, esophagus) should be monitored continuously, especially when a circulatory arrest is contemplated. Very thin thermocouples (Ga 40) placed in fine polyethylene catheters can be used for this purpose. The brain temperature of patients can be estimated by measuring the tympanic temperature with thermocouples.

Circuits

Depending on the site of the surgical intervention, several different circuits can be used. Partial bypass with closed-chest procedures,[507,512] venous gravity drainage, and a single pump allows the trauma of thoracotomy to be avoided. Several adequate types of heat exchangers are available. Various pumps can be used. The new pumps with pulsatile flow appear to be better for inducing higher tissue blood flows and an adequate perfusion. After the heart fails, extracorporeal circulation should be increased to the maximum rate allowed by the venous drainage and by a maximal central venous pressure of 10 mm Hg. In order to avoid the sudden vasoconstriction of the blood vessels leading to a decreased venous return, the blood should be progressively cooled, especially during the early phases of the perfusion cooling.

SUMMARY

Many different extracorporeal circuits can be used. Physiological considerations and the physiological applicability of the circuit constitute the primary factor to keep in mind before deciding which circuit is to be employed.

Oxygenation

Many types of oxygenators are being used today. Various film oxygenators,[518] screen oxygenators,[188] disc oxygenators,[391,523,525,541,542] bubble oxygenators,[21,132,190,191,393,565] and membrane oxygenators[312,313,315,406,407,409] are employed in experimental work or in clinical practice. Even miniaturized membrane oxygenators for small laboratory animals such as rats or hamsters are available (Fig. 3-7).[416,417,429] Bubble oxygenators probably damage blood more than the other types, especially at high-volume blood flows, and may lead to microembolization. Cooling may also be induced without oxygenators.[105]

SUMMARY

Many types of oxygenators are commercially available today, and all of them are being improved constantly. Presently the membrane-type oxygenators appear to damage blood less than the other types of oxygenators.

Priming Volume

Herparinized blood, diluted blood, or pure diluent may be used to start the extracorporeal perfusion. Low-molecular-weight dextran, glucose saline, or other diluent mixtures may be used for the priming volume.

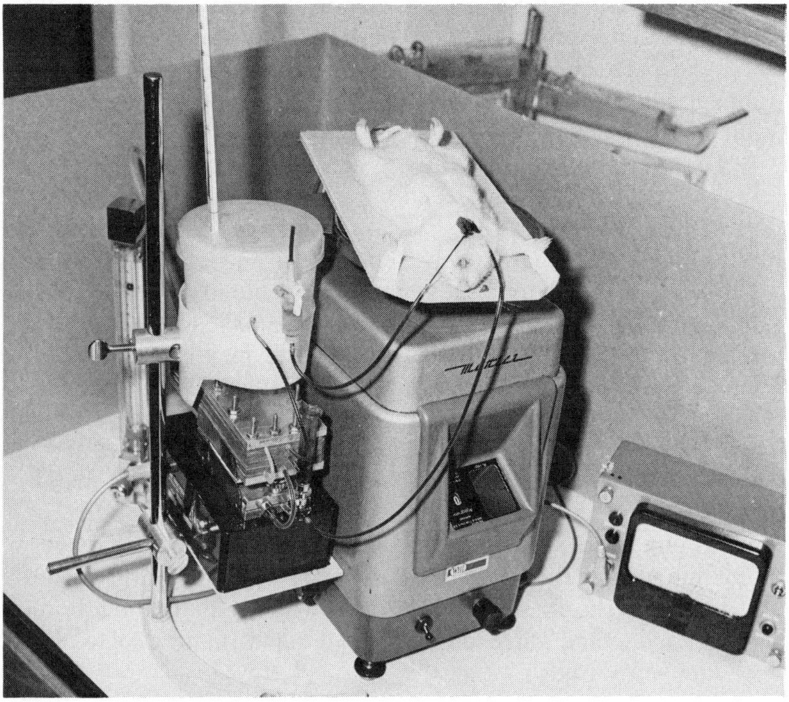

Fig. 3-7. Miniaturized membrane oxygenator for small laboratory animals.[416,417,429]

Heat Exchangers

Many types of heat exchangers are available,[117,214,254,264,268,279] and some of them are disposable.[459] Cooling due to the Peltier effect was also used as the basis for some of the miniaturized heat exchangers.[303] In order to achieve uniform hypothermia a combination of extracorporeal cooling with surface cooling is employed.[196,547]

Circulatory Support during Cooling

High-volume blood flow (60 ml/kg/min or higher) is recommended by many investigators.[483,536,537] Fast cooling for better protection of central vital organs, less developed metabolic acidosis[378] (especially during occlusion surgery),[377] and other advantages are mentioned when high-volume blood flows are employed. Some investigators suggest the use of perfusion flows that are even higher than those simply calculated on the basis of an oxygen need. However, the perfusion rate is often limited by the available venous drainage and the level of tolerable central venous pressure (maximum 8–10 mm Hg).

There are reports that the oxygen tension of the mixed blood remains in a normal range even with a decreased perfusion blood flow of 20 ml/ kg/min.[330] However, that still does not mean that all of the tissues are adequately perfused.

Some investigators advocate low blood flow perfusion rates[320,324,405,408] in order to decrease the damage to the blood. It is possible that low blood flow perfusion rates may even damage the heart sublethally (subendocardial necrosis), especially after a prolonged circulatory arrest.[88] Low blood flow perfusion rates may even lead to neurologic deficits and to damage of the central nervous system.[537] Such lesions cannot be prevented by dilution or by an increase of the carbon dioxide tension of the blood.

In our work[435] we have used high flow rates (above 60 ml/kg/min) during the cooling of dogs to a body temperature of 2 to 6 C. Survival of the dogs was 100 percent when hemodilution (priming volume: saline and glucose only, about 800 ml) and a high-volume flow rate were used.

SUMMARY

High blood flow rates during extracorporeal circulatory support appear to be more beneficial than low flow rates.

Ventricular Fibrillation

Ventricular fibrillation seldom appears during the cooling phase. If it does appear, the extracirculatory support should be immediately increased to compensate for the pumping action of the heart. During cooling, defibrillation of the heart is not needed. The heart will be arrested when the temperature of the heart is decreased below a temperature of 10 to 18 C.[193] This cold-induced cardioplegia is obviously the best method that one can use today for arresting the heart[73,452] though it is still not without some hazards.[474,522] Electrical pacing of the heart is not recommended because it usually decreases the cardiac output. It is important to note that during ventricular fibrillation and during a cold-induced cardiac arrest, the pressure in the pulmonary bed and in the left heart is increased (often to the level of the arterial pressure maintained by the extracorporeal circuit) and that decompression of the left heart is needed.[435] In our experiments, cannulation of the left ventricle with a large catheter that drains blood into the venous reservoir of the heart–lung machine, increased the survival of dogs cooled to a body temperature of 4 C (with 60 minutes circulatory arrest) from 40 to 100 percent. The dogs quickly recovered after rewarming and did not show any ill effects after the deep cooling and long-lasting circulatory arrest.

Cardioplegia with potassium citrate is dangerous at a high body temperature and should not be used. Some investigators believe that potassium, as a cardioplegic agent, is harmful even in hypothermic conditions. Deliberate ventricular fibrillation in hypothermia probably should not be employed (except in certain conditions as in the case of Wolfson's technique of brain cooling,[546] for instance, because it does not protect the heart more, although it does make it more manageable for surgery. Magnesium ions might have a protective effect during the cardiac arrest.[475,549] There are reports that prolonged cardioplegia does not lead to progressive elevation of the left atrial pressure,[274] but this finding has not been supported by sufficient experimental findings.

SUMMARY

Cooling appears to be the best method for arresting the heart. Ventricular fibrillation seldom occurs when adequate cooling or heating techniques are used. If it occurs, the ventricular fibrillation does not represent a major problem.

Hemodilution

Hemodilution induces a fast and uniform cooling and replaces priming blood. Hemodilution reduces the viscosity and probably brings about an improvement in the peripheral blood flow[72] and in the microcirculation. It appears likely that hemodilution decreases hemolysis of the blood and a denaturation of the fats. It also appears that blood proteins and blood-clotting mechanisms are preserved better during perfusion hypothermia with diluted blood than with nondiluted blood. The administration of low-molecular dextran (1 gm/kg) improves survival. This has been observed during surface cooling as well.[359] It has been reported that during perfusion cooling, hemodilution decreases blood sequestration, blood sludging, and cell aggregation.[40,324] Patients tolerate a dilution with a priming volume of 5 percent dextrose in saline well.[563] The same applies to dogs cooled to a body temperature of 4 to 8 C.[435] Some investigators use low-molecular dextran as priming solution.[561] There are reports that dilution increases the oxygen supply to tissues,[269,510] possibly by increasing the capillary circulation, and might be protective for postgastrointestinal bleeding.[509] Hemodilution can be brought to an extreme, and whole blood might be replaced with oxygenated Ringer's solution at a very low body temperature.[202,292] On the other hand, several investigators believe that there is no definite proof that hemodilution is beneficial. They state that the main difficulty associated with hemodilution is a rapid loss of the diluent from the vascular compartment. This eventually leads to a progressive reduction of the blood volume and to an eventual decrease in venous return.[528] It has been suggested that hemodilution might increase the postoperative bleeding.[245]

Pulmonary complications are sometimes noticed after hemodilution. In such cases, lungs show diffused atelectasis, alveolar congestion, and vascular occlusion. Contrary to this observation there are reports that the perfusion lung syndrome is somewhat decreased by hemodilution, though possibly not completely abolished. These pulmonary complications, observed with or without hemodilution, indicate the need for continuous monitoring of the central venous pressure, particularly the left atrial pressure, which should not exceed 8 to 10 mm Hg during the extracorporeal cooling. The blood volume loss observed after hemodilution with saline primer should eventually be replaced by whole blood, once the subject is rewarmed close to a normal body temperature. When circulatory arrest is performed, the diluted blood from the body may be easily collected in the extracorporeal venous reservoir and then replaced with donor blood.

It has also been suggested that additional amounts of blood or of fluids should be administered to the patient or to the experimental animal during the process of cooling in order to prevent vasoconstriction. Even more important is that large amounts of fluid should be given intravenously during the last stages of rewarming. It appears that this hypervolemia increases the success of perfusion cooling[435] and even surface cooling.

SUMMARY

Hemodilution is very beneficial during profound cooling and the early parts of the rewarming process.

Differential Cooling

During perfusion cooling the vital central organs cool faster than the peripheral tissues, especially during high-volume blood flows.[173] The cooling rate of tissue depends more on the volume flow of cold blood than on the thermal coefficient of the tissue.[342] The thermal gradients established this way do not produce cardiac arrhythmias[172] as it previously had been thought. The brain, which is more susceptible to anoxic damage than any other system, cools faster than peripheral tissues except for the heart. During high-volume blood flows the temperature of the brain may lag as much as 10 C behind the temperature of the esophagus or of the heart. It is likely that during the cooling phase there might be some temperature gradients in the brain itself.[560] Unfortunately, the direct measurements of cerebral temperatures in human patients are not practical. However, a thermocouple placed in the external auditory canal or retro-orbital space can be used to estimate the temperature and the rate of brain cooling. An important adjunct for accelerating the brain cooling is 5 or even 10 percent carbon dioxide added to the oxygen in the breathing mixture. Carbon dioxide induces cerebral vasodilation and greatly increases the volume blood flow and the rate of cooling of the brain[15,198,200,201,404] and prevents cerebral ischemia.[77,207]

SUMMARY

Many organs or parts of the body (heart, brain, lung, extremities, etc.) can be profoundly cooled while the rest of the body stays normothermic or is cooled only slightly.

Respiratory Support

Endotracheal intubation should be used during perfusion cooling. The tube must be cleaned frequently by suction, especially during the rewarming phase. During rewarming, only pure oxygen should be administered. This way the increased oxygen consumption of the organisms will be supported and the danger of anoxia and the appearance of high metabolic acidosis will be prevented.[207]

During circulatory arrest, the endotracheal tube should be clamped to maintain the lungs in a midinflated position or occasionally the lungs should be slightly ventilated (1–2/min). Unduly vigorous ventilation might easily damage the lung tissue during a circulatory arrest.

After complete rewarming, during a period of 2 to 3 hours, assisted respiration (at a reduced volume but at an increased rate) should be administered to prevent atelectasis and to ensure adequate oxygenation. Close to normal pO_2 and pCO_2 of the blood indicates proper respiratory support. These indicators should therefore be continuously monitored.

SUMMARY

Respiratory support is needed during the intial phases of cooling and during the last part of rewarming.

Acid–Base Balance

During cooling, alterations in the plasma and the tissue electrolytes always occur.[80,474] During this part of cooling, all animals and patients become acidotic.[20,300,392,467,469,493] Primarily this is caused by metabolic acidosis, which is a consequence of certain tissue oxygen debt.[528] Despite this rather common observation, there are reports that during cooling with high flow rates serious acidosis does not develop.[161,412,464] When perfusion cooling is combined with surface cooling the acidosis might even be developed to a small degree.[548] Bicarbonate[390] or buffers (Tris or THAM) should be used to correct both metabolic and respiratory acidosis.[34,257,365] The addition of 5 to 10 percent carbon dioxide appears to help maintain a more normal acid–base balance. In order to monitor the acid–base changes, frequent pH determinations taken at the same temperature (or corrected for the temperature decrease) are needed.[559] This applies especially to the rewarming process.

After rewarming, the pH of blood returns to normal. If acid–citrate–dextrose blood has been employed during perfusion cooling, however, attention must be called to the danger of a postoperative metabolic acidosis.[225] The pH measurements should therefore be continued for several hours after rewarming.

SUMMARY

An increased acidosis appears to occur naturally during cooling and disappears during the last part of rewarming. It is likely that this acidosis has an important protective role in hypothermia.

Circulatory Arrest

Extracorporeal circulatory support can be discontinued for a while during cooling when the body temperature is decreased to a very low level. The duration of safe circulatory arrest depends mainly on the depth of generalized cooling as well as on the depth of brain cooling. Complete cessation of the circulation, the ultimate goal of a surgeon, is rarely achieved.[105] The duration of circulatory arrest even in profound hypothermia is 1 or maybe 2 hours, but it may be somewhat extended by recirculating small amounts of blood for a short time. How long a circulatory arrest ("clinical death" in Russian literature) a deeply cooled organism can withstand is not known as yet. Determination of the length of safe circulatory arrest during a deep perfusion cooling has been the object of many studies.[32,89,218,284,318,413,442,532,533] Russian investigators have been interested in this problem. Professor Negovskii, a Russian leader in this field, wrote that "one of the most difficult problems facing researchers in the field of resuscitation is the prolongation of the period of clinical death with a complete and lasting recovery of vital functions."[372] Negovskii said that this can be done only when the body temperature of patients is greatly decreased.

A safe circulatory arrest of several minutes during profound cooling was reported in 1955 by Gollan et al.[209] Somewhat later, a safe circulatory arrest lasting 30 minutes was described.[88] At a body temperature of 25 C it appears possible to occlude the blood flow for 10 to 20 minutes[26,94,206,453] and possibly even for 30 minutes.[93,351] A circulatory arrest of up to 60 minutes can be achieved at a body temperature of 20[107] or 15 C.[487] Safe circulatory arrest lasting 60 to 80 minutes appears to be feasible when the body temperature of experimental animals is decreased to 5 to 10 C.[37,105,218,228,282,318,378–381,483,553] The cooling of dogs below a body temperature of 4 C permits a safe circulatory arrest of 1 to 1½ hours,[435] while deeper cooling of the dogs to a body temperature approaching 0 C extends the safe circulatory arrest to 1½ hours as Gollan[204] and Negre[376] have shown, or even to 2[454] or 2½ hours.[90,295] Deeply cooled patients[139] can withstand a circulatory arrest of 80 minutes equally well.

Young animals or young patients can withstand even longer periods of circulatory arrest. For instance, baby ground squirrels cooled to −4 C survive a total circulatory arrest of more than 11 hours without ill consequences.[418]

Negovskii observed long safe periods of circulatory arrest. He believed that the period of clinical death in dogs might be prolonged to 2 hours with subsequent complete restoration of their vital functions.

The oxygen tension of cerebral fluid, which reflects the mean oxygen tension of the brain tissue, falls to 0 mm Hg after 2 minutes of normothermic circulatory arrest. However, when the brain is cooled to a body temperature of 20 C the cerebral oxygen tension approaches 0 mm Hg after 12 to 15 minutes. At a brain temperature of 10 C, the oxygen tension of cerebral fluid does not reach 0 mm Hg even after a circulatory arrest of 40 minutes.[68] This finding is of importance because the brain has a very high metabolic rate. It does not have the ability to survive under marked oxygen debt and thus is very sensitive to anoxia.

SUMMARY

Profound hypothermia permits extended periods of circulatory arrest. Currently 2 hours of total circulatory arrest appears to be the safe limit that hypothermia brings to adult animals or patients. Infant animals or babies stand a total circulatory arrest much better and much longer than the adult animals or the adult patients.

Metabolic Features of Circulatory Arrest

The reason for permanent damage of vital functions after a long circulatory arrest is not known. It might be that the oxygen demand of cold tissues is still large enough to cause irreversible damage. If this should be the case, then an occasional low flow perfusion (with or without oxygen) or an occasional coronary perfusion could lead to a better recovery from a long-lasting circulatory standstill. There is, of course, the possibility that a washing out of the metabolites is more important than the supply of oxygen to the cold tissues. In such a case the problem of adequate irrigation of the metabolites from the tissues via a perfusate becomes more critical than anoxia itself.

High-energy phosphate levels are much less depleted in the hearts arrested in hypothermia than in normothermic hearts arrested by potassium or anoxia.[219,220] The same applies for glycogen. It appears that high-energy phosphate disappears 10 times slower in profound hypothermia than in normothermia. In dogs cooled to a body temperature of 10 C the increase in lactic acid is proportional to the duration of circulatory arrest.[377] However, the increase in lactic acid occurs much slower at lower body temperatures than in normothermic conditions.

It is interesting to note that the left ventricular stroke volume returns to the precooling level after rewarming from an extended circulatory arrest in deep hypothermia.[109,111,112,544] However, Russian investigators have demonstrated some changes in the activity of higher centers of the central nervous system after a circulatory arrest in profound hypothermia that lasted 30 minutes. During the first 2 weeks after resuscitation the conditioned reflex activity of the animals was suppressed, but later fully restored. Similar changes were observed after a 105-minute circulatory arrest in dogs whose brains were preferentially cooled,[546] though this technique was later improved so that only transient neurological signs were observed on monkeys after preferential brain cooling and 60 minutes of circulatory arrest.[545]

Though some investigators believe that "overenthusiastic application of cardioplegia and total circulatory arrest in hypothermia brought new problems,"[324] it is clear that the research in this field of endeavor will be continued. Imaginative approaches and better techniques are needed to overcome the existing dangers profound hypothermia sometimes brings forth. These dangers probably encompass some chronic subtle microscopic brain changes that have been described in animals surviving 1 hour or more of total circulatory arrest,[105] and maybe even some tissue in other organs. It has been proposed[105] that the brain damage observed after a circulatory arrest in profound hypothermia is the consequence of a rather inadequate protection from hypoxia during the period of arrest. However, there are some investigators who disagree with this point of view.

SUMMARY

It is not yet known why and exactly when the point of no return occurs during a long-lasting circulatory arrest in profoundly cooled animals or patients. Once these mechanisms are better known, it will be possible to appreciably extend the safe circulatory arrest that today can last 1 or 2 hours in adult organisms and up to 12 hours in newborn animals.

Rewarming

It is still unknown whether a slow or a fast rewarming is more beneficial for survival after induced hypothermia. Presently, most investigators tend to believe that a fast rewarming gives better protection. This is the view of the Russian school, too, based mainly on the surface-cooling experiments. It is suggested that for large experimental animals, the rate of rewarming should be about 1 C/min, somewhat faster than the rate of cooling. During rewarming, only pure oxygen (without the administration of CO_2) should be used. The blood volume and volume blood flow should not be increased appreciably until the heart starts its spontaneous pumping action. Further rewarming brings proper sinus rhythm. During rewarming, ventricles of large experimental animals and patients sometimes fibrillate. In children and in very young experimental animals this event rarely occurs. Instead of fibrillating, the ventricles start contracting spontaneously in the rhythm of the sino-atrial node throughout the whole period of rewarming.[532] If the ventricles fibrillate, they can easily be defibrillated with potassium, or even better with electric shocks. Reversion is especially easy during vigorous fibrillation and when the heart temperature is 28 C or higher, myocardial oxygenation is still adequate and cardiac muscle is not dilated. Shocks lasting 3 to 10 seconds are the most effective and probably the least damaging.

After a circulatory arrest, the cerebral blood flow is higher during rewarming than during cooling. During cooling, carbon dioxide is needed to make the flow more adequate. Better circulation during the rewarming is probably the consequence of vasodilating action of catabolytes released during hypothermic period.[135]

It has been suggested that the arterial blood pressure during the early phase of rewarming should remain below 60 mm Hg and should not exceed this value until the heart takes over the pumping action of the blood or partial heart–lung bypass is restored again. During rewarming, the blood temperature should not exceed 43 C. It is suggested that the head portion should be kept cooler than the rest of the body to prevent hypoxic brain damage during this critical part of the rewarming procedure. The limbs should also be kept cooler than the rest of the body, thereby decreasing the need for a high extracorporeal circulatory support.

The circulating blood volume should initially be kept at a low level, especially during rewarming to 28 to 30 C, until the heart is capable of starting its pumping action forcefully. It is advantageous to bring the blood volume to the normal value or even to increase it by 10 to 20 percent above the precooling level once the cardiac pumping action is fully restored.[435] During rewarming when the temperature of the central vital organs in the body reaches 33 to 34

C, the rewarming should be temporarily interrupted for 20 to 30 minutes, or even longer, until the cardiac output is fully stabilized at a normal or near normal level. At this time the arterial and especially the central venous pressure reflect the level of circulating blood volume and the status of the systemic circulation much better than other circulatory parameters. Unfortunately, if the heart or peripheral circulation does not recover rapidly enough during this last period of rewarming, death of the organism occasionally does result. The real causes of this "rewarming shock" are not yet known.

SUMMARY

It appears that fast rewarming is more beneficial than a slow rewarming. If nothing else, the duration of a long-lasting hypothermic bout is decreased this way. Hemodilution, and even more hypervolemia, during the last part of the rewarming process appears to be very beneficial.

After Rewarming

Exceptional care should be provided after rewarming. The rewarmed organism is extremely sensitive to either recooling or overheating. Continuous monitoring of the central venous pressure for several hours after rewarming is very important and appears to serve as the best index of the circulating blood volume, indicating eventual needs for additional transfusions. Systematic evaluation of the metabolic acid–base balance during the rewarming period is also important. Water drinking and urination are very good signs of the general well-being of the animal. Antibiotics should be given immediately after rewarming and then administered for 1 week. Other postoperative medications should be restricted to a minimum.

Disadvantages of Perfusion Hypothermia

Cooling affects tissue perfusion in numerous ways. It induces the possiblility of vasoconstriction, "sludging,"[457] aggregation of red blood cells,[230] sequestration of blood, increased blood viscosity, intravascular agglutination,[285,457] intravascular coagulation, hemolysis, and an increase in plasma hemoglobin.[564] Protein denaturation is also extensive in all types of perfusion cooling.[316] This phenomenon is most likely caused by the unnatural surface-tension forces existing in the extracorporeal circuits. Lethal as well as sublethal red blood cell damage has also been reported. Sometimes blood flow ceases in some small vessels of a deeply cooled organism which can lead to local tissue necrosis.

During partial bypass and during deep body cooling, the blood of the right and possibly of the left heart is probably moving to and fro through the pulmonary bed because of an incompetent pulmonary valve of the deeply cooled and thus placid right heart. The same probably applies to the mitral valve[540] and this might lead to a pulmonary hypertension. Left ventricular cannulas (introduced through the carotid artery) drain blood by gravity into venous reservoirs, completely eliminating this problem. In this case the left heart distention and pulmonary congestion are prevented, even in animals that are cooled to a body temperature of 4 to 8 C with 1 hour of circulatory arrest.[435]

Some of the changes observed during perfusion hypothermia are similar to those reported in traumatic shock. As in the case of shock, the main (and the least understood) problem of perfusion hypothermia is what is happening with the microcirculation in deeply cooled tissues. This is the problem that must await even a partial clarification in the future.

Coagulation[387,552] is often impaired during perfusion cooling. Mortality and morbidity are especially high after prolonged circulatory occlusions.[401] Platelets fall during perfusion cooling from 250,000 to 15,000 and then rise during rewarming to a value of 50,000 or 70,000. Antithrombin and fibrinolytic activity are also increased during cooling, leading to postoperative bleeding.[21] In addition, renal tubular nephrosis,[98] caused by deposition of fibrinogen and microemboli, has been described in a few cases. The use of fresh blood and neutralization of the heparin at the end of rewarming with protamine sulfate apparently eliminate these problems. Nevertheless, there are some investigators who believe that after rewarming, the neutralization of heparin is not necessary. An elevated central venous pressure should not be permitted to last too long. Gas emboli or, even more likely, solid emboli probably decrease the efficiency of brain cooling, something that should be avoided with an increased CO_2 tension in the respired air or perfused blood. Serotonin, released from platelets,[441] might occasionally lead to vasodilation and consequently to a decreased mean arterial blood pressure during the rewarming phase.

It has been suggested that low-molecular-weight dextran might decrease or even abolish many of the pathologic changes described above. However, it appears that other methods of diluting the blood are even more beneficial, as for instance, dilution with Ringer glucose.[435] Overdistention of the cardiac chambers and congestion or consolidation of the lungs might sometimes cause difficulties.[299] This especially happens in the case of a long-lasting circulatory arrest.

It is known that perfusion hypothermia is more dangerous to children than to adult patients. For this reason surface cooling, which is performed more easily in children anyhow, is today the technique of choice for the cooling of young patients.

SUMMARY

Various blood changes were reported during perfusion cooling. It is possible that these changes are related more to a specific cooling technique than to perfusion hypothermia itself.

Advantages of Perfusion Cooling

It has been said that experimental physiology and medical practice have seldom witnessed a better partnership than extracorporeal circulation combined with hypothermia. Both techniques are extremely useful but both have some important drawbacks. In clinical practice, normothermic extracorporeal circulatory support seldom reaches 70 to 80 percent of the needed cardiac output. Furthermore, long-lasting extracorporeal circulation damages the circulating blood to varying degrees. On the other hand, the beneficial effects of hypothermia are present only when the cooling is very profound. Such a profound cooling, especially of central vital organs, cannot easily be achieved with surface cooling. The combination of hypothermia with extracorporeal cooling solves many of these problems. Deep cooling decreases the need for a large extracorporeal circulatory support[65] because hypothermia decreases the metabolic demand for oxygen.[244] On the other hand, perfusion techniques permit a faster and much deeper cooling (especially of vital organs in the body) than when surface-induced hypothermia is employed.[317,318]

The solubility of oxygen in plasma is increased. Hypothermia decreases the pH of the blood, favorably changing the oxygen dissociation curve, though it might be that this effect is seen more in vitro than in vivo. More importantly, extracorporeal circulation damages the blood much less when the blood is cooled.[51,298] Denaturation of the proteins and hemolysis induced by extracorporeal circulation are also decreased in hypothermia. In hypothermia the danger of cerebral gas emboli induced at the interfaces in oxygenators is diminished. This is done probably because of an increased solubility of the gases in the cold blood. Furthermore, circulatory interruption is tolerated much longer in hypothermia, especially when the brain is cooled early and adequately.[324] Other advantages of deep hypothermia combined with extracorporeal circulation are the availability of a quiet and bloodless operative field and the possibility to arrest the heart for extended periods. The accumulation of acid metabolites is also diminished. In profound perfusion hypothermia the extracorporeal volume blood flow is diminished appreciably because the metabolic needs of the cooled tissues are decreased.[469] Perfusion cooling permits a reduction of the priming volume of donor blood, fewer passages of blood to the heart–lung machine with less damage to cellular and protein elements of the blood, and a decreased release of histamine, serotonin, and other vasoactive compounds released during extracorporeal circulatory support.[251] Of all these advantages the most important appears to be the protection against the hypoxic damage observed when profound hypothermia is combined with extracorporeal circulation.

However, besides all these advantages there are some risks in combining the two techniques.[324] One might expect, though, that progress in this field will eventually bring solutions to these problems and that the future will see an effective and better use of perfusion hypothermia in experimental work as well as in clinical practice.

SUMMARY

Both extracorporeal circulatory support and profound hypothermia have certain important drawbacks, though combination of extracorporeal circulation and hypothermia proved to be extremely useful.

Experimental and Clinical Use of Perfusion Hypothermia

The combination of hypothermia and extracorporeal circulation was found to be useful in experimental work,[71,83,98,124,203,210,276,287,308,354,403,408,413,435,497] and in clinical work as well.[33,52,54,57,84,85,104,118,119,128,139–141,145,146,148–152,167,186,213,217,289,290,301,332,345,352,361,365,383,390,391,411,469–471,476,482,486,533]

Perfusion hypothermia has been shown to increase the tolerance to experimentally induced myocardial infarction.[176,304,305,307,308] It has been successfully used also for treatment of congenital heart disease[149] and for the repair of aneurysms.[174] Perfusion hypothermia increases myocaradial contractility, lowers myocardium oxygen consumption, and increases cardiac efficiency after left cardiac failure.[211] This procedure permitted the restoration of cardiac output near to the normal level. It has been reported that pregnant women withstand core cooling well.[270]

Mild perfusion hypothermia (cooling to 28 C or less) was used first for cardiac surgery of short duration, such as for secundum atrial defects, pulmonary valvular stenosis, and valvular congenital aortic stenosis. Hypothermia of a similar or somewhat more profound degree has been used in interatrial and interventricular septal defects,[369] in congenital cardiac defects, pulmonary stenosis,[247] for correction of valvular lesions or mitral valve stenosis, and for tetralogy of Fallot.[222,227]

Perfusion hypothermia without an oxygenator was used for open-heart surgery also. Perfusion hypothermia was employed during the removal of cardiac tumors,[87] for correction of aneurysms,[69] for aortic valvulatomy,[42,187] and for mitral stenosis operations.[362]

Perfusion hypothermia of medium degree (arbitrarily defined as cooling to a body temperature of 20 C) was used for more complicated surgical problems.[562]

For very difficult and extended surgical procedures (anomalous venous drainage, Potts anastomoses, etc.) deep core cooling to a body temperature of 15 C or lower is needed.[228] Consequently, for complicated aortic valve surgery that may last 4 hours or more, profound perfusion hypothermia is suggested.[218] Partial bypass appears to be beneficial in the treatment of cardiogenic shock and in the resuscitation of some patients who are in danger of succumbing to an acute myocardial infarction.[329]

Hyperbaric oxygenation was used also in several instances in combination with perfusion hypothermia for complex intracardiac surgery.[39,445]

Extracorporeal circulation was used to cool animals successfully to 10 C[105] or to 0 to 5 C.[90,193,202,205,253,543] A sanguineous perfusion was successfully used in profound hypothermia also.[202,292]

SUMMARY

Perfusion hypothermia has been tried in many experimental as well as clinical situations. Some of them have been described here.

Clinical Application of Circulatory Arrest

Circulatory arrest, mostly in profound hypothermia, was first used experimentally[197,205,253,343,370,454] and then clinically for cardiac or for neurovascular surgery. Furthermore, profound perfusion hypothermia with circulatory arrest has been used for treatment of congenital cardiac malformations,[147,389] for the correction of congenital or acquired cardiac lesions,[263] for atrial septal defects, for traumatic aneurysm or fistula of the thoracic aorta,[78,155] as well as for other types of open-heart surgery.[154,263] Closed-chest circulatory arrest in profound hypothermia was used for operations involving intracranial aneurysms,[144] aortic aneurysms,[155] arteriovenous malformations, and excision of intracranial tumors.

Patients were cooled to a body temperature of 10 to 12 C with a full hour of circulatory arrest.[118,218,439] Dubost's group reported cooling in many patients to a body temperature of 10 C with complete circulatory arrest.[150] Patients who were cooled to a body temperature of 5 C with a circulatory arrest of 1 hour and 45 minutes recovered fully.[105]

Circulatory arrest is often used in children too for correction of heart lesions. However, in this case instead of core cooling, surface-cooling techniques were used,[134,358,477] though pump oxygenators, even in children, speed the rewarming process appreciably.[498]

SUMMARY

Circulatory arrest was used experimentally or clinically mostly for surgical interventions that have been discussed briefly here.

BIBLIOGRAPHY

1. Aldinger EE, Thrower WB, Gadsden RH: The effects of deep hypothermia on myocardial function and general metabolism. J Surg Res 3:178–184, 1963
2. Adolph EF: Some differences in responses to low temperatures between warm-blooded and cold-blooded vertebrates. Am J Physiol 166:92–103, 1951
3. Adolph EF, Klem S, Morrow LB: Reversible cessation of blood circulation in deep hypothermia. J Appl Physiol 13:397–405, 1958
4. Adolph EF, Nail RL: Vagal inhibition of the heart in deep hypothermia. J Appl Physiol 15:911–913, 1960
5. Anderson GL, Prewitt R Jr, Musacchia XJ: Myocardial correlates of helium-cold induction and maintenance in hypothermia. Am J Physiol 221:1760–1762, 1971
6. Andjus R, Pajevic J: Resistance of newborn rats to subzero body temperatures and the general problem of supercooling, in Symposium on Hypothermia: Proceedings 15th International Congress on Military Medicine and Pharmacology, Belgrade, 1957, p 72
7. Andjus RK, Smith AU: Revival of hypothermic rats after arrest of circulation and respiration. J Physiol 123:66-P–67-P, 1954
8. Andjus RK, Smith AU: Reanimation of adult rats from body temperatures between 0 and +2°C. J Physiol 128:446–472, 1955
9. Andrews PM, Panuska JA: Fractional distribution of cardiac output to the brains of unanesthetized normothermic and hypothermic rats. Am Zool 7:744, 1967
10. Andrews PM, Panuska JA, Felicetti CL, et al: Cardiovascular responses of the unanesthetized and unrestrained hypothermic rat. J Appl Physiol 27:539–543, 1969
11. Angelakos ET, Hegnauer AH: Myocardial contractility under hypothermia. Fed Proc 19:107, 1960
12. Angelakos ET, Laforet EG, Hegnauer AH: Ventricular excitability and refractoriness in the hypothermic dog. Am J Physiol 189:591–595, 1957
13. Arnovljevic V: Modification of the initial part of the ventricular complex in electrocardiography under the influence of low body temperatures. Glas Srp Akad Nauka (Med) 248:19–26, 1961
14. Austen WG: Cardiac hypothermia versus coronary perfusion during aortic occlusion. Surg Forum 15:206–208, 1964
15. Bacharach B, Snyder HM, Templeton JY: Effect of inhaling carbon dioxide on brain cooling during hypothermia. Surg Forum 12:186–187, 1961
16. Badeer H: Ventricular fibrillation in hypothermia. J Thorac Cardiovasc Surg 35:265–273, 1958
17. Badeer HS: Work capacity of the hypothermic heart. Am Heart J 63:839–840, 1962
18. Badeer HS: Effect of hypothermia on the contractile "capacity" of the myocardium. J Thorac Cardiovasc Surg 53:651–656, 1967
19. Baker RJ, St Ville JM, Suzuki F, et al: Evaluation of red cell equilibration in hemorrhagic shock. Arch Surg 90:538–544, 1965
20. Ballinger WF, Templeton JY, Vollenweider H, et al: Acidosis in patients

during hypothermia and biventricular bypass. J Cardiovasc Surg 3:323–326, 1962

21. Barnard CN, Terblanche J, Ozinsky J: Profound hypothermia and the helix reservoir bubble oxygenator. S Afr Med J 35:107–110, 1961
22. Battista AF: Phrenic and cardiac irregularities in the hypothermic cat. Arch Surg 95:30–37, 1967
23. Baum D, Dillard DH, Mohri H, et al: Metabolic aspects of deep surgical hypothermia in infancy. Pediatrics 42:93–105, 1968
24. Beavers WR, Covino BG: Relationship of potassium and calcium to hypothermic ventricular fibrillation. J Appl Physiol 14:60–62, 1959
25. Benichoux R, Kurtz M, Thibaut G, et al: Experimentation de l'association THAM—Serum adrenaline dans la cardioplegie par hypothermie profonde de contact. Anest Analg (Paris) 20:29–47, 1963
26. Benichoux R, Thibaut G, Marchal C, et al: THAM et hypothermie. J Cardiovasc Surg 4:556–565, 1963
27. Benzing G, Stockert J, DeForrest D, et al: Effect of myocardial ischemia on left ventricular function after hypothermic cardiopulmonary bypass. J Thorac Cardiovasc Surg 56:241–252, 1968
28. Berne RM: Myocardial function in severe hypothermia. Cir Res 2:90–95, 1954
29. Berne RM: Cardiodynamics and coronary circulation in hypothermia. Ann NY Acad Sci 80:365–383, 1959
30. Berne RM, Jones RD, Cross FS: Myocardial hypothermia in elective cardiac arrest. J Appl Physiol 12:431–436, 1958
31. Berne RM, Jones RD, Cross FS: Evaluation of selective cardiac hypothermia and potassium arrest of the heart. J Thorac Cardiovasc Surg 47:283–288, 1964
32. Bernhard WF, Gross RE: Extracorporeal circulation and profound hypothermia: A new surgical technique. Proceedings, 19th New England Cardiovascular Society, 1960–1961
33. Bernhard WF, Gross RE: The rationale of hypothermic cardioplegia in the management of congenital anomalies affecting the aortic valve, coronary arteries and proximal aortic arch. Ann Surg 156:161–172, 1962
34. Bernhard WF, Moore D, Gross RE: The management of metabolic lactic-acidosis accompanying prolonged hypothermic perfusion. Proceedings 20th New England Cardiovascular Society, 1961–1962
35. Bernhard WF, Schwarz HF, Hug G, et al: Alterations in myocardial metabolism subsequent to hypoxic and hypothermic cardiac arrest. Surg Forum 12:171–173, 1961
36. Bernhard WF, Schwarz HF, Mallick NP: Intermittent cold coronary perfusion as an adjunct to open heart surgery. Surg Gynecol Obstet 111:744–748, 1960
37. Bernhard WF, Schwarz HF, Mallick NP: Profound hypothermia as an adjunct to cardiovascular surgery. J Thorac Cardiovasc Surg 42:263–274, 1961
38. Bernhard WF, Schwarz HF, Mallick NP: Elective hypothermic cardiac arrest in normothermic animals. Ann Surg 153:43–51, 1961
39. Bernhard WF, Tank ES, Frittelli G, et al: The feasibility of hypothermic perfusion under hyperbaric conditions in the surgical management of infants with cyanotic congenital heart disease. J Thorac Cardiovasc Surg 46:651–664, 1963

40. Bernstein EF, Emmings FG, Mackey GC, et al: Effect of low molecular weight dextran on red blood cell charge during extracorporeal circulation. Trans Am Soc Artif Intern Organs 8:23–29, 1962
41. Bertho E: Production of cardiac arrest by an electrolyte solution. Can Med Assoc J 83:213–216, 1960
42. Bertho E, Bruneau J, Prive L, et al: Resection d'un anevrysme dissequant de l'aorte ascendante et bicuspidation des valvules aortiques au cours d'un syndrome de Marfan. Saguenay Med 10:1–10, 1963
43. Bigelow WG: Application of hypothermia to cardiac surgery. Minn Med 37:181–185, 1954
44. Bigelow WG, Callaghan JC, Hopps JA: General hypothermia for experiental intracardiac surgery. Ann Surg 132:531–539, 1950
45. Bigelow WG, Lindsay WK, Greenwood WF: Hypothermia: Its possible role in cardiac surgery: An investigation of factors governing survival in dogs at low body temperatures. Ann Surg 132:849–866, 1950
46. Bigelow WG, McBirnie JE: Further experiences with hypothermia for intracardiac surgery in monkeys and groundhogs. Ann Surg 137:361–365, 1953.
47. Bigelow WG, Mustard WT, Evans JG: Some physiologic concepts of hypothermia and their application to cardiac surgery. J Thorac Surg 28:463–480, 1954
48. Biorck G, Johansson B: Influence of anoxia on the hypothermic electrocardiogram of hedgehog and man. Cardiologia 30:344–348, 1957
49. Bjork VO: An artificial heart or cardiopulmonary machine; performance in animals. Lancet 2:491–493, 1948
50. Bjork VO: An effective blood heat exchanger for deep hypothermia in association with extracorporeal circulation but excluding the oxygenator. J Thorac Cardiovasc Surg 40:237–252, 1960
51. Bjork VO: Deep hypothermia without an oxygenator versus the use of the pump oxygenator for open heart surgery. Acta Chir Scand 119:351–356, 1960
52. Bjork VO: Methods for open heart surgery. Acta Chir Scand, Suppl 283:75–83, 1961
53. Bjork VO, Aletras H, Intonti F: The use of hypothermia in open heart surgery. J Cardiovasc Surg 3:182–194, 1962
54. Bjork VO, Gjessing J, Holmdahl MH, et al: Profound hypothermia in open heart surgery. Acta Anaesthesiol Scand 4:155–165, 1960
55. Bjork VO, Hogstrom S: Repeated circulatory arrest under hypothermia. Thorax 18:155–157, 1963
56. Bjork VO, Holmdahl MH: The oxygen consumption in man under deep hypothermia and the safe period of circulatory arrest. J Thorac Cardiovasc Surg 42:392–401, 1961
57. Bjork VO, Holmdahl MH: Deep hypothermia with extracorporeal circulation in open heart surgery. Nord Med 65:299–306, 1961
58. Bjork VO, Hultquist G: Contraindications to profound hypothermia in open-heart surgery. J Thorac Cardiovasc Surg 44:1–13, 1962
59. Blair E: Hypothermia—Physiologic rationale. Clin Pharmacol Ther 1:758–768, 1960
60. Blair E: Clinical Hypothermia. New York, McGraw-Hill, 1964, p 272

61. Blair E: A physiologic classification of clinical hypothermia. Surgery 58: 607–618, 1965
62. Blair E: Generalized hypothermia. Fed Proc 28:1456–1462, 1969
63. Blair E, Austin RR, Blount SG, et al: A study of cardiovascular changes during cooling and rewarming in human subjects undergoing total circulatory occlusion. J Thorac Cardiovasc Surg 33:707–718, 1957
64. Blair E, Cowley RA, Attar S, et al: The effect of hypothermia on circulatory reflexes in the human. Surg Gynecol Obstet 117:553–558, 1963
65. Blair E, Cowley RA, Singleton RT, et al: Role of hypothermia in intracardiac surgery. Circulation 22:725, 1960
66. Blair E, Montgomery AV, Swan H: Posthypothermic circulatory failure. I. Physiologic observations on circulation. Circulation 13:909–915, 1956
67. Blasius W, Albers C, Bach G, et al: On cardiac electrophysiology in hypothermia. Exp Med Surg 19:258–269, 1961
68. Bloor BM, Hellinger FR, Neville WE, et al: Oxygen tension of the brain and its modification by hypothermia. Second International Congress on Neurosurgery, Washington, D.C., 1961
69. Boba A: Hypothermia. Appraisal of risk in 110 consecutive patients. J Neurosurg 19:924–933, 1962
70. Boba A: An abnormal electrocardiographic pattern and its relation to ventricular fibrillation (observations during clinical and experimental hypothermia). Am Heart J 57:255–262, 1959
71. Bokeriia L, Marin A, Zalenikin M: Arresting the general circulation under experimental hyperbaric oxygenation and hypothermia. Grudn Khir 10: 58–63, 1968
72. Bolooki H, Goldberg RI, Antell HI, et al: Comparison of the effect of low molecular weight dextran on blood flow and peripheral resistance during extracorporeal circulation and hypothermia. J Thorac Cardiovasc Surg 54:216–221, 1967
73. Bonnabeau RC Jr., Sterns LP, Bilgutay A, et al: Cardiac temperature gradients with various types of cardioplegia during cardiopulmonary bypass. Surg Gynecol Obstet 116:569–574, 1963
74. Bonnabeau RC Jr, Sterns LP, Lillehei CW: Coronary artery resistance during prolonged profound selective hypothermia under cardiopulmonary bypass. Trans Am Soc Artif Intern Organs 10:43–51, 1964
75. Booker WM: Comparison of the action of adrenaline and nor-adrenaline against cocaine on the isolated perfused guinea pig heart during normothermia and hypothermia. Arch Int Pharmacodyn Ther 124:1–10, 1960
76. Borst HG, Schmidt-Mende M, Kovacicek S, et al: Oxygen consumption during extracorporeal hypothermia. Hypothermie profounde en Chirurgie Cardiaque, 1961–1962, p 212
77. Borst HG, Schmidt-Mende M, Kovacicek S, et al: Distribution of extracorporeal blood flow in normothermia and hypothermia. J Cardiovasc Surg 4:547–550, 1963
78. Borst HG, Schaudig A, Rudolph W: Arteriovenous fistula of the aortic arch: Repair during deep hypothermia and circulatory arrest. J Thorac Cardiovasc Surg 48:443–447, 1964

79. Bouchet M, Fredet M, Laborit MH, et al: Discussion planifiee sur les limites de l'arret circulatoire sous hypothermie profonde. Anesth Analg (Paris) 20: 67–92, 1963
80. Boyd JW, Webb WR: Alterations in tissue and serum electrolytes during hypothermic circulatory arrests. Clin Res 9:35, 1961
81. Brauer RW, Holloway RJ, Krebs JS, et al: The liver in hypothermia. Ann N Y Acad Sci 80:395–423, 1959
82. Brendel W, Albers C, Usinger W: Der Kreislauf in Hypothermie. Pfluegers Arch Ges Physiol 266:341–356, 1958
83. Brendel W, Hallwachs O, Usinger W: Sauerstoffverbrauch und Hamodynamik bei kombinierter Anwendung von Herz-Lungen Maschine und tiefer Hypothermie bis 10°C. Thoraxchirurgie 9:607–623, 1961-62
84. Brewer LA, King EL: Hypothermia in thoracic and thoracoabdominal surgery. Surv Anesthesiol 4:53–54, 1960
85. Brewer LA, King EL: Hypothermia in thoracic and thoraco-abdominal surgery: Use of light cooling as an adjunct to anesthesia in poor risk patients. Am J Surg 96:137–150, 1958
86. Brooks CMc: Hypothermia and the physiology of cardiac excitability, in Dripps RD (ed): The Physiology of Induced Hypothermia, Washington, National Academy of Sciences, 1956, pp 287
87. Bross W: Successful removal of pseudomyxoma from right atrium under hypothermia. J Cardiovasc Surg 6:234–237, 1965
88. Brown IW: Hypothermia combined with extracorporeal circulation, in Gibbon JH, Sabiston DC (eds): Surgery of the Chest. Philadelphia, Saunders, 1969, pp 708–746
89. Bucknam CA, Galindo A: Profound hypothermia by extracorporeal cooling. Surg Forum 11:412–414, 1960
90. Bucknam CA, Galindo A: Tolerance of circulatory arrest in deep hypothermia by extracorporeal cooling. J Neurosurg 18:339–347, 1961
91. Bullard RW: Maintenance of arterial pressure and cardiac output in the hypothermic rat. Fed Proc 15:28, 1956
92. Bullard RW: Cardiac output of the hypothermic rat. Am J Physiol 196:415–419, 1959
93. Burakovski V, Bukharin V, Gelshstein G: Experience in the use of the technique of excluding the heart from the circulation under hypothermia in clinical practice. Grudn Khir 9:15–21, 1967
94. Burakovski V, Gubler E: Exclusion of the heart from the circulation under great experimental hypothermia. Transactions of the 26th Congress on Surgery, Moscow, 1956, pp 177–183
95. Burdette WJ, Ashford TP: Response of myocardial fine structure to cardiac arrest and hypothermia. Ann Surg 158:513–525, 1963
96. Byon YK, Adolph EF: Oxygen in tissues during deep hypothermia. J Appl Physiol 16:827–830, 1961
97. Campkin V: Moderate hypothermia and circulatory arrest for neurosurgical operations. Br J Anaesth 37:528–532, 1965
98. Castberg T, Saurbrey J, Sivertsen U, et al: Extracorporeal circulation with hypothermia and sympathetic bloc. Acta Chir Scand 128:659–670, 1964

99. Cazzullo CL, Macchi V: Modificazioni elettrocardiografiche osservate in animali sottoposti ad ipotermia profonda artificiale. Folia Cardiol 13:235–256, 1954
100. Chevillard L, Giono H, Popovic V: Activite physiologique de rat refroidi. Effets cardiovasculaires de l'adrenaline. C R Soc Biol (Paris) 149:1925–1928, 1955
101. Clifton BS: Hypothermia in cardiac surgery. Med J Aust 1:641–647, 1960
102. Conn AW: Anaesthesia with hypothermia for open heart surgery in children. Can Anaesth Soc J 8:128–135, 1961
103. Conn AW, Allan D, Junkin I: Anesthesia with hypothermia for closure of atrial septal defects in children. Surv Anesthesiol 5:40–41, 1961
104. Connolly JE, Boyd RJ, Calvin JW: The protective effect of hypothermia in cerebral ischemia: Experimental and clinical application by selective brain cooling on the human. Surgery 52:15–24, 1962
105. Connolly JE, Roy A, Guernsey JM, et al: Bloodless surgery by means of profound hypothermia and circulatory arrest. Effect on brain and heart. Ann Surg 162:724–737, 1965
106. Connolly JE, Samson PC, Richards V, et al: Direct vision surgery of acquired aortic and mitral valvular stenosis under hypothermia. Surgery 45:181–197, 1959
107. Connolly JE, Stemmer EA: Blutleere Chirurgie in tiefer Hypothermie. Lang Arch Klin Chir 316:898–908, 1966
108. Cook WA, Webb WR: Pump oxygenators and hypothermia. Ann Thorac Surg 1:466–504, 1965
109. Cooper KE: The circulation in hypothermia. Br Med Bull 17:48–51, 1961
110. Cooper KE, Ross DN: Hypothermia in Surgical Practice. Philadelphia, Davies, 1960, p 116
111. Cooper T, Willman VL, Zafiracopoulos P, et al: Myocardial function after elective cardiac arrest during hypothermia. Surg Gynecol Obstet 109:423–426, 1959
112. Cooper T, Willman VL, Zafiracopoulos P, et al: Myocardial function after elective cardiac arrest during hypothermia. Surv Anesthesiol 5:1, 1961
113. Covino BG, D'Amato HE: Mechanism of ventricular fibrillation in hypothermia. Circ Res 10:148–155, 1962
114. Covino BG, Williams L: Excitability cycle of the ventricle in hypothermia. Am J Physiol 181:362–366, 1955
115. Cross CE, Rieben PA, Salisbury PF: Coronary vasomotor tonus in moderate hypothermia. Am J Physiol 203:825–828, 1962
116. Dahlen RW: Some effects of hypothermia on the cardiovascular system and ECG of rats. Proc Soc Exp Biol Med 115:1–4, 1964
117. DeGasperis A, Demetz A, Donatelli R: An ultrarapid heat exchanger for profound hypothermia. J Thorac Cardiovasc Surg 45:343–352, 1963
118. DeGasperis A, Demetz A, Donatelli R: Profound hypothermia and cardiocirculatory arrest for intracardiac surgery. J Thorac Cardiovasc Surg 45:353–361, 1963
119. DeGasperis A, Donatelli R, Rovelli F: Sulla correzione chirurgica acuore aperto delle malformazioni cardiache. Acta Tertii Europae de Cordis Scentia Conventus, Roma, 1960, p 179

120. Deleze J: Possible reasons for drop of resting potential of mammalian heart preparations during hypothermia. Circ Res 8:553–557, 1960
121. Delin NA, Hoyt RK, Schenk WG Jr: Cardiac performance in hypothermic woodchucks (*Marmota monax*). J Cardiovasc Surg 8:427–441, 1967
122. Delin NA, Kjartansson KB, Pollock L, et al: Redistribution of regional blood flow in hypothermia. J Thorac Cardiovasc Surg 49:511–516, 1965
123. Delin NA, Pollock L, Kjartansson KB, et al: Cardiac performance in hypothermia: An experimental study of left ventricular power, oxygen consumption and efficiency in dogs. J Thorac Cardiovasc Surg 47:774–790, 1964
124. Delorme EJ: Experimental cooling of the blood stream. Lancet 2:914–915, 1952
125. Delorme EJ: Hypothermia in dogs. Technical report. ONRL 83:53, 1952
126. Delorme EJ: Controlled hypothermia. Postgrad Med J 31:456–462, 1955
127. Delorme EJ: Hypothermia. Br Med Bull 11:221–225, 1955
128. Derra E: Erfahrungen mit Operationen an dem aus dem Kreislauf ausgeschalteten Herzen unter Verwendung von Hypothermie und der extracorporalen Zirkulation. Wien Med L Wochenschr 110:33–38, 1960
129. Derrick JR: Technique of applying right ventricular outflow patch with the use of hypothermia. J Thorac Cardiovasc Surg 43:701–702, 1962
130. Desbaillets P, Rivier JL, Mahaim C, et al: Etat actuel de la chirurgie a coeur ouvert a l'hospital cantonal de Lausanne. Cardiologia 38:152–157, 1961
131. DeWall RA, Lillehei CW: Simplified total body perfusion: (reduced flows, moderate hypothermia, and hemodilution). JAMA 179:430–434, 1962
132. DeWall R, Lillehei CW, Hodges P, et al: Description of the helical reservoir bubble-type pump oxygenator for hemodilution hypothermic perfusions. Dis Chest 44:113–120, 1963
133. Dillard DH, Mohri H, Hessel EA, et al: Correction of total anomalous pulmonary venous drainage in infancy utilizing deep hypothermia with total circulatory arrest. Circulation 35–36, Suppl 1:105–110, 1967
134. Dillard DH, Mohri H, Merendino KA: Correction of heart disease in infancy utilizing deep hypothermia and total circulatory arrest. J Thorac Cardiovasc Surg 61:64–69, 1971
135. Dogliotti AM, Ciocatto E, Querci M, et al: Extracorporeal circulation in deep hypothermia: An experimental study: Blood changes and hemodynamic changes: Behavior of cerebral blood flow. Int Surg 35:302–318, 1965
136. Doherty JE, Hara M: The effect of citrate infusion on the electrocardiogram of the hypothermic and normothermic dog. Am Heart J 61:225–235, 1961
137. Drew CE: Profound hypothermia in cardiac surgery. Br Med Bull 17:37–42, 1961
138. Drew CE: Profound hypothermia in cardiac surgery. Lond Clin Med J 7:15, 1966
139. Drew CE, Anderson IM: Profound hypothermia in cardiac surgery. Report of three cases. Lancet 1:748–750, 1959
140. Drew CE, Anderson JM, Howart D, et al: Recent modifications in use of profound hypothermia in surgery of congenital heart disease. Br Heart J 34:964, 1972
141. Drew CE, Keen G, Benazon DB: Profound hypothermia. Lancet 1:745–747, 1959

142. Drucker WR: The influence of hypothermia on metabolism during hemorrhagic shock. Surg Forum 11:136–138, 1960
143. Drucker WR, Kaye M, Kendrick R, et al: Metabolic aspects of hemorrhagic shock. Surg Forum 9:49–54, 1959
144. Dubost C: Anevrysme carotido-caverneux opere sous hypothermie profonde avec arret circulatoire. Acad Chir 32:8–9, 1966
145. Dubost C, Blondeau P: The association of the artificial heart lung with deep hypothermia in open heart surgery. J Cardiovasc Surg 1:85–93, 1960
146. Dubost C, Blondeau P, Passelecq J, et al: L'association du coeur poumons artificiel et de l'hypothermie profonde dans la chirurgie a coeur ouvert. Actial Cardiol Int 2:95–101, 1959
147. Dubost C, Blondeau P, Piwnica A: L'association du coeurpoumons artificiel et de l'hypothermie profonde avec arret circulatoire total dans le traitement des cardiopathies congenitales. Ann Chir 14:1025–1056, 1960
148. Dubost C, Blondeau P, Piwnica A: L'association du coeur-poumon artificiel et de l'hypothermie profonde dans la chirurgie a coeur ouvert. Cardiologia 38:158–171, 1961
149. Dubost C, Blondeau P, Piwnica A: The treatment of congenital heart disease by the association of artificial heart-lung and profound hypothermia with total circulatory arrest. J Cardiovasc Surg 3:80–93, 1962
150. Dubost C, Blondeau P, Piwnica A: Extracorporeal circulation during profound hypothermia with prolonged total circulatory arrest. J Cardiovasc Surg 3:286–293, 1962
151. Dubost C, Blondeau P, Weiss M, et al: L'association du coeur-poumons artificiels et de l'hypothermie profonde dans la chirurgie a coeur ouvert. Mem Acad Chir 86:146–156, 1960
152. Dubost C, Blondeau P, Weiss M, et al: Association du coeur-poumon artificiel et de l'hypothermie profonde dans la chirurgie a coeur ouvert. Acta Cardiol 16:319, 1961
153. DuBouchet N, Prochiant E, Latscha B: L'arret cardiaque provoque par hypothermie profonde, sa superiorite sur les autres techniques. Anesth Analg (Paris) 19:239–250, 1962
154. Dubourg MM, Fontan F, Trarieux M, et al: Hypothermie profonde nuancee, selection restrictive des arrets circulatoires. Anesth Analg (Paris) 20:49–52, 1963
155. Dumanian AV, Hoeksema TD, Santschi DR, et al: Profound hypothermia and circulatory arrest in the surgical treatment of traumatic aneurysm of the thoracic aorta. J Thorac Cardiovasc Surg 59:541–545, 1970
156. Ebert PA, Austen WG, Greenfield LJ, et al: Direct and reflex effects of hypoxia, hypotension and hypothermia on the heart. Am J Med Res Eng Electron 3:162–168, 1964
157. Ebert PA, Austen WG, Greenfield LJ, et al: Direct and reflex effects of hypoxia, hypotension and hypothermia on the heart. Surv Anesthesiol 10:99–101, 1966
158. Egerton N, Egerton WS, Kay JH: Neurologic changes following profound hypothermia. Ann Surg 157:366–374, 1963
159. Elder ME, Malinin TI, Panuska JA: Activity of the isolated mammalian heart during cooling and rewarming. Cryobiology 4:262, 1967-8

160. El-Fiky SBI, Katzung BG: Effects of hypothermia and pronethalol on ionic correlates of ouabain arrhythmias in dogs. Circ Res 24:43–50, 1969
161. Ellison RG, Ellison LT, Brackney EL et al: Metabolic alterations of individual organs during cardiopulmonary bypass and profound hypothermia. Surg Forum 12:175–177, 1961
162. Ellison RG, Singal SA, Moretz WH, et al: Further studies on myocardial metabolism during elective cardiac arrest and hypothermia. Surg Forum 11:198–200, 1960
163. Ellison RG, Singal SA, Moretz WH, et al: Role of hypothermia in the protection of myocardial metabolism during cardiopulmonary by-pass and elective cardiac arrest. Dis Chest 40:87–93, 1961
164. Emiroglu F: Fibrillation in normothermic and hypothermic rabbit heart and effect of adrenaline. Arch Int Physiol Biochem 73:55–64, 1965
165. Emiroglu F, Gokhan N, Cirpili E: The sensitivity of chemoreceptors of the dog during progressive hypothermia. Arch Int Physiol Biochem 70:41–48, 1962
166. Emslie-Smith D, Sladden GE, Stirling GR: The significance of changes in the electrocardiogram in hypothermia. Br Heart J 21:343–351, 1959
167. Enenki MV, Bednarik MB: The apparatus for deep hypothermia and the experiments with extracorporeal deep hypothermia during operations of heart disease. Refrig Sci Tech, Suppl 4:411, 1965
168. Fava E, Querci M, Marchiaro G: La neuroleptoanalgesia quale mezzo di induzione per la ipotermia moderata di superficie. Rass Int Clin Ter 44:782, 1964
169. Feldman E, Rubin B, Surks SN: Beneficial effects of hypothermia after cardiac arrest. JAMA 173:499–501, 1960
170. Felicetti CL, Panuska JA, Joyce RA: Blood pressure and heart rate in unrestrained rats during progressive hypothermia. Am Zool 6:304, 1966
171. Fineberg C, Foris N, Camishion RC: Revascularization of the dog myocardium. II. Acute ligation of the left circumflex coronary artery with and without hypothermia. Arch Surg 85:717–719, 1962
172. Fisher B, Fedor EJ: Cardiac temperature gradients during extracorporeal perfusion and profound hypothermia. Proc Soc Exp Biol Med 106:275–277, 1961
173. Fisher B, Fedor EJ, Smith JW: Temperature gradients associated with extracorporeal perfusion and profound hypothermia. Surgery 50:758–764, 1961
174. Flick WF, Hollerman FJ, Feldt RH, et al: Aneurysm of aortic cannulation site. Successful repair by means of peripheral cannulation, profound hypothermia, and circulatory arrest. J Thorac Cardiovasc Surg 61:419–423, 1971
175. Floyd WL, Dillon ML, Weissler AM: Observations on left ventricular function in hypothermia. Clin Res 8:181, 1960
176. Freese JW, Lesage AM, Young WG Jr, et al: The effect of core induced hypothermia of 25°C and 7°C on dogs with myocardial infarction. Trans Am Soc Artif Intern Organs 6:218–226, 1960
177. Freundl H, Hennersdorf G, Hochrein H: Adaptationsvorgange unter Hypothermie bei Druckbelastung des Herzens. Arch Kreislaufforsch 65:14–28, 1971
178. Friedman EW, Davidoff D, Fine J: Effect of hypothermia on tolerance to hemorrhagic shock, in Dripps RD (ed): The Physiology of Induced Hypothermia. Washington, National Academy of Sciences, 1956, pp 369–380

179. Friedman EW, Davidoff D, Fine J: Hypothermia in hemorrhagic shock. Am J Physiol 185:521–527, 1956
180. Galindo A, Baldwin M: Profound hypothermia and ventricular fibrillation during neurosurgery. Ann Surg 156:30–40, 1962
181. Galindo A, Sprouse JH: The effect of anesthesia on cardiac excitability produced by single pulse electrical stimulation. Anesth Analg 41:659–669, 1962
182. Galindo A, Sprouse JH: The influence of epidural anesthesia on cardiac excitability in profound hypothermia. Can Anaesth Soc J 11:614–620, 1964
183. Galindo A, Sprouse JH, Aubry U, et al: Anesthesia and ventricular fibrillation in deep hypothermia. Proceedings of the First European Congress on Anesthesiology, Vienna, 1962, p 140
184. Galletti P, Brecher GA: Heart and Lung Bypass. New York, Grune & Stratton, 1969, p 391
185. Gerbode F, Johnston JB, Sader AA, et al: Complete correction of tetralogy of Fallot. Arch Surg 82:793–800, 1961
186. Gibson P, Simpson JA: Clinical use of hypothermia combined with cardiopulmonary bypass. Br Med J 1:592–595, 1962
187. Gilbert JW, Morrow AG, Braunwald E: The results of open commissurotomy in acquired calcific aortic stenosis: Clinical and hemodynamic studies in patients operated upon with general hypothermia. Ann Surg 151:1–10, 1960
188. Gleichmann U, Lohr B, Ringler W, et al: Carbon dioxide exchange in the vertical-screen oxygenator (Mayo-Gibbon type) with addition of 3 percent CO_2 in combination with moderate hypothermia. J Thorac Cardiovasc Surg 45:628–634, 1963
189. Glitsch HG: Uber das Membranpotential des Meerschweinchenverhofes nach Hypothermie. Pfluegers Arch Ges Physiol 307:29–46, 1969
190. Goetz RH: Vertical bubble oxygenation with built-in heat exchanger requiring no priming volume for total body hypothermia. J Cardiovasc Surg 4:791–794, 1963
191. Goetz RH, Vilmos P, Mallonga E, et al: Vertical bubble oxygenator with built-in heat exchanger requiring no additional priming volume for total body hypothermia. Surg Forum 14:264–266, 1963
192. Goldberg LI: Effects of hypothermia on contractility of the intact dog heart. Am J Physiol 194:92–98, 1958
193. Gollan F: Cardiac arrest of one hour duration in dogs during hypothermia of 0°C followed by survival. Fed Proc 13:57, 1954
194. Gollan F: Physiological effects of artificial heart valves. Trans Am Soc Artif Intern Organs 2:71–73, 1956
195. Gollan F: Physiology of cardiac surgery. Beaumont Lecture, 1958, Springfield, Thomas, 1958, p 108
196. Gollan F: Physiology of cardiac surgery. Hypothermia, extracorporeal circulation and extracorporeal cooling. J Mich Med Soc 58:53–76, 1959
197. Gollan F: Physiology of deep hypothermia by total body perfusion. Ann NY Acad Sci 80:301–314, 1959
198. Gollan F: Hemodynamique-coeur: The role of capillary flow in deep hypothermia. Ann Chir Thorac Cardiovasc 1:539–543, 1962
199. Gollan F: Development of hypothermic perfusion since 1897. Minn Med 46: 245–248, 1963

200. Gollan F: Carbon dioxide, waste product or elixir? J Mt Sinai Hosp NY 32: 132–152, 1965
201. Gollan F: Criteria and requirements of adequate body perfusion, in Best AN (ed): Heart Substitutes. Springfield, Thomas, 1969, pp 1–11
202. Gollan F: Adequacy of anemic and hypoxemic perfusion, in Malinin Th, Zeppa R, Gollan F, Callahan AB (eds): Reversibility of Cellular Injury due to Inadequate Perfusion. Springfield, Thomas, 1973, pp 407–425
203. Gollan F, Blos P, Schuman H: Studies on hypothermia by means of pump oxygenator. Am J Physiol 171:331–340, 1952
204. Gollan F, Blos P, Schuman H: Exclusion of heart and lung from circulation in the hypothermic, closed-chest dog by means of a pump oxygenator. J Appl Physiol 5:180–190, 1952
205. Gollan F, Grace JT, Schell MW, et al: Left heart surgery in dogs during respiratory and cardiac arrest at body temperatures below 10°C. Surgery 38: 363–372, 1955
206. Gollan F, Kory RC: Coronary flow and coronary occlusion in hypothermic dogs during bypass of heart by means of a pump oxygenator. 19th International Physiology Congress, 1953
207. Gollan F, McDermott J, Winkler J, et al: Induced respiratory acidosis for perfusion hypothermia with venous blood. Trans Am Artif Intern Organs 10:52–56, 1964
208. Gollan F, Phillips R, Grace JT, et al: Cardiac arrest in dogs below 13°C without ventricular fibrillation. Fed Proc 14:60, 1955
209. Gollan F, Phillips R Jr, Grace JT, et al: Open left heart surgery in dogs during hypothermic asystole with and without extracorporeal circulation. J Thorac Surg 30:626–630, 1955
210. Gollan F, Tysinger DS, Grace JT, et al: Hypothermia of 1.5°C in dogs followed by survival. Am J Physiol 181:297–303, 1955
211. Gollan F, White WP, McDermott J: The therapeutic effect of mild perfusion hypothermia on acute cardiac decompensation. The Physiologist 8:319, 1965
212. Goodyer A: Effects of hypothermia and pyrexia on left ventricular function in the intact animal. Am J Cardiol 15:206–212, 1965
213. Gordon AS: The surgical management of congenital supravalvular, valvular, and subvalvular aortic stenosis using deep hypothermia. J Thorac Cardiovasc Surg 43:141–156, 1962
214. Gordon AS: Heat exchangers as hypothermia inducers in heart surgery. Ann Rev Med 13:75–86, 1962
215. Gordon AS: Cerebral blood flow and temperature during deep hypothermia for cardiovascular surgery. J Cardiovasc Surg 3:299–307, 1962
216. Gordon AS, Jones JC, Luddington LG, et al: Deep hypothermia for intracardiac surgery: Experimental and clinical use without an oxygenator. Am J Surg 100:332–337, 1960
217. Gordon AS, Meyer BW, Jones JC: Open heart surgery using deep hypothermia without an oxygenator. J Thorac Cardiovasc Surg 40:787–812, 1960
218. Gordon AS, Meyer BW, Jones JC: Intracardiac surgery under deep hypothermia without a mechanical oxygenator. Circulation 22:757, 1960
219. Gott VL, Bartlett M, Johnson JA, et al: High energy phosphate levels in the human heart during potassium citrate arrest and selective hypothermic arrest. Surg Forum 10:544–547, 1959

220. Gott VL, Bartlett M, Long DM, et al: Myocardial energy substances in the dog heart during potassium and hypothermic arrest. J Appl Physiol 17:815–818, 1962
221. Greenberg JJ, Edmunds LH Jr, Brown RB: Myocardial metabolism and post arrest function in the cold and chemically arrested heart. Surgery 48:31–42, 1960
222. Greer A, Carey J, Zuhdi, N: Hypothermic circulation with a temperature-regulating pump oxygenator. Ann Surg 26:770–772, 1960
223. Greer AE, Carey JM, Zuhdi N: Hemodilution principle of hypothermic perfusion—A concept obviating blood priming. J Thorac Cardiovasc Surg 43:640–648, 1962
224. Gribbe P, Hirvonen L, Lind J, et al: Cineangiocardiographic observations in hypothermic dogs. Cardiologia 39:341–362, 1961
225. Grigor KC: Metabolic alkalosis and acid urine following open-heart surgery with cardiopulmonary bypass. Br J Anaesth 40:943–960, 1968
226. Grigor KC, Hutchison JRS, Welsh TM: Controlled water immersion hypothermia in cardiac surgery. Anesthesia 18:336–342, 1963
227. Gross RE, Bernhard WF, Litwin SB: Closure of Potts anastomoses in the total repair of tetralogy of Fallot. J Thorac Cardiovasc Surg 57:72–82, 1969
228. Guiot G, Piwnica A, Vourc'h G, et al: Anevrysme carotido-caverneux opere sous hypothermie profonde avec arret circulatoire. Acad Chir (Paris) 92:224–228, 1966
229. Gukevich E: Exclusion of the cerebral circulation under hypothermia. Eksp Khir 1:30–34, 1958
230. Gupta S, Basu AK: Rapid hypothermia and intravascular aggregation in total body perfusion. Acta Chir Scand 128:678–682, 1964
231. Guz A, Kurland GS, Freedberg AS: Relation of coronary flow to oxygen supply. Am J Physiol 199:179–182, 1960
232. Hall FG, Salzano JV: Effects of graded hemorrhage on cardiopulmonary functions of hypothermic dogs. J Surg Res 4:329–333, 1964
233. Hall P, Bjorkman G, Johansson B, et al: The influence of hypothermia on the microscopical picture of different organs in rabbits. Acta Pathol Microbiol Scand 49:151–155, 1960
234. Hallman GL, Cooley DA: False aortic aneurysm following division and suture of a patient ductus arteriosus: Successful excision with hypothermia. J Cardiovasc Surg 5:23–28, 1964
235. Hamel AL, Moe JH: Effect of total ischemia on hind limbs of dogs subjected to hypothermia. Surgery 55:274–280, 1964
236. Han J, Moe GK: Nonuniform recovery of excitability in ventricular muscle. Circ Res 14:44–60, 1964
237. Hanson AT, Haxholdt BF, Husfeldt E, et al: Measurement of coronary blood flow and cardiac efficiency in hypothermia by use of radioactive krypton 85. Scand J Clin Lab Invest 8:182–188, 1956
238. Hanson A, Johansson BW: Myocardial lactate concentration in guinea pigs, normothermic and hypothermic hedgehogs, in a hibernating and a non-hibernating state. Acta Physiol Scand 53:137–141, 1961
239. Hardin RA, Scott JB, Haddy FJ: Effect of cardiac cooling on coronary vascular resistance in normothermic dogs. Am J Physiol 199:163–166, 1960

240. Hegnauer AH, D'Amato HE: Oxygen consumption and cardiac output in the hypothermic dogs. Am J Physiol 178:138–142, 1954
241. Hegnauer AH, Flynn J, D'Amato H: Cardiac physiology in dog during rewarming from deep hypothermia. Am J Physiol 167:69–75, 1951
242. Hehre FW: Hypothermia for operations during pregnancy. Anesth Analg 44:424–428, 1965
243. Heimbecker RO, Lajos TZ: Ice-chip cardioplegia. Arch Surg 84:130–140, 1962
244. Heimbecker RO, Young WE, Sanford DC: Experimental studies on the production of deep hypothermia by means of a pump oxygenator and heat exchanger with a note on the clinical application. Can J Surg 3:79–85, 1959
245. Hellstrom G, Bjork VO: Hemodilution with rheomacrodex during total body perfusion. J Thorac Cardiovasc Surg 45:395–401, 1963
246. Hennersdorf G, Freundl H, Schoffel R, et al: Uber die digitalis-und hypothermiebedingten Kontractilitatsanderungen des isolierten Warmbluterherzens bei akuter Belastiengsadaptation. Z Kreislaufforsch 58:1088–1100, 1969
247. Hessel EA, Dillard DH, Winterscheid LC, et al: Surgical treatment of pulmonic stenosis with intact ventricular septum with the use of cardiopulmonary bypass. J Thorac Cardiovasc Surg 49:796–812, 1965
248. Hickey MD, Shanahan WR, Gaffney JD, et al: Experimental and clinical experiences with profound hypothermia. J Cardiovasc Surg 3:327–328, 1962
249. Hirose T, Madden RE: Optimal coronary flow in the bypassed normothermic and hypothermic heart. J Thorac Cardiovasc Surg 48:82–93, 1964
250. Hoff HE, Geddes LA: Potential changes in the heart caused by cooling. J Appl Physiol 7:416–424, 1955
251. Hollenberg M, Pruett R, Thal A: Vasoactive substances liberated by prolonged bubble oxygenation. J Thorac Cardiovasc Surg 45:402–411, 1963
252. Holobut W, Stazka W: On dynamic heart efficiency in hypothermia. Acta Physiol Pol 13:621–629, 1962
253, Holt MH, Macalalad F, Lewis FJ: Autogenous oxygenation with cardiac bypass, hypothermia, and an atrioventricular clamp. J Thorac Cardiovasc Surg 40:536–548, 1960
254. Horecky J: Apparatus for heat exchange in local perfusions. Rozhl Chir 44:51–63, 1965
255. Horecky J, Popovic P, Popovic V: Physical and biochemical characteristics of artificial circulation. Proceedings of the 7th Cardiosurgical Conference, Bratislava, 1971, pp 157–162
256. Horecky J, Sujansky E, Pivkova A: The possibilities of influencing the distribution of perfusion volume during deep hypothermia in extracorporeal circulation. Rozhl Chir 45:173–183, 1966
257. Horecky J, Sujansky E, Pivkova A, et al: Total Bypass ohne Thorakotomie mit tiefer Hypothermie Experimentelle Unteresuchungen. Thor Vask Chir 15:204–209, 1967
258. Horiuchi T, Koyamada K, Honda T, et al: Clinical experience of open-heart surgery by means of hypothermia and heart-lung machine. Tohoku J Exp Med 83:146–158, 1964
259. Horiuchi T, Koyamada K, Ishitoya T, et al: Radical operation under hypothermia for ventricular septal defect in infancy. A report of 64 consecutive cases. J Cardiovasc Surg 8:85–92, 1967

260. Horiuchi T, Koyamada K, Matano I, et al: Radical operation for ventricular septal defect in infancy. J Thorac Cardiovasc Surg 46:180–190, 1963
261. Howat DDC: Die Rolle des Anaesthesisten bei der tiefen Hypothermie. Anaesthesist 17:245–253, 1968
262. Hufnagel CA, Conrad PW: The direct approach for the correction of aortic insufficiency. JAMA 178:275–279, 1961
263. Hufnagel CA, Conrad PW, Schanno J, et al: Profound cardiac hypothermia. Ann Surg 153:790–796, 1961
264. Hufnagel CA, Schanno JF, Pifarre R, et al: A versatile heat exchanger for use in extracorporeal bypass systems. J Cardiovasc Surg 2:158–164, 1961
265. Hunter J: Methods of induction and effect of "cardiac arrest" in relationship to the hypothermic state, in Temperature—Its Measurement and Control in Science and Industry, Vol 3. Princeton, Van Nostrand-Reinhold, 1963, pp 485–494
266. Hunter J, Hurley DA: The influence of respiratory and renal factors on cardiac activity during deep hypothermia. Can J Biochem Physiol 41:551–560, 1963
267. Hurley EJ, Lower RR, Dong E, et al: Clinical experience with local hypothermia in elective cardiac arrest. J Thorac Cardiovasc Surg 47:50–65, 1964
268. Hurt RL: Apparatus for profound hypothermia by the Drew technique. Lancet 1:783, 1962
269. Ikeda S, Medina H, Clowes GHA Jr: Oxygen consumption during total perfusion with diluted blood at normal and hypothermic temperatures. Surg Forum 15:212–213, 1964
270. Jaluvka VL: Die Problematik der Anwendung der Hypothermie und des extralorporalen Kreislaufes bei den schwangeren Frauen. Zentralbl Chir 89:1622–1627, 1964
271. Johansson B, Hall P: Electrocardiographical and microscopical heart studies in hypothermic rats, mice, rabbits, guinea pigs, dogs and hedgehogs. Cardiologia 35:171–178, 1959
272. Johansson BW, Huttunen M: Influence of dextran of low and high molecular weight on the electrocardiogram of hypothermic dogs. Am J Cardiol 12:792–794, 1963
273. Johnson P, Lesage A, Floyd WL, et al: Prevention of ventricular fibrillation during profound hypothermia by quinidine. Ann Surg 151:490–495, 1960
274. Johnston JB, Nield JM, Pritchard GR, et al: Studies of left atrial pressure during cardioplegia produced by profound hypothermia using the closed chest technique. Thorax 20:234–237, 1965
275. Jude JR, Haroutunian LM, Folse R: Hypothermic myocardial oxygenation. Am J Physiol 190:57–62, 1957
276. Juvenelle AA, Lind J, Wegelius C: A new method of extracorporeal circulation. Am Heart J 47:692–736, 1954
277. Kahler RL, Goldblatt A, Braunwald E: Circulatory effects of profound hypothermia during extracorporeal circulation. Am J Physiol 202:523–526, 1962
278. Kalisnik M: Histological studies in hypothermia. I. "Vasa plasmatica" in profound lethargic hypothermia in rats. Jubil Zbornik Med Fak (Yugosl) 1945–55:39–48, 1956
279. Kaplan A, Carrol F, Fisher B: A gas-type heat exchanger for induction of profound hypothermia and rewarming. J Thorac Cardiovasc Surg 43:388–391, 1962

280. Kaplan A, Fisher B: Prevention of fibrillation during hypothermia by pericardial space perfusion. Arch Surg 77:319–330, 1958
281. Karow AM Jr, Shlafer M, Sims R: Contractile and ultrastructural effects of hypothermia and of high pressure on rat hearts during ischemia. J Surg Res 11:571–583, 1971
282. Kazanskii Y, Makarenko T, Karpukhin V: Hypothermia in surgical practice, in Current Problems in Anesthesiology. Moscow, 1957, pp 13–36
283. Keatinge WR: Mechanism of adrenergic stimulation of mammalian arteries and its failure at low temperatures. J Physiol 174:184–205, 1964
284. Keen G, Dowlatshahi K: The effects of circulatory arrest during profound hypothermia upon human myocardial fine structure. Cardiovasc Res 4:348–354, 1970
285. Keen G, Gerbode F: Observations on the microcirculation during profound hypothermia. J Thorac Cardiovasc Surg 45:252–260, 1963
286. Kendrick JE, Turner KA: Carotid sinus depressor reflexes during hypothermia. Am J Physiol 207:777–781, 1964
287. Kenyon NM, Litwak RS, Beck HJ, et al: Preliminary observations in isolated hypothermic cardiac asystole. Surg Forum 10:567–570, 1959
288. King H, Bounous G: Cardiac input in hypothermia. Surg Gynecol Obstet 107:753–757, 1958
289. Kirklin JW, Dawson B, Devloo RA, et al: Open intracardiac operations: Use of circulatory arrest during hypothermia induced by blood cooling. Ann Surg 154:769–776, 1961
290. Kirklin JW, Devloo RA: Hypothermic perfusion and circulatory arrest for surgical correction Tetralogy of Fallot with previously constructed Potts anastomosis. Dis Chest 39:87–91, 1961
291. Kitlak W, Kintzel HW: Elektrokardiographische Untersuchungen Fruhgeborener wahrend langanhaltender Hypothermie. Arch Kinderheilkd 176:17–26, 1967-8
292. Klebanoff G, Phillips J: Temporary suspension of animation using total body perfusion and hypothermia. A preliminary report. Cryobiology 6:121–125, 1969-70
293. Koivikko A: Experimental hypothermia in neonatal lambs. Poor cardiac response to increased oxygen consumption during shivering. Acta Physiol Scand 78:571–573, 1970
294. Kolder H, Horres AD, Brecher GA: Influence of temperature on development of rigor mortis in dog hearts. Circ Res 13:218–222, 1963
295. Kondo Y, Kuwahara O, Don Turner M: Prolonged suspended animation in puppies. Cryobiology 10:512, 1973
296. Kondratovich MA: The reflex control of vascular tone during hypothermia. Biull Eksp Biol Med 50:65–69, 1960
297. Kondratovich MA: The effect of hypothermia on the excitability of the vascular interoceptors. Fiziol Zh (Kyev) 7:221–225, 1961
298. Konikova A, Pogosova A, Portnoi V: The interrelationship between proteins of organs and of the blood plasma in extracorporeal circulation in the dog with normal temperature and with hypothermia. Eksp Khir Anesteziol 12:64–68, 1967
299. Krasna IH, Shuster M, Baronofsky ID: A study of left atrial pressures in profound hypothermia. Surgery 49:375–380, 1961

300. Krauss H, Zimmermann WE, Feyen M: Veranderungen des Saure-Basen-Haushaltes, der arteriellen Blutgase und des Exzess Laktats (Sauerstoffschuld) bei Herzoperationen mit extrakorporaler Perfusion and leichter Hypothermie (28° bis 34°C) und deren therapeutische Beeinflussung. Thoraxchirurgie und Vaskul Chirurgie 14:262–285, 1966
301. Kreuzer H, Bostroem B, Gleichmann U, et al: Das Verhalten der Myocardtemperaturen wahrend der extrakorporalen Zirkulation bei verschiedenen Arten des Kaltestillstandes. Thoraxchirurgie und Vaskul Chirurgie 10:435–446, 1962-3
302. Krieger EM: Reflex bradycardia in hypothermic rats. Acta Physiol Lat Am 11:127–134, 1961
303. Krog J, Smith RE: Miniature Peltier heat exchanger for extracorporeal circulation. J Appl Physiol 22:354–357, 1967
304. Kuhn LA: Extracorporeal circulatory support in cardiac disease. Am J Cardiol 10:149–153, 1962
305. Kuhn LA, Apter R, Weinrauch H, et al: Hemodynamic and metabolic effects of skin and blood-stream cooling in experimental myocardial infarction with shock. Am J Cardiol 12:795–801, 1963
306. Kuhn LA, Turner JK: Alterations in pulmonary and peripheral vascular resistance in immersion hypothermia. Circ Res 7:366–374, 1959
307. Kuhn LA, Weiser F, Beck AR, et al: Effects of hypothermia and closed-chest extracorporeal circulation in myocardial infarction with shock. Clin Res 9:142, 1961
308. Kuhn LA, Weiser F, D'Aria J, et al: Hemodynamic and metabolic effects of hypothermia and extracorporeal circulation in experimental myocardial infarction and shock. Circ Res 10:916–924, 1962
309. Kuprilanov IA: Open heart surgery under hypothermia. Vestn Khir 82:81–93, 1959
310. Lacquet LK: Emploi actuel de l'hypothermie en chirurgie cardiaque. Acta Chir Belg 63:827–830, 1964
311. Lacroix E, Leusen I: The influence of immersion hypothermia and rewarming on oxygen consumption and glycogen content of rat heart. Arch Int Physiol Biochem 67:222–226, 1959
312. Lande AJ, Parker B, Kaster R: A new membrane pump-oxygenator for prolonged support. JAMA 204:529, 1968
313. Lande AJ, Parker B, Subramanian V, et al: Methods for increasing the efficiency of a new dialyzer-membrane oxygenator. Trans Am Soc Artif Intern Organs 14:227–232, 1968
314. Laurent D, Sprovieri L, Dubost C: External defibrillation: A simple method of cardiac resuscitation after profound hypothermia and total circulatory standstill without thoractomy. Trans Am Soc Artif Intern Organs 8:333–343, 1962
315. Lee WH, Krumhaar D, Derry G, et al: Comparison of the effects of membrane and non-membrane oxygenators on the biochemical and biophysical characteristics of blood. Surg Forum 12:200–202, 1961
316. Lee WH Jr, Krumhaar D, Fonkalsrud EW, et al: Denaturation of plasma proteins as a cause of morbidity and death after intracardiac operations. Surgery 50:29–39, 1961
317. Lesage AM, Sealy WC, Brown IW Jr, et al: Hypothermia and extracorporeal

circulation. Experimental studies of profound hypothermia of 10–20°C. Arch Surg 79:607–613, 1959

318. Lesage MA, Sealy WC, Young WG Jr, et al: Experimental studies on profound hypothermia induced and reversed with a pump oxygenator. Ann Surg 156:831–844, 1962
319. Lesage AM, Sealy WC, Young WG Jr.: Deep hypothermia in the rat. Studies on survival and tolerance to circulatory arrest. Technical Document Report AAL-TDR-62-43, 1963, pp 1–12
320. Lesage MA, Tsuchioka H, Young WG, et al: Tolerance of dogs to deep hypothermia. Arch Surg 89:677–684, 1964
321. Lewis FJ, Taufic M: Closure of atrial septal defects with the aid of hypothermia: Experimental accomplishments and the report of one successful case. Surgery 33:52–59, 1953
322. Lewis FJ, Varco RL, Taufic M: Repair of atrial septal defects in man under direct vision with the aid of hypothermia. Surgery 36:538–556, 1954
323. Lillehei CW, Todd DB, Levy MJ, et al: Partial cardiopulmonary bypass, hypothermia, and total circulatory arrest. J Thorac Cardiovasc Surg 58:530–544, 1969
324. Long DM Jr, Folkman MJ, McClenathan JE: The use of low molecular weight dextran in extracorporeal circulation, hypothermia, and hypercapnea. J Cardiovasc Surg 4:617–641, 1963
325. Long DM Jr, Sterns LP, DeRiemer RH, et al: Subtotal and total replacement of aortic valve with plastic valve prostheses: Experimental investigation and successful clinical application utilizing selective cardiac hypothermia. Surg Forum 10:660–665, 1959
326. Lopez-Belio M, Tasaki G, Balagot R, et al: Effect of hypothermia during cardiopulmonary bypass on peripheral resistance. Alteration by dilute blood perfusate and by chlorpromazine. Arch Surg 81:283–290, 1960
327. Lynch HF: Red blood cell distribution in the hypothermic ground squirrel. J Appl Physiol 14:990–994, 1959
328. Lynch HF, Adolph EF: Blood flow in small blood vessels during deep hypothermia. J Appl Physiol 11:192–196, 1957
329. MacFarlane JK, Scott HJ, Cronin RFP: Effects of left heart bypass in experimental cardiogenic shock. J Thorac Cardiovasc Surg 57:214–224, 1969
330. Mahoney EB, DeWeese JA, Harris PD, et al: Tissue oxygen tension during total body perfusion and hypothermic cardiac arrest. J Thorac Cardiovasc Surg 44:658–666, 1962
331. Mahoney EB, DeWeese JA, Jones TI, et al: Coronary artery perfusion with oxygenated whole blood in open cardiac surgery under hypothermia. Bull Soc Int Chir 17:34–40, 1958
332. Mahoney EB, Manning JA DeWeese JA, et al: Clinical results of correction under hypothermia of atrial septal defects and pulmonary valvular stenosis. J Thorac Cardiovasc Surg 38:292–308, 1959
333. Malhotra CL, Anand BK, Singh B, et al: External cardiac excitation as cause of ventricular fibrillation during hypothermia and its prevention by acetylcholine. Indian J Med Res 48:198–207, 1960
334. Malmejac J: L'hypothermie profonde en chirurgie. Assoc Fr Chir 64:371–386, 1962

335. Malmejac J: Hypothermie profonde sans circulation extra-corporeale. Ann Chir Thorac Cardiovasc 1:1–18, 1962
336. Malmejac J, Malmejac C: Circulation coronaire et rythme idioventriculaire en hypothermie a 19–20°C. C R Soc Biol 153:1322–1324, 1959
337. Malmejac J, Malmejac C: Sur l'limportace des conditions physicochimiques de fibrillation cardiaque en hypothermie a 16°–18°C. J Physiol (Paris) 53:415–417, 1961
338. Malmejac J, Malmejac C, Fredenucci R: Influence de l'adrenaline sur la circulation coronaire en hypothermie a 19°–20°C. C R Soc Biol 153:782–784, 1959
339. Malmejac J, Malmejac C, Fredenucci R, et al: Circulation coronaire limite permettant la defibrillation electrique apres 45 a 50 minutes de fibrillation ventriculaire en hypothermie. J Physiol (Paris) 52:161–162, 1960
340. Malmejac J, Malmejac C, Laville C, et al: Action cardiaque de l'adrenaline en hypothermie profonde. C R Soc Biol 157:956–960, 1963
341. Mangiardi JL, Aiken JE, Behrer A, et al: Coronary blood flow during moderate and profound hypothermia. J Cardiovasc Surg 6:349–355, 1965
342. Mangiardi J, Ponder E: Coefficient of thermal conduction-homogenized tissues: Thermal conduction and the rate of blood flow. Nature 196:1203, 1962
343. Manteuffel-Szoege L: New observations concerning the hemodynamics of deep hypothermia. J Cardiovasc Surg 3:316–319, 1962
344. Manteuffel-Szoege L: Hemodynamic disturbances in normo- and hypothermia with excluded heart and during acute heart mucle failure. J Cardiovasc Surg 4:551–555, 1963
345. Marchand P, DuPlessis L, Beckerling C, et al: Extracorporeal hypothermia without thoracotomy: An experimental study in the use of cold for neurosurgery and cancericidal perfusions. Br J Surg 51:305–314, 1964
346. Marshall JM, Willis JS: The effects of temperature on the membrane potentials in isolated atria of the ground squirrel, *Citellus tridecemlineatus*. J Physiol 164:64–76, 1962
347. Martinez JB, Kass I, Hoffman MS: Factors involved in recovery of a patient after prolonged ventricular fibrillation during hypothermia. J Thorac Surg 36:749–756, 1958
348. Mazzella H, Mullin RG, Tavella H: Circulatory reflexes during induced hypothermia. Arch Int Pharmacodyn 122:419–427, 1959
349. McConnell JA, Dodds WA, Graves HB: The value of hypothermia in surgery of the abdominal aorta. Can Anaesth Soc J 10:5–17, 1963
350. McKain JM, Poepsel HF, Badame JM, et al: Control of cardiac activity by ischemia and hypothermia. Arch Surg 82:511–514, 1961
351. Mellina D, Pollara C: Ricerchi sperimentali: Sulla chirurgia del cuore esangue (ipotermia locale del cuore assoc. ad ipotermia gener). Minerva Chir 11:923–928, 1956
352. Meshalkin E, Fufin V, Obukhov V: On increasing the possibilities of surgical treatment of interventricular septal defects with the use of hypothermia. Grudn Khir 10:8–11, 1968
353. Michael CR, Menaker M: The effect of temperature on the isolated heart of the bat, *Myotis lucifugus*. J Cell Comp Physiol 62:355–358, 1963
354. Miller DR, Hallaba MAS, Steegmann AT: Effect of profound hypothermia

with circulatory arrest in dogs.: Special reference to changes in cerebrovascular permeability. Ann Surg 161:272–285, 1965

355. Miller FS, Miller JA Jr: Body temperature and tolerance of asphyxia in newborn kittens. Bull Tulane Univ Med Fac 24:197–210, 1965
356. Miller JA, Gribbe P, Von Hedenberg C, et al: Deep hypothermia and generalized vasoconstriction in white mice. Anat Rec 136:244, 1960
357. Mohri H, Barnes RW, Winterscheid LC et al: Challenge of prolonged suspended animation: A method of surface-induced deep hypothermia. Ann Surg 168:779–787, 1968
358. Mohri H, Dillard DH, Crawford EW: Method of surface-induced deep hypothermia for open-heart surgery in infants. J Thorac Cardiovasc Surg 58:262–270, 1969
359. Mohri H, Hessel EA, Nelson RJ, et al: Use of rheomacrodex and hyperventilation in prolonged circulatory arrest under deep hypothermia induced by surface cooling. Method for open heart surgery in infants. Am J. Surg 112:241–250, 1966
360. Mohri H, Merendino KA: Hypothermia with and without a pump oxygenator, in Gibbon IH, Sabiston DC, Spencer FC (eds): Surgery of the Chest. Philadelphia, Saunders, 1969, pp 643–673
361. Moll J: Deep hypothermia and extracorporeal circulation in open heart surgery. Pol Tyg Let 18:121–127, 1963
362. Moll J: Die tiefe Hypothermie bei der Behandlung der Restenose der Mitralis. Zentralbl Chir 90:1342–1345, 1965
363. Mollaret P: Les ultimes possibilites de la reanimation ou les frontieres actuelles entre vie et mort. Anesth Analg (Paris) 20:1–15, 1963
364. Monroe RG, Strang RH, LaFarge CG, et al: Ventricular performance, pressure-volume relationships, and O_2 consumption during hypothermia. Am J Physiol 206:67–73, 1964
365. Moore D, Bernhard WF: Efficacy of 2-amino-2-hydroxymethyl-1,3 propanediol (Tris buffer) in management of metabolic lacticacidosis accompanying prolonged hypothermic perfusions. Surgery 52:905–912, 1962
366. Mouritzen CV, Andersen MN: Myocardial temperature gradients and ventricular fibrillation during hypothermia. J Thorac Cardiovasc Surg 49:937–944, 1965
367. Mouritzen CV, Andersen MN: Mechanisms of ventricular fibrillation during hypothermia. J Thorac Cardiovasc Surg 51:585–589, 1966
368. Mundth ED, Sokol DM, Levine FH, et al: Preservation of myocardial function during extended periods of coronary ischemia. Surg Forum 20: 176–178, 1969
369. Mustard WT, Baird RJ, Trusler GA: The use of hypothermia in the closure of atrial septal defects in children. Surgery 50:301–308, 1961
370. Nagarajan TM, Talwar JR, Kapur BML, et al: Protective role of halothane, hyperoxaemia and hypothermia during experimental venous inflow occlusion. Indian J Med Res 52:979–987, 1964
371. Nayler WG, Wright JE: Effect of epinephrine on the mechanical and phosphorylase activity of normo- and hypothermic hearts. Circ Res 13:199–206, 1963

372. Negovskii VA: Resuscitation and Artificial Hypothermia. New York, Consultants Bureau, 1962, p 286
373. Negovskii V, Soboleva V: The pattern of extinction and restoration of the vital functions during lethal exsanguination under hypothermia. Arkh Patol 18:58–70, 1956
374. Negovskii VA, Soboleva V, Gurvich NL, et al: Restoration of vital functions in monkeys after mortal exsanguination in hypothermic conditions. Biull Eksp Biol Med 48:30–33, 1959
375. Negovskii VA, Soboleva V, Gurvich NL, et al: Deep hypothermia as a method of prolonging the clinical death periods. Bull Exp Biol Med 11:39–43, 1963
376. Negre E, DuCailar J, Thevenet A, et al: Correction des canaux atrioventriculaires sous hypothermie profonde. Ann Chir Thorac Cardiovasc 2:1–4, 1963
377. Neville WE, Kameya S, Oz M, et al: Profound hypothermia and complete circulation interruption. Arch Surg 82:108–119, 1961
378. Neville WE, White RJ, Verdura J: Relationship of flow rate, "excess lactate," and buffer base during closed chest profound hypothermic perfusion with a pump oxygenator. Surgery 55:281–290, 1964
379. Niazi SA, Lewis FJ: Tolerance of adult rats to profound hypothermia and simultaneous cardiac standstill. Surgery 36:25–32, 1954
380. Niazi SA, Lewis FJ: Resumption of heart beat in dogs, after standstill at low temperatures. Surg Forum 5:113–115, 1955
381. Niazi SA, Lewis FJ: Profound hypothermia in the dog. Surg Gynecol Obstet 102:98–106, 1956
382. Niazi SA, Lewis FJ: Profound hypothermia in the monkey with recovery after long periods of cardiac standstill. J Appl Physiol 10:137–138, 1957
383. Niazi SA, Lewis FJ: Profound hypothermia in man. Ann Surg 147:264–266, 1958
384. Nielsen KC, Owman C: On the control of ventricular fibrillation during hypothermia. Commun Dept Anat U Lund, Sweden 6:1–13, 1965
385. Nielsen KC, Owman C: Control of spontaneous ventricular fibrillating during induced hypothermia in cats by acute cardiac sympathectomy. Acta Physiol Scand 76:73–81, 1969
386. Nielsen KC, Owman C, Rosengren E: Effort of cardiac catecholamine depletion through sympathectomy on spontaneous ventricular fibrillation during induced hypothermia in cats. Experientia 24:1215–1217, 1968
387. Nilsen NO, Christensen A: The influence of extracorporeal circulation combined with hypothermia on the thrombocytes. Acta Chir Scand 127:297–302, 1964
388. O'Brien LJ: Negative diastolic pressure in the isolated hypothermic dog heart. Circ Res 8:956–960, 1960
389. Obukhova VP: Study of several immunohematologic indices in children with congenital heart defects in late periods following surgery with artificial circulation and hypothermia. Kardiologia 11:80–83, 1971
390. Ogata T, Osborn JJ, Kerth WJ, et al: Metabolic changes in deep perfusion hypothermia for cardiac surgery. J Thorac Cardiovasc Surg 45:610–617, 1963
391. Osborn JJ, Bramson ML, Gerbode F, et al: A rotating disk blood oxygenator

and integral heat-exchanger of improved inherent efficiency. J Thorac Cardiov Surg 39:427–437, 1960
392. Osborn JJ, Ross K, Bramson ML, et al: Hypothermia, blood pH and blood-gas solution. Clin Res 8:138, 1960
393. Overbeck W: Extracorporeal circulation combined with deep hypothermia. Surgery 49:763–767, 1961
394. Overton RC, DeBakey ME: Experimental observations on the influence of hypothermia and autonomic blocking agents on hemorrhagic shock. Ann Surg 143:439–447, 1956
395. Oz M, Kameya S, Neville W, et al: Relationship of blood volume, systemic peripheral resistance, and flow rate during profound hypothermia. Trans Am Soc Artif Intern Organs 6:204–217, 1960
396. Pace-Floridia A, Galindo A: Cardiac arrhythmia induced by negative phase in artificial ventillation. Anesthesiology 29:382–383, 1968
397. Paintal AS: The responses of chemoreceptors at reduced temperatures. J Physiol 217:1–18, 1971
398. Pantelic D, Vajs E, Debijadji R: ECG changes during posthaemorrhagic hypotension in precooled dogs. Q J Exp Physiol 45:229–234, 1960
399. Pantzer JG, Shumacker HB Jr: Observations on coronary sinus flow. Am J Surg 102:657–660, 1961
400. Pantzer JG, Shumacker HB, Bounous G: Vasopressors, vasodilators, and coronary sinus flow. Surgery 51:779–785, 1962
401. Parulkar GB, Dhruva AJ, Panday SR, et al: A technique of hypothermic perfusion combined with intravenous oxygenation. Surgery 58:395–403, 1965
402. Passelecq J, Blanc J, Dubost C: L'anesthesie et la reanimation per operatoire en chirurgie cardique sous hypothermie moderee. Revue de 200 cas. Presse Med 70:1677–1680, 1962
403. Patterson RH, Bronson SR: Profound hypothermia for intracranial surgery: Laboratory and clinical experiences with extracorporeal circulation by peripheral cannulation. Ann Surg 156:377–393, 1962
404. Payne WS, Theye RA, Kirklin JW: Effect of carbon dioxide on rate of brain cooling during induction of hypothermia by direct blood cooling. J Surg Res 3:54–57, 1963
405. Peirce EC: The value of a low flow pump oxygenator combined with hypothermia. Trans Am Soc Artif Intern Organs 2:28–40, 1956
406. Peirce EC: Postassium reversion, hypothermic ventricular fibrillation. J Thorac Cardiovasc Surg 48:996–1006, 1964
407. Peirce EC, Dabbs CH: Metabolic acidosis and oxygen consumption before, during, and following total cardiopulmonary bypass with and without hypothermia. Surg Forum 10:597–601, 1959
408. Peirce EC, Dabbs CH, Rogers WK, et al: Reduced metabolism by means of hypothermia and the low flow pump oxygenator. Surg Gynecol Obstet 107:339–352, 1958
409. Peirce EC, Kent KM, Sinclair SH: Alpha and beta receptor activity in intermediate hypothermia. Clin Res 15:58, 1967
410. Penefsky ZJ: Effects of hypothermia and stretch on contraction and relaxation of cardiac muscle. Am J Physiol 214:730–736, 1968

411. Perasalo O, Halonen PT, Telivuo L, et al: Hypothermia with extracorporeal circulation. Acta Chir Scand 122:230–234, 1961
412. Pierucci L Jr, Haupt GJ, Templeton JY: Studies in profound hypothermia. Trans Am Soc Artif Intern Organs 6:197–203, 1960
413. Piwnica A, Weiss M, Lenfant C, et al: Circulatory arrest and deep hypothermia induced with a pump oxygenator system and a heat exchanger. J Cardiovasc Surg 1:74–84, 1960
414. Pokrovskii VM: Temperataure analysis of the properties of the heart. Biull Eksp Biol Med 68:9–11, 1969
415. Pool JL, Kessler LA: Mechanism and control of centrally induced cardiac irregularities during hypothermia. I. Clinical observations. J Neurosurg 15:52–64, 1958
416. Popovic P, Horecky J, Popovic V: Circulation extracorporelle chez le rat blanc en hypothermie. J Physiol (Paris) 58:594, 1966
417. Popovic P, Horecky J, Popovic V: Hypothermic cardiopulmonary bypass in white rats. Ann Surg 168:298–301, 1968
418. Popovic P, Popovic V: Survival of newborn ground squirrels after supercooling or freezing. Am J Physiol 204:949–952, 1963
419. Popovic P, Popovic V: Survival of young rats after supercooling to −3°C. Cryobiology 2:23, 1965
420. Popovic P, Popovic V: Protective effects of differential hypothermia, in Musacchia XJ, Saunders JF (eds): Depressed Metabolism. New York, Am Elsevier, 1969, pp 499–524
421. Popovic V: L'hibernation artificielle du spermophile (*Citellus citellus*). Arch Sci Biol (Belgrade) 4:37–43, 1952
422. Popovic V, Arnovljevic V, Popovic P: Electrocardiographic changes during prolonged hypothermia in rats. Glas Acad Serbe Sci 230:13–41, 1958
423. Popovic V: Lethargic hypothermia in hibernators and nonhibernators. Ann NY Acad Sci 80:320–331, 1959
424. Popovic V: Physiological characteristics of rats and ground squirrels during prolonged lethargic hypothermia. Am J Physiol 199:467–471, 1960
425. Popovic V: Survival time of hypothermic white rats (15°C) and ground squirrels (10°C). Am J Physiol 199:463–466, 1960
426. Popovic V: Cardiac output in hibernating ground squirrels. Am J Physiol 207:1345–1348, 1964
427. Popovic V: Tissue perfusion in hypothermia, in Malinin TI, Zeppa R, Gollan F, Callahan RA (eds): Reversibility of Cellular Injury due to Inadequate Perfusion. Springfield, Thomas, 1972, pp 422–425
428. Popovic V, Arnovljevic V, Popovic P: Electrocardiographic changes during prolonged hypothermia in rats. Glas Acad Serbe Sci 230:13–41, 1958
429. Popovic V, Horecky J, Popovic P: A miniaturized pump oxygenator for evaluation of peripheral circulatory changes induced by long-term weightlessness in rats. Space Life Sci 2:113–115, 1970
430. Popovic V, Kent KM: 120-day study of cardiac output in unanesthetized rats. Am J Physiol 207:767–770, 1964
431. Popovic V, Kent KM: Cardiovascular responses in prolonged hypothermia. Am J Physiol 209:1069–1074, 1965
432. Popovic V, Kent KM: Factors limiting survival in hypothermic animals.

Proceedings of the International Microcirculation Conference, Cambridge, 1966, pp 63–64
433. Popovic V, Kostolny I, Larose JH, et al: Enhanced perfusion in microwave heated part of hypothermic lung. J Physiol (Paris) 63:386–389, 1971
434. Popovic V, Kostolny I, Novicic D, et al: Selective embedding of I-131 albumin in microwave heated part of hypothermic lung. Proceedings of the 7th Cardiosurgical Conference, Bratislava, 1971, pp 247–254
435. Popovic V, Kostolny I, Pass K, et al: Survival of extracorporeally cooled dogs after one hour circulatory arrest. Cryobiology 8:390, 1971
436. Postel AH, Reid LC, Hinton JW: Effect of hypothermia in irreversible hemorrhagic shock. Circ Res 4:594–598, 1956
437. Postel AH, Reid LC, Hinton JW: The therapeutic effect of hypothermia in experimental hemorrhagic shock. Ann Surg 145:311–316, 1957
438. Purpura DP, Pool JL, Housepian EM, et al: Hypothermic potentiation of centrally induced cardiac irregularities. Anesthesiology 19:27–37, 1958
439. Rehder K, Kirklin JW, MacCarty CS, et al: Physiologic studies following profound hypothermia and circulatory arrest for treatment of intracranial aneurysm. Ann Surg 156:882–889, 1962
440. Remensnyder JP, Austen WG: Diastolic pressure-volume relationships of the left ventricle during hypothermia. J Thorac Cardiovasc Surg 49:339–351, 1965
441. Replogle R, Levy M, DeWall RA, et al: Catecholamine and serotonin response to cardiopulmonary bypass. J Thorac Cardiovasc Surg 44:638–648, 1962
442. Rheinlander HF, Wallace HW: The effects of coronary artery perfusion on myocardial metabolism during hypothermic cardiac arrest. Surgery 52:47–54, 1962
443. Rheinlander HF, Wallace WH, Robeles AJM: The effects of hypothermia on the metabolism of the post-arrested canine heart. J Cardiovasc Surg 6:126, 1965
444. Riberi A, Grice PF, Shumacker HB Jr: Ventricular fibrillation in the hypothermic state. II. The effect of sino-auricular node blockade in preventing ventricular fibrillation at low degrees of body temperature. Am Surg 21: 1084–1090, 1955
445. Richards V, Pinto D, Coombs P: Considerations and uses of hyperbaric oxygen therapy in surgery. Am J Surg 106:114–127, 1963
446. Riley PA, Barila TG, Hughes CW: Ventricular fibrillation in hypothermic dogs as influenced by thiopental, pentobarbital and succinylcholine. Anesthesiology 17:277–283, 1956
447. Rittenhouse EA, Ito CS, Mohri H, et al: Circulatory dynamics during surface-induced deep hypothermia and after cardiac arrest for one hour. J Thorac Cardiovasc Surg 61:359–369, 1971
448. Rittenhouse EA, Mohri H, Morgan BC, et al: Electrocardiographic changes in infants undergoing surface-induced deep hypothermia for open-heart surgery. Am Heart J 79:167–174, 1970
449. Rittenhouse EA, Mohri H, Reicherbach D, et al: Morphological alterations in vital organs after prolonged cardiac arrest at low body temperature. Ann Thorac Surg 13:564–574, 1972

450. Rivkin LM, Uhley HN: Electrocardiographic alterations induced by incisions in the distal conduction system. Surg Forum 11:202–204, 1960
451. Roe BB, Stoney AJ: Ventricular function after myocardial ischemia at various levels of hypothermia. J Cardiovasc Surg 4:483–488, 1963
452. Roe BB, Weirich WL: Total and regional hypothermia with extracorporeal circulation. Circulation 22:800, 1960
453. Ross DN: Problems associated with the use of hypothermia in cardiac surgery. Proc R Soc Med 50:76–78, 1957
454. Rush BF, Wilder RJ, Fishbein R, et al: Effects of total circulatory standstill in profound hypothermia. Surgery 50:40–49, 1961
455. Russ C, Lee JC: Metabolic response of intact dog heart to prolonged hypothermia. J Einstein Med Cent 12:58–62, 1964
456. Russ C, Lee JC: Effect of hypothermia on myocardial metabolism. Am J Physiol 208:1253–1258, 1965
457. Sachs D, Derry GH, Krumhaar D, et al: Chemical and hypothermic inhibition of intravascular sludging in extracorporeal circulation. Ann Surg 160: 183–188, 1964
458. Salisbury PF, Cross CE, Rieben PA: Integrative study of the circulation in moderate hypothermia. Am J Cardiol 12:184–193, 1963
459. Salmon PA, Buckley JJ, Assimacopoulos CA: A simple disposable heat exchanger for blood transfusions. Surgery 52:784–787, 1962
460. Sanger PW, Robicsek F, Daugherty HK, et al: Topical cardiac hypothermia in lieu of coronary perfusion. J Thorac Cardiovasc Surg 52:533–541, 1966
461. Sarajas HSS: Myocardial damage induced by immersion hypothermia. Am J Cardiol 13:355–366, 1964
462. Sarajas HSS, Nilsson TE: Beobachtungen uber die Patholegie der experimentellen Hypothermie beim Hunde. Verh Dtsch Ges Inn Med 60:119–124, 1954
463. Schafer PW, Hughes CW, Barila TG: Tolerance of hypothermic normal dog's heart to ventricular fibrillation. Arch Surg 70:723–728, 1955
464. Schlosser V, Grote G: Blood gas and acid-base metabolism with the use of blood and blood substitutes in artificial circulation during hypothermia. Surgery 55:440–445, 1964
465. Schlosser V, Streicher HJ: Studies of the length of time the heart will tolerate ischemia in normo- and hypothermia. J Thorac Cardiovasc Surg 48:430–435, 1964
466. Schmidt RF, Chang JJ: Aktionspotential und Mechanogramm von Purkinje-Faden in tiefer Temperatur. Pfluegers Arch Ges Physiol 272:393–399, 1960-1
467. Schmitz T: Die metabolische Acidose bei Anwendung der extrakorporalen Zirkulation und Hypothermie. Klin Wochenschr 42:1252, 1964
468. Schumer W: Moderate hypothermia in controlled hemorrhage in dogs: Physiochemical response of the microcirculation. Am Surg 32:347–354, 1966
469. Sealy WC, Brown IW, Young WG: A report on the use of both extracorporeal circulation and hypothermia for open heart surgery. Ann Surg 147:603–613, 1958
470. Sealy WC, Brown IW, Young WG, et al: Hypothermia. Low flow extracorporeal circulation and controlled cardiac arrest for open heart surgery. Surg Gynecol Obstet 104:441–450, 1957

471. Sealy WC, Brown IW, Young WG, et al: Hypothermia and extracorporeal circulation for open heart surgery: Its simplification with heat exchanger for rapid cooling and rewarming. Ann Surg 150:627–639, 1959
472. Sealy WC, Lesage AM, Young WG: Tolerance of the profoundly hypothermic dog to complete circulatory standstill. Proc Soc Exp Biol Med 102:691, 1959
473. Sealy WC, Lesage AM, Young WG: Vascular responses during hypothermia. Technical Documentary Report AAL-TDR-63-19, 1963, p 64
474. Sealy WC, Young WG, Brown IW, et al: Potassium, magnesium, and neostigmine for controlled cardioplegia. Arch Surg 77:33–38, 1958
475. Sealy WC, Young WG, Lesage AM, et al: Observations on heart action during hypothermia induced and controlled by a pump oxygenator. Ann Surg 153:797–814, 1961
476. Searles PW, Sadove MS, Julian OC: Hypothermia in surgery for major vascular graft. Ill Med J 109:235–239, 1956
477. Seelye ER, Harris EA, Squire AW, et al: Metabolic effects of deep hypothermia and circulatory arrest in infants during cardiac surgery. Br J Anaesth 43:449–459, 1971
478. Sellick BA: Factors limiting the use of conventional hypothermia alone in open cardiac surgery. Acta Chir Belg 63:823–826, 1964
479. Shumacker HB, Riberi A, Boone RD, et al: Ventricular fibrillation in hypothermic state. IV. Role of extrinsic cardiac innervation. Ann Surg 143:223–229, 1956
480. Shumway NE, Lower RR: Topical cardiac hypothermia for extended periods of anoxic cardiac arrest. Surg Forum 10:563–566, 1959
481. Siebecker KL, Kimmey JR, Kraemer RJ, et al: The prevention and treatment of cardiac arrhythmias during hypothermia. Anesth Analg 42:527–533, 1963
482. Simpson JA, Gibson P, Bloomfield DA: Profound hypothermia in cardiac surgery: A preliminary report. Med J Aust 1:647–650, 1960
483. Smith TK, Spencer DC, Derrick JR: Experimental considerations of deep hypothermia in animals. Am Surg 28:259–265, 1962
484. Sommerville W: The effect of hypothermia on atrial fibrillation and other arrhythmias. Surv Anesthesiol 6:4–5, 1962
485. Speicher CE, Ferrigan L, Wolfson SK, et al: Cold injury of myocardium and pericardium in cardiac hypothermia. Surg Gynecol Obstet 114:659–665, 1962
486. Spencer FC, Eiseman B, Norton LW, et al: Coronary artery patch graft: Experiment with cardiopulmonary bypass and hypothermia. Arch Surg 86: 81–86, 1963
487. Spohn K, Kolb E, Heinzel J, et al: Tiefe Hypothermie unter 20°C. Die Methode von Watanabe, Okamura and Ishikawa. Ihre Leistungsfahigkeit bei Operationen am offenen Herzen im Tierversuch. Arch Klin Chir 290:365, 1959
488. Spohn K, Kolb E, Heinzel J, et al: Tiefe Hypothermie unter 28°C ohne extrakorporalen Kreislauf zur langdauernden Operation am eroffneten Herzen. Zentralbl Chir 86:213–230, 1961
489. Sprouse JH, Galindo AH, Morrow AG: Influence of various drugs and anesthetic agents on cardiac excitability in man. Anesthesiology 24:141–142, 1963
490. Spurr GB, Barlow G: Influence of prolonged hypothermia and hyperthermia on myocardial sodium, potassium, and chloride. Circ Res 7:210–218, 1959

491. Starkov PM: The Problem of Acute Hypothermia. London, Pergamon Press, 1960, p 310
492. Stephen CR, Dent SJ, Hall KD, et al: Physiologic reactions during profound hypothermia with cardioplegia. Anesthesiology 22:873–881, 1961
493. Stephen CR, Dent SJ, Sealy WC, et al: Anesthetic and metabolic factors associated with combined extracorporeal circulation and hypothermia. Am J Cardiol 6:737–746, 1960
494. Sterns LP, Bonnabeau RC, Lillehei CW: Coronary resistance changes with hypothermic perfusion. J Thorac Cardiovasc Surg 51:579–584, 1966
495. Stinson EB, Dong E, Angell WW, et al: Myocardial hypothermia for cardiac transplantation. Laval Med 41:195–198, 1970
496. Stoney RJ, Roe BB: Ventricular function after induced, intermittently ischemic ventricular fibrillation: Effect of moderate hypothermia. J Thorac Cardiovasc Surg 48:838–843, 1964
497. Su CS, Hardin R, King H: The use of hypothermia with cardiopulmonary bypass for open heart surgery: An experimental study. Surgery 44:1079–1082, 1958
498. Subramanian S, Wagner H, Vlad P, et al: Surface-induced deep hypothermia in cardiac surgery. J Pediatr Surg 6:612–617, 1971
499. Sumbera J, Braveny P, Kruta V: Effects of temperature on the duration and velocity of myocardial contraction in normal and low calcium media. Arch Int Physiol Biochem 75:261–276, 1967
500. Suzuki M, Penn I: A reappraisal of the micorcirculation during general hypothermia. Surgery 58:1049–1060, 1965
501. Svanes K, Zweifach BW, Intaglietta M: Effect of hypothermia on transcapillary fluid exchange. Am J Physiol 218:981–989, 1970
502. Swan H, Paton BC: The current status of hypothermia in cardiovascular surgery. Prog Cardiovasc Dis 4:228–258, 1961-62
503. Swan H, Paton BC: Deep hypothermia in congenital heart disease. J Cardiovasc Surg 3:294–298, 1962
504. Swan H, Sawyer DC: Prevention of ventricular fibrillation during experimental hypothermia: Failure of sodium diphenylhydantoin. Arch Surg 95: 23–26, 1967
505. Swan H, Zeavin I, Blount SG Jr, et al: Surgery by direct vision in the open heart during hypothermia. JAMA 153:1081–1085, 1953
506. Swan H, Zeavin I, Holmes JH, et al: Cessation of circulation in general hypoermia. I. Physiology changes and their control. Ann Surg 138:360–376, 1953
507. Swenson EW, Choudhury JD, Gollan F: Profound hypothermia by partial perfusion in the closed chest dog. Trans Am Soc Artif Intern Organs 8: 328–332, 1962
508. Szegi J, Rausch J: Wirkung von Strophanthin auf normale und gekuhlte Herz-Lungen-Praparate von Katzen. Acta Physiol Hung 13:79–87, 1957
509. Taguchi K, Sasaki N, Matsuura Y, et al: Clinical experiences with hemodilution in total cardiopulmonary bypass. An analysis of 650 patients. Surgery 63:252–260, 1968
510. Tanaka T, Inoue T, Paton BC: Oxygen availability during hypothermic perfusions using diluted blood. Surg Forum 13:138–140, 1962

511. Tanche M, Chatonnet J: Modifications apportees par l'hypothermie a l'excitabilite des commandes nerveuses extra-cardiaques chez le chien; I. Accelerateurs cardiaques. Anesth Analg Reanim 16:833–840, 1959
512. Telivuo LJ, Laitinen EA, Vinkkula L: Left heart bypass in normo- and hypothermia. An experimental study on dogs and a clinical report. Ann Chir Gynecol Fenn 54:5–39, 1965
513. Terry HR Jr, Michenfelder JD, Daw EF: Hypothermia by extracorporeal circulation for neurosurgery: An anesthetic technic. Anesth Analog (Cleve) 41:241–248, 1962
514. Thauer R: Ergebnisse experimenteller Kreislaufuntersuchungen bei Hypothermie. Thorax Chirurgie 3:522–538, 1956
515. Thauer R: The circulation in hypothermia of nonhibernating animals and men, in Hamilton WF (ed): Handbook of Physiology, American Physiology Society 3. Baltimore, Waverly Press, 1965, pp 1899–1920
516. Thauer R, Albers C, Behmann FW, et al: Circulatory dynamics in hypothermia, in Symposium sur l'hypothermie, 15th Congress International Military Medicine and Pharmacy, Beograd, 1959, pp 58–71
517. Thauer R, Brendel W: Hypothermie. Prog Surg 2:73–271, 1962
518. Theye RA, Kirklin JW: Vertical film oxygenator performance at 30°C and oxygen levels during rewarming. Surgery 54:569–572, 1963
519. Thomas AN, Hall AD, Blaisdell FW, et al: Survival after prolonged induced circulatory arrest, hyperbaric oxygenation and hypothermia. Proceedings of the 3rd International Conference on Hyperbaric Medicine, 1966, pp 382–390
520. Torres JC: Ventricular conduction and refractoriness during hypothermia. Circ Res 18:323–329, 1966
521. Tsifutis A, Burton RM, Goldring D: The effect of hypothermia and anoxia upon oxygen consumption and contractility of human and rat heart muscle. Am Heart J 79:88–95, 1970
522. Ungar I, Eglajs J, Buhl T, et al: A study of three methods of inducing cardiac arrest in dogs maintained on total body perfusion by means of a pump-oxygenator; namely, localized hypothermia, potassium, and anoxia. Trans Am Soc Artif Intern Organs 7:237–251, 1961
523. Urschel HC, Greenberg JJ: Differential cardiac hypothermia for elective cardioplegia. Ann Surg 152:845–855, 1960
524. Urschel HC, Greenberg JJ, Hufnagel CA: Elective cardioplegia by local cardiac hypothermia. N Engl J Med 261:1330–1332, 1959
525. Urschel HC Jr, Greenberg JJ, Roth EJ: Rapid hypothermia: An improved extracorporeal method. J Thorac Cardiovasc Surg 39:318–329, 1960
526. Ushiyama J, McC Brooks C: Hypothermia and minimal gradient requirements for excitation of cardiac muscle. Am J Physiol 200:718–722, 1961
527. Vadot L, Estanove S, Gounod R, et al: Calcul de l'arret circulatoire admissible en hypothermie. Anesth Analg (Paris) 20:61–65, 1963
528. Verdura J, Neville WE, White RJ: The hypoxic acidosis of profound hypothermia with extracorporeal perfusion and total circulatory arrest. Surg Forum 14:420–422, 1963
529. Veroft R, Delbrouck F: L'arret cardiaque par hypothermie selective. Acta Chir Belg 62:278–294, 1963

530. Villamil A, Franco RJ, Clavijo J, et al: Electrocardiographic changes in artificial hibernation. Am Heart J 53:365–379, 1957
531. Watanabe A, Okamura H, Takahashi T, et al: Etude experimentale de la reanimation cardiaque apres interruption circulatoire prolongee pratiquee a tres basse temperature. Pathol Biol 7:1017–1026, 1959
532. Weiss M, Piwnica A, Lenfant C, et al: Arret circulatoire sous hypothermie profonde, obtenue grace a un systcm pompe oxygenateur et un echangeur thermique. Rev Fr Clin Biol 5:65, 1960
533. Weiss M, Piwnica A, Lenfant C, et al: Deep hypothermia with total circulatory arrest. Trans Am Soc Artif Intern Organs 6:227–239, 1960
534. Westin B, Sehgal N, Assali NS: Hemodynamic alterations during hypothermia in dogs. Clin Res 9:86, 1961
535. Westin B, Sehgal N, Assali NS: Regional blood flow and vascular resistance during hypothermian dog. Am J Physiol 201:485–491, 1961
536. Whalen RE, Brown IW Jr, Smith WW, et al: Cinefluorographic and hemodynamic studies of cardiopulmonary bypass with hypothermia. Clin Res 10:183, 1962
537. Whalen RE, Brown IW Jr, Smith WW, et al: Perfusion hypothermia studies in dogs: Cinefluorographic and hemodynamic studies. Arch Surg 86:118–125, 1963
538. White DC, Nowell NW: The effect of alcohol on the cardiac arrest temperature in hypothermic rats. Clin Sci 28:395–399, 1965
539. Wilber CG, Zeman FJ: Response of the guinea pig heart to hypothermia. Ohio J Sci 68:229–233, 1968
540. Wilder RJ, Rush BF, Fishbein RH, et al: Cardiac dynamics during partial bypass for profound hypothermia (4°C). Surg Forum 12:173–175, 1961
541. Wilder RJ, Rush BF, Ravitch MM: Destruction of canine red blood cells by the disc oxygenator—Protective effect of hypothermia. Surg Forum 13: 118–119, 1962
542. Wilder RJ, Rush BF, Ravitch MM: Protective effect of hypothermia on canine whole blood during extracorporeal circulation. Ann Surg 160:1057–1061, 1964
543. Wilder RJ, Rush BF, Yaycioglu Y, et al: Survival and physiologic studies with profound hypothermia (0° to 8°C) and a pump-oxygenataor in dogs. Surgery 49:629–635, 1961
544. Willman VL, Howard HS, Cooper T, et al: Ventricular function after hypothermic cardiac arrest. Arch Surg 82:120–127, 1961
545. Wolfson SK Jr, Icoz MV, Luber S: Preservation of conditioned responses in primates after total circulatory arrest withh preferential cerebral hypothermia. Surg Forum 16:409–411, 1965
546. Wolfson SK Jr, Inouye WY, Kavianian A: Preferential cerebral hypothermia for circulatory arrest. Surgery 57:846–855, 1965
547. Wolfson SK Jr, Yalav E, Eisenstat S: An isothermic technique for profound hypothermia and its effect on metabolic acidosis. J Thorac Cardiovasc Surg 45:466–475, 1963
548. Wolfson SK Jr, Yalav EH, Eisenstat S: Temperature differentials and metabolic acidosis in profound hypothermia. JAMA 183:674–676, 1963
549. Wright JS, Osborn JJ, Perkins HA, et al: Heparin levels during and after hypothermic perfusion. J Cardiovasc Surg 5:244–250, 1964

550. Yeh TJ, Ellison LT, Ellison RG: Hemodynamic and metabolic responses of the whole body and individual organs to cardiopulmonary bypass with profound hypothermia. J Thorac Cardiovasc Surg 42:782–792, 1961
551. Young WG, Sealy WC, Brown IW, et al: Metabolic and physiologic observations on patients undergoing extracorporeal circulation in conjunction with hypothermia. Surgery 46:175–184, 1959
552. Yver J: Surveillance biologique de la coagulation et de la fibrinolyse dans la chirurgie cardiaque avec circulation extra-corporelle et hypothermie profonde. These, Paris, 1962
553. Zellos S, Gillespie JF, Hufnagel CA: Observations on the effect of low pO_2 in extreme hypothermia in dogs. J Cardiovasc Surg 7:133–147, 1966
554. Ziegelhoffer A, Fedelesova M, Hubka M, et al: Observation of metabolic changes of the isolated hypothermic heart during resuscitation with coronary perfusion, obtained in dogs "in vivo" after a hypothermic cardiac arrest. Bratisl Lek Listy (Czech) 46:361–366, 1966
555. Zimny ML, Romano CC, Haydel R: ATPase and succinate dehydrogenase in hearts of hypothermic ground squirrels and rats. Cryobiology 9:61–65, 1972
556. Zimny ML, Sherman M, Romano CC: Ultrastructural modifications of the intercalated disc during hypothermia in the rat and the ground squirrel. Cryobiology 4:317–328, 1967-8
557. Zindler M: Kunstliche Hypothermie fur "offene" Operationen angeborener Herzfehler, in Kremer K (ed): Die chirurgische Behandlung der angeboren Fehlbildungen. Stuttgart, Thieme, 1961, pp 248–292
558. Zindler M, Dudziak R, Euniki S, et al: Surface hypothermias for heart operation with circulatory arrest. Int Anesthesiol Clin, Eur Trends Anesth 3: 733–755, 1965
559. Zingg W: The control of the acid-base balance during open-heart surgery. Can Anaesth Soc J 11:123–146, 1964
560. Zingg W, Kantor S: Observations on the temperatures in the brain during extracorporeal differential hypothermia. Surg Forum 11:192–193, 1960
561. Zuhdi N, Carey J, Sheldon W, et al: Hemodilution, low flow rates and moderate internal hypothermia for extracorporeal circulation. Concepts obviating the use of blood for priming. Angiology 14:571–575, 1963
562. Zuhdi N, McCollough B, Montroy J, et al: Prolonged simple aortic occlusion during hypothermic perfusion as an aid to open heart surgery—Clinical application. Postgrad Med 28:507–509, 1960
563. Zuhdi N, McCollough B, Carey J, et al: Hypothermic perfusion for open heart surgical procedures. Report on the use of a heart-lung machine primed with 5% dextrose in water, inducing hemodilution. J Int Coll Surg 35:319–326, 1961
564. Zuhdi N, McCollough B, Carey J, et al: Double helical reservoir heart-lung machine. Arch Surg 82:320–325, 1961
565. Zuhdi N, McCollough B, Craig N, et al: Apparatus for hypothermic perfusion—Clinical application. Am Surg 26:446–450, 1960

4

Respiration

LUNG FUNCTION IN HYPOTHERMIA

During progressive cooling some physiological functions cease earlier than others. While all processes can be reinstated with rewarming, the temporary cessation of some may damage the cooled organism sooner than the cessation of others. One of these processes, lung ventilation, becomes critical in the early phase of cooling and ceases at a higher body temperature than the others. In experimental hypothermia ventilation failure appears to be the primary cause of death.[21,32] Circulatory failure becomes the critical function for survival at a somewhat lower body temperature if ventilation is mechanically supported.

One observes several distinctly different phases of lung ventilation according to the depth of cooling. The first phase, observed during mild cooling, is associated with increased lung ventilation and increased lung performance. It is characterized by the maximal involvement of the temperature regulatory mechanisms,[19] while the organism if fighting to preserve a normal or near-normal body temperature. Deep anesthesia, and to a lesser degree fast core cooling, can decrease or maybe even abolish this hypermetabolic and hyperventilatory phase.

Hypothermic and normothermic animals react to an increased

CO_2 concentration in essentially the same manner.[36] The impulse frequency of phrenic and vagal volleys increases continuously during progressive cooling.[5]

The regulation of respiration in surface-cooled animals is adequate at a body temperature of 26 C.[2,41] Progressively deeper cooling will eventually depress lung ventilation.[33] During the second phase of cooling the respiratory rate and minute ventilation of lungs decrease, as well as the $PaCO_2$.[39] The pulmonary AV temperature difference[43] is greatly increased. Nevertheless, it appears that the depression of respiration during a more profound cooling cannot be attributed to any alterations in the excitability of the peripheral nervous mechanisms. Excitability of the chemoreceptors is retained in hypothermia.[7] In small laboratory animals the regulation of respiration is adequate even at a body temperature of 15 to 20 C.[19,23]

The third phase of cooling is characterized by the inadequate ventilation of the lungs. Assisted—positive or negative—pressure breathing is recommended. It appears that negative pressure breathing rather than positive pressure breathing might be more suitable in hypothermia.[3] During positive pressure breathing the anatomical dead space is increased[38] but the physiological dead space might be either enlarged[37] or remain unchanged.[38] However, artificial positive pressure breathing keeps a high pO_2 in the tissues in surface-cooled animals even at a body temperature of 10 C.[1]

Respiratory acidosis is regularly observed during surface or core-cooling. This phenomenon has been described in detail in Chapter 2.

During profound cooling there is a slight increase in blood oxygenation.[12,27] The function of an isolated perfused dog lung for gas exchange is equal or better in hypothermia than at a normal body temperature.[12] Surface activity of the lungs remains unchanged after hypothermic perfusion.[15] Therefore, it appears that in perfusion hypothermia there is no failure of oxygen to reach tissues.[1,4]

During rewarming mechanical ventilatory support is useful for both surface-cooled[13,34] and core-cooled[31] animals.

SELECTIVE LUNG COOLING

Selective cooling of the blood in the pulmonary circuit ("selective pulmonary hypothermia"[11]) can be induced by separately perfusing the pulmonary from the systemic circulation. This selective pulmonary hypothermia increases the pulmonary arterial pressure and pulmonary vascular resistance[11] in a way similar to that observed during surface cooling.[40]

Selective cooling of only one lung was successfully achieved by forcing ice-cold oxygenated fluorocarbon fluid into the lung while ventilating the other with oxygen. This technique of differential hypothermia[30] allows the lung to be cooled to a temperature of 5 to 10 C in a normothermic thoractomized dog. Local warming of the "tumor"-designated area in the cold lung is achieved by microwave energy. This leads to an increased blood flow and an increased embedding of anticancer drugs in the warm tissue.[30]

OXYGEN CONSUMPTION

The oxygen consumption is increased during the initial part of progressive cooling. This increase is much smaller if the experimental animal is deeply anesthetized or core cooled[42] (Fig. 4-1). In core-cooled animals the oxygen consumption is decreased due to a rapid decrease in the body temperature, especially the temperature of the vital organs. The body temperature at which the oxygen consumption begins to decrease without anesthesia is around 32 to 33 C. Smaller animals and younger animals decrease their oxygen consumption and their lung ventilation at somewhat lower body temperatures than large animals or man.

During the second phase of cooling, the oxygen consumption steadily decreases and eventually passes through the basal metabolic rate (BMR) level. For rats this happens at a body temperature of 25 C, for guinea pigs around 28 C, and for unanesthetized human beings probably at a body temperature around 32 C. In man, anesthetized and cooled to a body temperature of 30 C, the oxygen consumption is decreased to 70 percent of the normothermic value.[35] At a body temperature of 25 C the oxygen consumption is about 50 percent of the normothermic value. When the body temperature of dogs is decreased to a temperature of 17 C, the oxygen consumption is decreased to 10 to 15 percent of the normothermic values. In rats this same decrease in oxygen consumption is observed at a body temperature of 17 to 20 C.

During cooling the level of oxygen consumption depends not

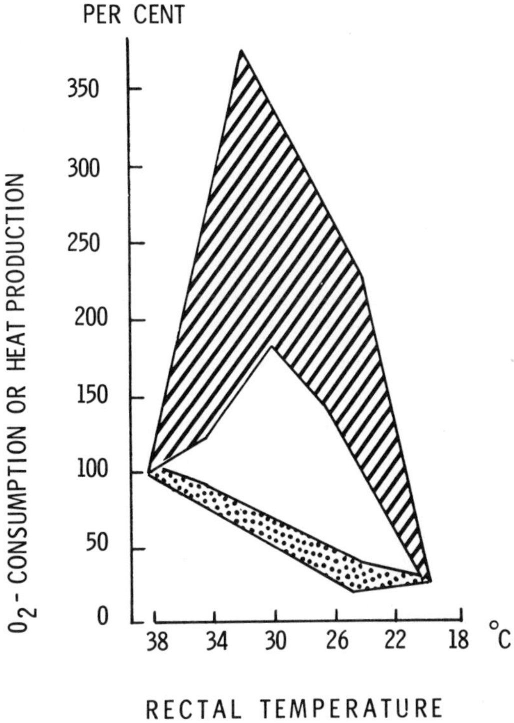

Fig. 4-1. Oxygen consumption or heat production of dogs and other experimental animals during progressive cooling, expressed in percent of the normothermic values.[42] Stripped area: during cooling with little or no anesthesia. Dotted area: after deep anesthesia.

only on the body temperature but also on the species used and on the temperature adaptation of that particular animal.[8,10] The amount of oxygen consumed depends not only on the temperature of the internal vital organs, or hypothalamus, but also on the temperature of the skin.

During the cooling of experimental animals (without the use of drugs), temperature regulation mechanisms are active until a very low body temperature is reached. In rats this is about 20 C. Shivering persists even in profound cooling, but decreases in intensity. Some shivering is present even at a body temperature of 18 to 22 C (if not suppressed by drugs).[25]

Young animals recover from asphyxia and are able to respire spontaneously after rewarming, even 2.5 hours after the cessation of cardiac activity.[14] Supercooled newborn ground squirrels fully recover without ill effects after 11 hours of respiratory and circulatory arrest.[18] Oxygen toxicity is decreased in hypothermia.[29]

The oxygen consumption of an artificially cooled hibernator is many times greater than the oxygen consumption of the same hibernator while in hibernation.[20] After a small stimulus that induces arousal from hibernation, the oxygen consumption of a hibernator increases 10 to 20 times in 4 to 5 minutes while the body temperature is still unchanged.[22,24,25] This is why cooling to a very low body temperature induces a cold narcosis in a nonhibernator but not in a hibernator. A hibernating hibernator reacts to operative procedures even at a body temperature close to the freezing point.[9]

ANESTHESIA

A rectilinear decrease in the anesthetic requirements is observed during progressive decreases in body temperature. For halothane a 10 C decrease in body temperature decreases the anesthetic requirements to about 40 percent.[17] During fast core cooling, the physical anesthesia of cold replaces chemical anesthesia. For this reason short-acting anesthetics are recommended when core cooling is used.

The toxicity of most, if not all, anesthetic agents is increased in hypothermia. Rats cooled and kept at a body temperature of 15 C for 5 to 6 hours can be recovered. A nontoxic injection of sodium pentobarbital (40 mg/kg) decreases this survival time to only 30 minutes.[26]

BREATHING ORGANIC LIQUIDS IN HYPOTHERMIA

During a rapid decompression gas bubbles appear in the body of an organism, a fact that was described as early as 1670 by Robert Boyle. The problem of decompression sickness that might lead to ischemic anoxia is observed during escape from a submarine or sudden decompression in an airplane. It has been speculated that this problem might be solved if man were to breathe a noncompressible fluid such as liquid fluorocarbon. Liquid fluorocarbon dissolves about 40 to 60 times more oxygen than water. It can support the respiration of mammals for short periods of time even at normal atmospheric pressure. When totally submerged in an oxygenated fluorocarbon fluid, rats, mice, and hamsters can survive much longer than when submerged in oxygenated water. The fluorocarbon liquid will support respiration of the mammals because these liquids dissolve much more oxygen than water.[6,16] Hypothermia lengthens the safe duration of fluorocarbon breathing.[6] Submerged hamsters, body temperature 4 C, recover even after 24 hours of fluorocarbon breathing.[28]

Summary

Ventilation is the first critical process that stops during progressive cooling. It can cause the death of the cooled organism if mechanical ventilation is not introduced. Initially oxygen consumption increases during progressive cooling due to temperature-regulating mechanisms. These mechanisms are abolished by profound anesthesia or fast core cooling. Most anesthetics are more toxic in hypothermia than in normothermia and last much longer due to a decreased metabolism of the tissues that disintegrate them.

BIBLIOGRAPHY

1. Adolph EF, Naberschíng A, Orchard DP: Ventilation of lungs in deeply hypothermic rats. J Appl Physiol 16:819–826, 1961
2. Blair E, Esmond WG, Attar S, et al: The effect of hypothermia on lung function. Ann Surg 160:814–823, 1964
3. Bryce-Smith R, Epstein HG, Glees P: Physiological studies during hypothermia in monkeys. J Appl Physiol 15:440–444, 1960
4. Byon YK, Adolph EF: Oxygen in tissues during deep hypothermia. J Appl Physiol 16:827–830, 1961
5. Cirpili E: Research on the nervous regulation of respiration in hypothermia. J Med Fac Istanbul, Monograph Series No. 34, Istanbul, 1964, pp 13–38
6. Clark LC Jr, Gollan F: Survival of mammals breathing organic liquids equilibrated with oxygen at atmospheric pressure. Science 152:1755–1756, 1966
7. Emiroglu F, Gokhan N, Cirpili E: The sensitivity of chemoreceptors of the dog during progressive hypothermia. Arch Int Physiol Biochim 70:41–48, 1962
8. Giaja J, Popovic V: L'energetique des homeotherms refroidis par rapport a leur taille. Glas Acad Serbe Sci 200:177–181, 1951

9. Giaja J, Popovic V: Reaction de l'hibernant et de non-hibernant refroidi aux agressions operatoires. C R Acad Sci (Paris) 237:1360–1362, 1953
10. Giaja J, Popovic V: Sur les modifications de l'intensite des echanges de l'organisme refroide. C R Acad Sci (Paris) 236:1700–1701, 1953
11. Goetz RH, Rohman M, Goetz VM, et al: Hemodynamic effects of selective pulmonary hypothermia. J Thorac Cardiovasc Surg 45:574–584, 1963
12. Haupt GJ, Myers RN, Forte IE, et al: Lung gas exchange in dogs during profound hypothermia. Trans Am Soc Artif Intern Organs 9:225–229, 1963
13. Hillman H, Rogers P: Recovery of spontaneous respiration in rats following hypothermia. J Physiol 204:87–88P, 1969
14. Kondo Y, Kuwahara O, Don Turner M: Prolonged suspended animation in puppies. Cryobiology 10:512, 1973
15. Miller DR, Kuenzig MC: Pulmonary changes following normothermic and profound hypothermic perfusion in dogs. J Thorac Cardiovasc Surg 56:717–731, 1968
16. Modell JH, Gollan F, Giammona ST, et al: Effect of fluorocarbon liquid on surface tension properties of pulmonary surfactant. Chest 57:263–265, 1970
17. Munson ES: Effect of hypothermia on anesthetic requirement in rats. Lab Anim Care 20:1009–1113, 1970
18. Popovic P, Popovic V: Survival of newborn ground squirrels after supercooling or freezing. Am J Physiol 204, 949–952, 1963
19. Popovic V: Contribution a l'etude de la thermogenese de l'homeotherme refroidi. Monogr Acad Serbe Sci 199:1–156, 1952
20. Popovic V: L'hibernation artificielle du spermophile (*Citellus citellus*). Arch Sci Biol (Belgrade) 4:37–43, 1952
21. Popovic V: Mecanisme de la mort de l'homeotherme refroidi. Acta Med Yugosl 7:40–62, 1953
22. Popovic V: L'effet de la temperature de millieu sur l'intensite de la consommation d'oxygene pendant l'hibernation. Glas Acad Serbe Sci 208:43–52, 1953
23. Popovic V: De L'hypothermie lethargique prolongee. Arch Sci Physiol (Paris) 9:219–229, 1955
24. Popovic V: La calorification de reveil de l'hibernant. Arch Sci Physiol (Paris) 11:29–35, 1957
25. Popovic V: Lethargic hypothermia in hibernators and nonhibernators. Ann NY Acad Sci 80:320–331, 1959
26. Popovic V: Survival time of hypothermic white rats (15°C) and ground squirrels (10°C). Am J Physiol 199:463–466, 1960
27. Popovic V: Physiological characteristics of rats and ground squirrels during prolonged lethargic hypothermia. Am J Physiol 199:467–471, 1960
28. Popovic V, Baughman JE: Longer survival of golden hamsters breathing an organic liquid after cooling. Cryobiology 8:305–306, 1971
29. Popovic V, Gerschman R, Gilbert DL: Effect of high oxygen pressure on ground squirrels in hypothermia and hibernation. Am J Physiol 206:49–50, 1964
30. Popovic V, Kostolny I, Larose JH, et al: Enhanced perfusion in microwave heated part of hypothermic lung. J Physiol (Paris) 63:386–389, 1971
31. Popovic V, Kostolny I, Pass K, et al: Survival of extracorporeally cooled dogs after one hour circulatory arrest. Cryobiology 8:390, 1971
32. Prewitt RL, Anderson GL, Musacchia XJ: Evidence for a metabolic limitation

of survival in hypothermic hamsters. Proc Soc Exp Biol Med 140:1279–1283, 1972
33. Regan MJ, Eger IE: Ventilatory responses to hypercapnia and hypoxia at northermia and moderate hypothermia during constant-debt halothane anaesthesia. Anesthesiology 27:624–633, 1966
34. Rogers PD, Hillman H: Increased recovery of rats' respiration following profound hypothermia. J Appl Physiol 29:58–63, 1970
35. Rolly G: Etude de la consommation d'oxygene pendant l'hypothermie moderee provoquee. Acta Anaesthesiol Belg 16:135–141, 1965
36. Salzano J, Hall FG: Effect of hypothermia on ventilatory response to carbon dioxide inhalation and carbon dioxide infusing in dog. J Appl Physiol 15:397–401, 1960
37. Salzano J, Hall FG: Influence of vagal blockade on respiratory and circulatory functions in hypothermic dogs. J Appl Physiol 17:833–836, 1962
38. Salzano J, Hall FG: Cardiopulmonary effects of continuous pressure breathing in hypothermic dogs. J Appl Physiol 20:669–674, 1965
39. Sodipo JO, Lee DC: Comparison of ventilation responses to hypercapnia at normothermia and hypothermia during halothane anaesthesia. Can Anaesth Soc J 18:426–433, 1971
40. Stern S, Braun K: Pulmonary arterial and venous response to cooling: Role of alpha-adrenergic receptors. Am J Physiol 219:982–985, 1970
41. Terzioglu M: Respiratory and acid base balance adjustments in acute hypothermia. Med Bull Istanbul Univ 1:18–35, 1968
42. Thauer R: The circulation in hypothermia of nonhibernating animals and men, in Hamilton WF (ed): Handbook of Physiology. Washington, American Physiological Society, 1965, pp 1899–1920
43. Zikria BA, Ferrer JM, Malm JR: Pulmonary hypothermia in dogs. J Appl Physiol 24:707–710, 1968

5

Gastrointestinal System, Kidney, and Endocrine Hypothermia

GASTROINTESTINAL SYSTEM IN HYPOTHERMIA

Cooling Techniques

Both generalized and localized hypothermia can be induced by cooling a particular part of the gastrointestinal system. A deep generalized hypothermia can be induced by peritoneal dialysis with ice-cold saline. Generalized body cooling is also induced through gastric balloon cooling.[75,78] In this case the stomach is cooled more than the other parts of the body. The deep "gastrointestinal" hypothermia could permit a circulatory arrest of 30 minutes.[103] Because of the greater blood flow through the gastrointestinal area than through the cooled skin, "gastrointestinal cooling" is appreciably faster than surface cooling. Gastronintestinal cooling is beneficial because it removes the excess K^+ from the blood which accumulates during the hypothermic exposure.[54] If only the stomach is cooled and the rest of the body kept warm (surface rewarming, microwave rewarming), one might call this kind of cooling "gastric hypothermia."

Physiology of Gastric and Intestinal Cooling

It is well known that enzyme secretion depends on the oxygen consumption of a gland. Therefore, enzyme secretion depends on the temperature of that gland as well. When the stomach is cooled to a temperature of 17 to 20 C there is a marked depression of acid and pepsin secretion.[111] Cooling to a temperature of 30 C or lower decreases the enzyme activity of duodenal juice.[108] Pancreatic insulin secretion is depressed in hypothermia.[14,22] The temperature coefficient of insulin secretion is very high. Reduced secretion could lead to an altered carbohydrate metabolism and to a severe deficit of carbohydrate utilization. It appears that the glucose disappearance rate is not appreciably altered in hypothermia. The blood flow through the hypothermic pancreas[14,26,108] or hypothermic mesenteric area[6] is decreased also. The volume, but not the concentration, of excreted bile is decreased in hypothermia.[105,196] Both active and passive ionic transport are preserved during profound cooling of the liver.[65] Secretory function of an isolated canine stomach is well preserved after a 24-hour storage to a temperature of 4 C.[63]

Clinical Application

Due to the reduced blood flow through the gastrointestinal region during cooling, generalized hypothermia was successfully used in treatment of massive gastrointestinal hemorrhages,[36,72] or for an extended interruption of blood flow in the liver.[76] Generalized hypothermia has been used in the management of gastrointestinal hemorrhage, especially when the precise origin of the bleeding was unknown. Bleeding was controlled even in patients who needed large quantities of transfused blood.

Localized gastric cooling[47,91] was also often successful for the control of massive gastric hemorrhage.[7,21,40,111,112] In the United States, however, this technique was never widely accepted. Russian surgeons are using gastric hypothermia extensively for massive gastrointestinal hemorrhages,[85] and gastric cooling is often used in other European countries.

Local hypothermia has been successfully used to control bleeding in the large bowel.[6] Local cooling of the bowel appears to be more effective than generalized cooling in decreasing ammonia production.[4]

Peritonitis[62] or acute pancreatitis is successfully treated with localized cooling[108] or with a generalized cooling.[25,92] The localized cooling of an experimentally induced strangulated groin hernia gives a considerable degree of protection.[15]

During the cooling of children, the level of immunoreactive insulin is low despite the hyperglycemia induced by the administration of glucose.[9] After rewarming this process is fully reversible.[9] Similar results were obtained in experimental work,[11] which suggests the need for caution when glucose is given. Excessive glucose administration to the hypothermic patient may cause an excessive hyperosmolarity.

Summary

Gastric or peritoneal cooling can be used successfully as techniques for the induction of generalized hypothermia, or for the induction of localized gastric or intestinal hypothermia. Glandular secretion, mobility of the gastrointestinal tract, and blood flow through gastrointestinal areas are depressed by hypothermia. This last fact was used clinically for the treatment of gastric ulcers, massive gastrointestinal hemorrhages, and acute pancreatitis.

KIDNEY IN HYPOTHERMIA

Physiology

Though the cardiac output decreases during progressive hypothermia, the renal blood flow appears to be increased in mild hypothermia and only decreases when the kidney temperature is low.[17,34] There are reports of an increased kidney vascular resistance.[80] The same pattern occurs in urine flow which first increases and then decreases only in profound hypothermia.[59] Glomerular filtration is continuously decreased during progressive hypothermia.[77] Active tubular transport mechanisms are directly affected by cooling,[102] leading to a voluminous isosmotic reabsorption,[115] but not to the active reabsorption of sodium and water.[97] In general, kidney reabsorption is decreased, though distal segmental reabsorption is even increased.[17] The volume of urine is not reduced much in the early stages of hypothermia. Reabsorption of bicarbonates is decreased.[17,58] Thus it is clear that hypothermia affects the various renal functions in dissimilar fashions.[17,46,57]

In hibernation the urine flow is diminished.[79] Cation transport is less sensitive to the temperature decrease in hibernating animals than in nonhibernators.[121]

Renal functions recover after rewarming. Complete, but slow recovery of these functions was seen if the hypothermic episode was extended.

Kidney Preservation

Cooling protects the kidney from ischemia.[19,28,113] Apparently there is a threefold increase in ischemic tolerance of the kidney after profound cooling.[56] This protective role of cooling was successfully used to extend the functional viability of kidneys harvested for transplantation.

Perfused kidneys can be successfully used for transplantation after 24 hours of cold storage, sometimes combined with hyperbaric oxygenation. This has been proved both in experimental[41,64,67,69,83,96,104,107] and in clinical situations.[71,90]

New techniques extended the functional viability of kidneys to 3,[12,49] 5,[50] or even 7 days.[122] Kidneys for transplantation are also obtained from cadavers.[20,100]

Clinical Application

Hypothermia is used for surgical interventions involving the prostate,[29,68] the kidneys, and the urinary system.[35,38,74] Regional renal hypothermia has been used by urologists for several years.[68,82,118,119] Profound cooling of the kidney provides the surgeon with a bloodless field.[39,95,119]

In order to decrease the temperature of a kidney localized cooling can be used[24,28,81,82,117] instead of complicated generalized cooling only. Localized kidney hypothermia was successfully used for the treatment of massive renal hemorrhage.[55,56] Uremia leads to a spontaneous hypothermia[30] but hypothermia has a protective effect on uremia.[32]

A short-lasting but pronounced diuresis[114] and probably an increased release of adrenergic agents[42] are observed in patients after rewarming from profound hypothermia.

Summary

During progressive cooling various renal functions are affected in a dissimilar fashion. A decrease in the body or kidney temperature of several degrees slows down some renal processes, but increases others. In profound hypothermia all renal processes are decreased or even temporarily abolished. Generalized hypothermia or localized cooling protects the kidney. This fact was used for long-term cold perfusions of harvested kidneys for transplantation or for surgical interventions.

ENDOCRINE GLANDS

A slight decrease in the body temperature of a homeotherm usually leads to a pronounced "stress response."[94] Deep hypothermia decreases the release of all hormones.[13]

Hypothermia of 24 to 26 C decreases the neurosecretion of the hypothalamic–hypophyseal axis and leads to the depletion of neurosecretory material. This decreased neurosecretion is probably caused by an impairment in the microcirculation of the cooled tissues.[94] During progressive hypothermia the arterial blood pressure decreases more in hypophysectomized than in normal rats.[51,52] Initially, cooling increases the release of growth hormone; sometimes this increase is induced mainly by the technique of anesthesia.[10]

It appears that during mild hypothermia the hypothalamo–pituitary–thyroid axis is well preserved[123] as well as the hypothalamo–pituitary–adrenal interaction.[93] In man, mild hypothermia is not a stimulus for the release of thyreotropic hormone.[123] Hypothermia decreases ACTH secretion.

The thyroid has an increased activity during the initial stages of cooling,[101] and the plasma protein-bound iodine is increased,[31] but when the body temperature is decreased to 15 C or lower the uptake of labeled iodine is inhibited.[89] The moderate hypothermia (31 C) which develops during preoptic warming in animals leads to an increase in the protein-bound iodine as soon as hypothalamic warming is interrupted.[2] Thyroid secretion is arrested in profound hypothermia if the temperature-regulating mechanisms are blocked prior to cooling.[5] Thyroidectomy was performed without ill consequences in a thyrotoxic patient kept at 34 C for 4 days.[43]

The sensitivity of smooth muscles to norepinephrine[33,116] and the vasoconstrictor effect of epinephrine are reduced at a low body temperature. A temperature of 5 C prevents norepinephrine from having any electrochemical or mechanical effect. Interruption of the early stages of depolarization is probably caused by the profound depression of energy metabolism.[60]

Hypothermia decreases norepinephrine release after nerve stimulation,[61] though to a smaller degree than after the administration of sympathicomimetic amines.[116] It seems that hypothermia acts directly on nerve conduction and on the release of norepinephrine from the nerve endings. Nerve conduction is blocked when the temperature of the body or of the nerve is decreased below 8 C. At body temperatures above this critical temperature, the somewhat prolonged nerve conduction observed probably does not have any physiological significance.[116]

It has been reported that the plasma epinephrine is either decreased[99] or increased[44,45] in hypothermia. If the concentration of epinephrine administered in hypothermia is increased, it should indicate a longer lifetime. The secretion of epinephrine is completely interrupted when the body temperature is below 17 C.[70]

It has been suggested that a study of hormones, particularly catecholamines, is of importance for open heart surgery combined with hypothermia.[99] Administration of epinephrine increases the incidence of fibrillation.[3,27]

Local hypothalamic cooling in unanesthetized baboons[31] leads to cold defense responses which include the increased urinary secretion of both epinephrine and norepinephrine.

It is possible that the depletion of the epinephrine contents in the adrenals[23,84] causes the inability to rewarm spontaneously after a long-lasting profound hypothermia. Adrenalectomized hibernators do not enter into hibernation. Once cooled they cannot arouse from hypothermia.[89,109,110] It is still unknown why the animals survive after being rewarmed from a prolonged hypothermia (body temperature 15 C) lasting 5 to 6 hours (biological survival),[87] but die during rewarming if this same hypothermia lasts 6 hours or longer (clinical survival).[86,88]

The differential physiological effects of cooling on hormonal action were described by Agid and his collaborators. Epinephrine administered to rats cooled to a body temperature of 17 C has a hyperglycemic action. Glucagon, whose mode of action is similar to epinephrine, has no biochemical effect at this low body temperature.[1] The hyperglycemia observed in hypothermia is brought on by an increased adrenal activity[73] during the initial stages of cooling.

The plasma corticosteroid level, induced by surface or core cooling,[16,18,31,37] is increased in hypothermia or in accidental hypothermia.[98] However, there are reports of an unchanged[8] or decreased level of adrenocortical hormones.[48]

Administration of renin or of angiotensin II increases the arterial blood pressure in hypothermia.[53]

After migration to the scrotum, the testes of mammals need a low temperature. This low temperature is not necessary for normal testis functioning in birds.[120]

Hypothermia was successfully used to reduce the amount of blood loss in early puerperal periods.[66]

Summary

Initial phases of cooling affect endocrine glands, in most cases decreasing their function, but leaving secretion of some hormones unchanged or even increased. Profound cooling interrupts the function of the endocrine glands temporarily. After rewarming all functions eventually return to a normal level.

BIBLIOGRAPHY

1. Agid R, Murat JC: Action differentielle de la temperature sur l'activite hyperglycemiante du glucagon et de l'adrenaline: Etude chez le rat en hypothermie profonde. C R Acad Sc 270:3272–3275, 1970
2. Andersson B, Ekman L, Gale CC, et al: Blocking of the thyroidal response to cold by local warming of the preoptic region. Acta Physiol Scand 56:94–96, 1962
3. Angelakos ET, Daniels JB: Effect of catecholamine infusions on lethal hypothermic temperatures in dogs. J Appl Physiol 26:194–196, 1969
4. Barker CF, Peskin GW: The effect of general and local intestinal hypothermia on the production and absorption of ammonia. Surgery 59:1092–1098, 1966
5. Bard P, Woods JW: Thyroid activity during hypothermia produced without the use of drugs. Bull Johns Hopkins Hosp 107:163–174, 1960
6. Barker CF, Nance FC, Nelson HM, et al: Local hypothermia for the control of bleeding in the large bowel and measurements of inferior mesenteric blood flow during colonic cooling. Am J Surg 109:84–88, 1965
7. Barker CF, Nance FC, Peskin GW: Regional hypothermia for massive bleeding. Surgery 56:624–627, 1964

8. Barlow G, Spurr GB, Bowe RL: Circulating levels of 17-hydroxycorticosteroid in prolonged hypothermia. J Appl Physiol 14:777–780, 1959
9. Baum D, Dillard DH, Porte D: Inhibition of insulin release in infants undergoing deep hypothermic cardiovascular surgery. N Engl J Med 279:1309–1314, 1968
10. Baum D, Gale CC, Dillard DH: Plasma growth hormone in the infant undergoing deep hypothermic cardiovascular surgery. Proc Soc Exp Biol Med 128:70–75, 1968
11. Baum D, Porte D: Alpha-adrenergic inhibition of immunoreactive insulin release during deep hypothermia. Am J Physiol 221:303–311, 1971
12. Belzer FO, Ashby BS, Dunphy JE: Twenty-four hour and seventy-two hour preservation of canine kidneys. Lancet 11:536–539, 1967
13. Bigelow WG, Sidlofsky S: Hormones in hypothermia. Br Med Bull 17:56–60, 1961
14. Blackard WG, Nelson NC, Labat JA: Insulin secretion in hypothermic dog. Am J Physiol 212:1185–1187, 1967
15. Boerema WJ, Catchpole BN, Finlay-Jones LR: The prophylactic value of cooling strangulated herniae locally. Br J Surg 57:306–308, 1970
16. Boulouard R, Buzalkov R: Influence de la mise en hypothermie et du rechauffement sur le taux des hormones cortico-surrenaliennes du plasma chez le rat. Ann Endocrinol 24:157–167, 1963
17. Boylan JW, Hong SK: Regulation of renal function in hypothermia. Am J Physiol 211:1371–1378, 1966
18. Carveth SW, McGoon DC, Mattox VR, et al: Effect of surgery with and without whole body perfusion on plasma 17-hydroxycorticosteroids in man. Ann Surg 161:105–111, 1965
19. Cockett ATK: The kidney and regional hypothermia. Surgery 50:905–910, 1961
20. Couch NP, Wilson RE, Hager EB, et al: Transplantation of cadaver kidneys: Experience with 21 cases. Surgery 59:183–188, 1966
21. Crampton RS, Coli JR, Yerys P, et al: Experience with gastric hypothermia for active upper gastrointestinal tract hemorrhage. Surgery 55:607–611, 1964
22. Curry DL, Curry KP: Hypothermia and insulin secretion. Endocrinology 87:750–755, 1970
23. Davidovic V, Petrovic VM: Effect of prolonged hypothermia on spontaneous warming and on the catecholamine level in the adrenal glands and the heart of rats. J Physiol (Paris) 63:36A, 1971
24. Drobner VL: Capsule for local hypothermia of the kidney. Eksp Khir Anesthesiol 16:81–82, 1971
25. Eichelter P: Influence of hypothermia on the course of experimental pancreatitis. Arch Surg 94:280–285, 1967
26. Eichelter P, Worthington GS: The influence of hypothermia on pancreatic secretion and blood flow. Arch Surg 96:883–886, 1968
27. Emiroglu F: Fibrillation in normothermic and hypothermic rabbit heart and effect of adrenaline. Arch Int Physiol Biochem 73:55–64, 1965
28. Fegen JP, Albert DJ, Persky L: Regional hypothermia in acute renal ischaemia: A re-evaluation of the optimal renal temperature. Br J Urol 42:273–276, 1970

29. Franks DP, Cockett AT: Local hypothermia of urinary bladder during transurethral surgery. Anesthesiology 22:15–19, 1961
30. Freeman RM: The role of magnesium in the pathogenesis of uremic hypothermia. Clin Res 17:52, 1969
31. Gale CC, Jobin M, Proppe DW, et al: Endocrine thermoregulatory responses to local hypothalamic cooling in unanesthetized baboons. Am J Physiol 219: 193–201, 1970
32. Garrell SL: Hypothermia in uremia. N Engl J Med 283:1001, 1970
33. Gaskell P, Hoeppner DL: The effect of local temperature on the reactivity to noradrenaline of digital vessels. Can J Physiol Pharmacol 45:93–102, 1966
34. Gil-Rodriguez JA, O'Gorman P: Renal function during profound hypothermia. Br J Anaesth 42:557, 1970
35. Goriunov VG: Renal hypothermia and its application in urologic surgery. Urol Nefrol 33:74–78, 1968
36. Gowen GF, Lindenmuth WW: General hypothermia for managing gastrointestinal hemorrhage. JAMA 175:29–33, 1961
37. Grad B, Rafizadeh F: Plasma corticosterone, hemoglobin, creatinine and blood urea nitrogen levels, and urinary corticosteroid amounts in mice made hypothermic by exposure to 10°C. Can J Physiol Pharmacol 49:657–665, 1971
38. Hanley HG: Renal hypothermia in complicated nephrolithomy. J Urol 99: 517–520, 1968
39. Hanley HG: An improved system of local renal hypothermia. Br J Urol 42: 540–544, 1970
40. Herman G, Karsh HB, Kauvar AJ: Gastric cooling in the management of massive upper gastrointestinal hemorrhage. Gastroenterology 47:513–516, 1964
41. Herrmann TJ, Turcotte JG: Preservation of canine kidneys. Arch Surg 98: 121–127, 1969
42. Hinshaw LB, Masucci FD, Brake CM, et al: Renal vascular response to hypothermia. Proc Exp Biol Med 118:623–627, 1965
43. Hoffenberg R, Louw JH, Voss TJ: Thyroidectomy under hypothermia in a pregnant patient with thyroid crisis. Lancet 2:687–689, 1961
44. Holobut W: Content of catechol hormones: Adrenaline and noradrenaline in peripheral blood in moderate hypothermia. Acta Physiol Pol 14:563–572, 1963
45. Holobut W, Stazka W: Variations de la teneur en adrenaline et noradrenaline du plasma au cours de l'hypothermie et de l'etat de chock chez le chien. Abst 22 Int Congr Physiol Sci 483, Leiden, 1962
46. Hong SK, Boylan JW: Renal concentrating operation in hypothermic dogs. Am J Physiol 196:1150–1154, 1959
47. Hubbard TB: A method of gastric hypothermia. Surgery 59:670–672, 1966
48. Hume DH, Egdahl RH: Effect of hypothermia and of cold exposure on adrenal cortical and medullary secretion. Ann NY Acad Sci 80:435–444, 1959
49. Humphries AL, Russell R, Stoddard LD, et al: Three-day kidney perfusion: Perfusion of kidneys with hypothermic, diluted blood or plasma. Surgery 63: 646–652, 1968
50. Humphries AL, Russell R, Stoddard L, et al: Successful five-day kidney preservation. Perfusion with hypothermic, diluted plasma. Invest Urol 5: 609–619, 1968

51. Hunter J, Haist RE: A study of blood pressure responses during hypothermia in hypophysectomized rats. Can J Physiol Pharmacol 42:209–215, 1964
52. Hunter J, Haist RE: A study of the effects of pitressin and serotonin in the maintenance of blood pressure in the hypophysectomized hypothermic rat. Can J Physiol Pharmacol 42:217–224, 1964
53. Hunter J, Hurley DA: The influence of respiratory and renal factors on cardiac activity during deep hypothermia. Can J Biochem Physiol 41:551–560, 1963
54. Iversen JG: Peritoneal dialysis of cooled rats. J Physiol 210:23P, 1970
55. James PM, Michie A: Local hypothermia for massive renal hemorrhage. Surgery 56:1134–1136, 1964
56. Jones WR, Politano VA: The effects of renal artery occlusion on renal function under normothermia and regional hypothermia. J Urol 89:535–540, 1963
57. Kanter GS: Renal clearance of sodium and potassium in hypothermia. Can J Biochem Physiol 40:113–122, 1962
58. Kanter GS: Bicarbonate excretion during hypothermia. Can J Biochem Physiol 41:91–96, 1963
59. Karim F, Reza H: Effect of induced hypothermia and rewarming on renal hemodynamics in anesthetized dogs. Life Sci 9:1153–1163, 1970
60. Keatinge WR: Mechanism of adrenergic stimulation of mammalian arteries and its failure at low temperatures. J Physiol 174:184–205, 1964
61. Kirpekar SM, Prat JC, Yamamoto H: Dependence of norepinephrine (NE) release from spleen on metabolic energy. Fed Proc 28:415, 1969
62. Kolde H, Weidemann H: Anwendung der kontrollierten Hypothermie bei schwerster Peritonitis. Chirurgie 26:179–181, 1955
63. Kowalewski K, Jirsch DW, Kolodej A: Secretory function of canine stomach in vitro after prolonged hypothermic and hyperbaric preservation. Surg Gynecol Obstet 136:225–233, 1973
64. Ladaga LG, Nabseth DC, Besznyak I, et al: Preservation of canine kidneys by hypothermia and hyperbaric oxygen. Long-term survival of autografts following 24-hour storage. Ann Surg 163:553–558, 1966
65. Lambotte L: Persistence of active and passive ionic transport during low-temperature liver preservation. Surgery 73:8–14, 1973
66. Landau IaM: Use of local hypothermia for reducing the amount of blood loss in the placental and early puerperal periods. Akush Ginekol (Moskva) 47:76, 1971
67. Lokkegaard H, Gyrd-Hansen N, Iversen-Hansen R, et al: Kidney preservation with pulsatile and non-pulsatile hypothermic serum perfusion. Acta Med Scand 188:245–255, 1970
68. Madsen PO, Bohlman DC, Madsen RE: Local hypothermia during transurethral surgery. Anesth Analg 44:734–736, 1965
69. Makin GS, Howard JM: Hyperbaric oxygenation and profound hypothermia to preserve canine kidneys. Arch Surg 91:568–571, 1965
70. Malmejac J, Malmejac C, Fredenucci R, et al: Resistance du system adrenalino-secreteur a l'ischemie sours hypothermie controlee a 17°–18°C. C R Soc Biol (Paris) 153:1776–1778, 1959
71. Manax WG, Bloch JH, Largiader F, et al: Organ perfusion before transplantation with particular reference to the kidney. Surgery 57:528–534, 1965
72. Mark JBD, Gaisford WD, Knauer CM, et al: Further experience with general

body hypothermia in the treatment of massive gastrointestinal hemorrhgage. Am J Surg 116:286–292, 1968
73. McComiskey DM, Beaton JR: A note on metabolic effects of hypothermia in adrenalectomized rats. Can J Biochem Physiol 41:2038–2041, 1963
74. Metzner MJ: Simplified renal hypothermia as adjunct to conservative renal surgery. Br J Urol 44:126–127, 1972
75. Mitchell JW, Myers GE, Hutchinson WJ, et al: An experimental and analytical investigation of an internal cooling technique. J Appl Physiol 28:695–699, 1970
76. Mito M, Tamaki A, Kin T, et al: Experimental studies on differential hypothermia of the liver. J Surg Res 5:207–212, 1965
77. Morales P, Carbery W, Morello A, et al: Alterations in renal function during hypothermia in man. Ann Surg 145:488–499, 1957
78. Moss G: Systemic hypothermia via gastric cooling. Arch Surg 92:80–82, 1966
79. Moy RM: Renal function in the hibernating ground squirrel *Spermophilus columbianus*. Am J Physiol 220:747–753, 1971
80. Munday KA, Noble AR: Renin secretion in the hypothermic dog. J Physiol 206:38P–39P, 1970
81. Palmer JM, Connolly JE: Intrarenal arteriovenous fistula: Surgical excision under selective renal hypothermia with kidney survival. J Urol 96:599–605, 1966
82. Palmer JM, Guernsey JM, Connolly JE: An experimental study of selective renal hypothermia. Am J Surg 106:224–232, 1963
83. Pegg DE, Green CJ: Renal preservation by hypothermic perfusion. Cryobiology 10:56–66, 1973
84. Petrovic VM, Davidovic V: Effet de l'hiberation et de l'hypothermie prolongee sur le rapport adrenaline-noradrenaline dans le surrenal chez le spermophile. J Physiol (Paris) 58:589, 1966
85. Petrov BA, Korenev NN: Local gastric hypothermia in gastroduodenal hemorrhage. Surgery 67:574–576, 1970
86. Popovic V: Lethargic hypothermia in hibernators and nonhibernators. Ann N Y Acad Sci 80:320–331, 1959
87. Popovic V: Survival time of hypothermic white rats (15°C) and ground squirrels (10°C). Am J Physiol 199:463–466, 1960
88. Popovic V: Physiological characteristics of rats and ground squirrels during prolonged lethargic hypothermia. Am J Physiol 199:467–471, 1960
89. Popovic V, Vidovic V: Les glandes surrenales et le sommeil hibernal. Arch Sci Biol (Belgrade) 33:17, 1951
90. Reisner GS, Kerby C: A simple hypothermic hyperbaric perfusion system for kidney storage. N Z J Surg 40:91–93, 1970
91. Rider JA, Puletti EJ, Moeller HC: Biochemical and pathologic changes after gastric hypothermia. Clin Res 12:107, 1964
92. Romanov AI: Use of hypothermia in the treatment of acute pancreatis. Vestn Khir 104:43–45, 1970
93. Saakov BA: Secretory activity of the hypothalamo-hypophysis-adrenal system in hypothermia. Biull Eksp Biol Med 67:25–28, 1969
94. Sarajas HS, Karlsson LK, Hirvonen JI: Subcommissural and hypothalamo-hypophyseal neurosecretion in relation to fluid and electrolyte imbalances in hypothermic rat. Ann Acad Sci Fenn Ser A 106/9:1–10, 1967

95. Schiosuhwili TI: Local hypothermia during surgery of a "dry" kidney. Z Urol Nephrol 64:503–507, 1971
96. Scott DF, Morley AR, Swinney J: Canine renal preservation following hypothermic perfusion and subsequent function. Br J Surg 56:688–691, 1969
97. Slotkoff LM, Eisner GM, Lilienfield LS: Sodium and water reabsorption in the cold kidney. Circulation 28:806–807, 1963
98. Sprunt JG, Maclean D, Browning MCK: Plasma corticosteroid levels in accidental hypothermia. Lancet 1:324–326, 1970
99. Stepanyan YP, Bukharin VA, Chernyavskaya MA: Investigation of catecholamines in various organs of dogs under conditions of deep hypothermia. Bull Exp Biol Med 9:56–60, 1963
100. Sterling WA, Pierce JC, Hutcher NE, et al: A comparison of hypothermic preservation with hypothermic pulsatile perfusion in paired human kidneys. Surg Forum 22:229–230, 1971
101. Sundsten JW, Matheson GK: Changes in "core" temperature and thyroid activity in response to hypothalamic cooling in the baboon (*Papio doguera*). Anat Rec 154:429, 1966
102. Terblanche J, Isaacson LC, Eales L, et al: Renal function during and immediately after profound hypothermia. Surgery 50:869–876, 1961
103. Trinkle JK, Franz JL, Furman RW, et al: Circulatory arrest during deep hypothermia, induced by peritoneal dialysis. Arch Surg 103:648–649, 1971
104. Turner MD, Hicks FF, Hicks JS, et al: The use of metabolic inhibitors in hypothermic kidney storage. J Surg Res 9:665–669, 1969
105. Vanlerenberghe J, Bar N: Action de l'hypothermie sur la cholerese du foie de rat perfuse. J Physiol (Paris) 55:352–353, 1963
106. Vanlerenberghe J, Trupin-Bar N, Guislain R, et al: Action de l'hypothermie sur la fonction biliaire. J Physiol (Paris) 59:111–138, 1967
107. Van Zyl JJW, Van Zyl JA, de Klerk JN, et al: A new hyperbaric hypothermic kidney preservation unit. Invest Urol 6:89–93, 1968/69
108. Veghelyi PV, Kemeny TT, Zsinka AT, et al: Pancreatic function in hypothermia. Nature 200:478, 1963
109. Vidovic V, Popovic V: Role of the adrenal and the thyroid during wintersleep of the ground squirrel. Arch Sci Biol (Belgrade) 5:171–189, 1953
110. Vidovic V, Popovic V: Studies on the adrenal and thyroid glands of the ground squirrel during hibernation. J Endocrinol 11:125–133, 1954
111. Wangensteen OH, Root HD, Jenson CB, et al: Depression of gastric secretion and digestion by gastric hypothermia: Its clinical use in massive hematemesis. Surgery 44:265–274, 1958
112. Wangensteen SL: Intragastric cooling for upper gastrointestinal hemorrhage. Surg Clin N Am 42:1171–1180, 1962
113. Weiss M: Rein et hypothermie. Actualites nephrologiques de l'hopital Necker. Paris, Publ Flammarion, 1962, pp 201–236
114. Weiss M, Guery J, Bidet L: A propos du fonctionnement renal apres les operations a coeur ouvert sous hypothermie profonde et arret circulatoire. Ann Chir Thorac Cardiovasc 1:1–8, 1962
115. Weiss M, Hinglais J, Bidet L: Contribution a l'etude du fonctionnement renal sous hypothermie profonde. I. Caracteres des urines au cours d'une hypothermie a 18°C associee a une circulation extra-corporelle. Rev Fr Etud Clin Biol 7:744–747, 1962

116. Wennmalm A, Hedqvist P, Stjarne L: Effects of hypothermia on norepinephrine release and effector response in isolated perfused cat spleen. Circ Res 27:39–44, 1970
117. Wickham JE: Regional renal hypothermia. Ann R Coll Surg Engl 48:99–113, 1971
118. Wickham JEA: A system of regional renal hypothermia. Br J Surg 58:866, 1971
119. Wickham JEA, Mathur VK: Hypothermia in the conservative surgery of renal disease. Br J Urol 43:648–657, 1971
120. Williams DD: A histological study of the effects of subnormal temperature on the testis of the fowl. Anat Rec 130:225–242, 1958
121. Willis JS: Cold resistance of kidney cells of mammalian hibernators cation transport vs respiration. Am J Physiol 214:923–928, 1968
122. Woods JE: Successful three to seven day preservation of canine kidneys. Arch Surg 102:614–616, 1971
123. Woolf PD, Hollander CS, Mitsuma T, et al: Accidental hypothermia: Endocrine function during recovery. J Clin Endocrinol Metab 34:460–466, 1972

6

Nervous System

"Slow down, look around."

EXCITATION AND METABOLISM OF NERVOUS TISSUE

During cooling the conductivity of an isolated nerve decreases and eventually disappears at a body temperature of about 5 to 10 C. This decrease in conduction velocity during cooling is roughly linear.[39,46] The neurons seem to contain less chloride in hypothermia, indicating a relative repolarization.[40] Localized cooling of the cuneate nucleus of the synaptic transmission to a temperature of 25 to 30 C greatly increases field potential. The excitability of the postganglionic fibers is increased during cooling.[82] Thus during cooling one observes first hyperresponsiveness and hyperreflexia, then later, reversible descending CNS paralysis. The synaptic transmission is also reduced during cooling because of an increased synaptic delay.[10] However, there are reports that the excitability of both pre- and postsynaptic fibers is decreased during cooling.[11] In any case a profound decrease is observed when the temperature is reduced below 20C.[10]

The reflexes that disappear last during progressive cooling are usually those which appear first during the ontogenetical development. The cortical functions are abolished first.[134] Locomotion, voluntary movements, and other processes associated with higher nervous functions disappear before vision and hearing, then cold narcosis takes over. Corneal and papillary reflexes disappear last.

During the initial phase of cooling the EEG does not change except for occasional appearance of epileptic electric potentials.[69] Below a temperature of 30 C the EEG changes proportionately with the body temperature.[16,41] The EEG amplitude at a body temperature of 22 C is only 10 percent of that observed at a normal body temperature. In rabbits, at a brain temperature below 22 C, one observes only low voltage activity.[144] Even during localized intracerebral cooling, one observes low-voltage cortical activity.[84] The various types of electrical potentials are affected differentially during brain cooling.[22] The effect of pCO_2 on the EEC is greatly decreased in hypothermia.[73]

The brain becomes isoelectric at a temperature of 23 C.[79] During cooling the isoelectrical point is found at the same body temperature (around 20 C) in nonhibernators[117] as in hibernators. Profound hypothermia brings a state of cold or physical anesthesia. In children the EEG disappears at a lower body temperature than in adults,[27] suggesting that the same low body temperature causes fewer physiological changes. This physiological difference is probably the reason that young animals and children can tolerate profound and prolonged hypothermia better than adults.

The NA–K transport in the nervous tissues of mammalian hibernators is decreased less by low temperatures than that of the nonhibernators.[61] Perhaps this is why the excitability of the nerves and the muscles is still present at a very low body temperature in hibernators while in nonhibernators it does not exist. Hibernators can survive lower body temperatures.

Immediately after rewarming, the K content in the brain of rats cooled to 0 C is decreased while the content of Na and H_2O is increased. Twelve hours later the K, Na, and H_2O contents are normal again. These changes, found immediately after cooling, are similar to those which occur in cerebral edema and can probably be explained by a temperature-induced preferential inhibition of the active transport.[137] High-energy phosphates and glycogen of the brain are maintained or even elevated in hypothermic animals.[158,175] At low temperatures the decrease in the ATP concentration of the brain does not exceed 10 percent. Hypothermia protects the ATP concentration of the brain during circulatory arrest.[57,79] After a long-lasting circulatory arrest in hypothermia, there is 3 to 4 times more cerebral ATP than after a normothermic arrest.[79] Contrary to these findings in hibernating hibernators the Na^+ and K^+ of the brain stay unchanged when compared to the normothermic state.[61] The same applies to Na–K–ATPase of the brain in hibernators.[62]

Hypothermia increases concentration of glutamin and aspartic acid[158] and increases the brain content of γ-aminobutyrate (GABA) also with a concomitant fall in the brain glutamate. Since similar changes are encountered in states such as natural hibernation or in hypoxia, it seems possible that the hypothermia-induced alterations in the brain amino acid pools are traceable to depressed brain metabolism per se.[116] In hypothermic rats the brain level of glucose as well as lactates is increased.[143] The rate of cerebrospinal fluid formation in profound hypothermia is decreased.[53]

After a long-lasting circulatory arrest in profound hypothermia and eventual rewarming the electrical activity of the brain is not changed.[9,58,60,99,146]

Baby ground squirrels were cooled to a body temperature of 4 to 8 C below freezing point. At this supercooled state their respiration and electrical or mechanical activity of the heart are absent. Still these animals have survived at this body temperature for 8 to 12 hours. After reanimation the animals did not show any ill effects from the profound cooling.[131]

After rewarming, an isolated and supercooled cat's brain (at a temperature of −20 C for 6 days and in 15% glycerol) shows spontaneous electrical discharges,[152] indicating great resistance of the cold brain to anoxia.

During the cooling of the brain to temperatures of 37, 27, and 20 C, the oxygen requirements of the brain decrease linearly with the decreasing temperature at a rate of 5 percent for each degree.[6] The oxygen consumption and blood flow of the brain are decreased to 50 percent at a temperature of 18 C. A 10 C decrease in temperature of the brain leads to a 50 percent decrease in metabolism,[95] which is similar to the metabolic changes in the rest of the body. Q_{10} of the brain is 2.2, similar to other tissues.[95]

During cooling, the cerebral blood flow decreases at about the same rate as the oxygen consumption of the brain.[14,70,164] The brain appears to be perfused well until a temperature of 12 C or even lower.[77] As in normothermia, carbon dioxide induces cerebral vascular dilatation in hypothermia.

Brain metabolism has been studied after tracheal occlusion at 15 C body temperature (induced hypothermia). The survival time (ST_{50} judged on the basis of the duration of the postocclusion respiratory movements) was 9, 24, and 54 minutes, respectively, in adult rats, ground squirrels and neonatal rats. In adult rats and ground squirrels the revival time was 25 and 51 minutes, respectively.[12]

The volume of the brain decreases during cooling.[45,141] It appears that extracellular space of the brain (impedance technique) is decreased below a brain temperature of 20 C.[77] There are several reports that hypothermia protects against cerebral edema[38] or cerebral ischemia.[124,133,156] Contrary to this, however, there are indications of cold swelling of the brain.[32,68,91] This might happen in profoundly cooled rats, even during an extracorporeal circulatory support.[90] Higher nervous activity is decreased in rats cooled to 20 C.[8]

During cooling of the body the cerebrospinal pressure is also decreased. Experimentally induced high intracranial pressure in dogs can be decreased by brain cooling.[89]

Profound cooling of rats does not lead to any histologic changes of the brain or peripheral nerves.[24]

The "blood–brain barrier," probably a series of morphologic and functional components that determine the rate of uptake of substances by the mammalian brain, is preserved intact during cooling, but partial disruption of this system occurs in profound hypothermia.[56] This disruption appears to occur at a specific "critical" brain temperature except in hibernators, which can withstand the lowering of the brain temperature to 0 C. During localized microwave rewarming of segments of the brain, the blood–brain barrier is protected by generalized mild hypothermia.[154]

Summary

During cooling the metabolic excitability and the conductivity of nervous tissue decrease in the same fashion as in the other tissues of the hypothermic body. Eventually one nervous process after the other temporarily ceases. Phylogenetically the youngest reflexes disappear first, others disappear at lower body temperatures, and cold narcosis then takes over. During cooling the cerebral circulation follows the metabolic needs. Perfusion of the brain seems adequate until brain temperatures become extremely low. After rewarming, all processes of the brain return to the normal level, some of them probably with a slight delay.

PROTECTIVE ROLE OF COOLING

The nervous system is more susceptible to anoxia than any other tissue or organ system in the body. The nervous system cannot develop any oxygen debt. The total permissible circulatory arrest of the brain is determined by this anoxic intolerance and is rather short. There are very few early findings that hypothermia might induce brain damage and change in reaction time,[25] but new experimental or clinical research has shown no brain impairment even with deepest cooling associated with long circulatory arrest and disappearance of EEC tracings. When the brain is cooled, there is a decrease in the oxygen consumption and a greater protection against anoxia during the decreased circulation or even during 1 to 2 hours of complete arrest.[31,43,106,167] Cooling to a temperature of 28 C expands the safe circulatory arrest from 7 to 90 minutes.[122] It is interesting to note that the biological survival of the brain is almost the same for all species of mammals, as well as for man.

The protective role of hypothermia is demonstrated further in preserving energy-rich compounds in the brain[83] and in the treatment of asphyxia neonatorum.[97] Profound cooling permits young animals to survive anoxic exposure several times longer. The longest anoxic survival in neonates is at a body temperature of 15 C.[96] However, there are reports that shallow cooling decreases pO_2 of arterial blood in babies.[48,98,151] It appears that this applies to old animals or old patients as well.[72] Hypothermia protects against mortality in experimental brain injury, even if it is applied 3 hours after the injury.[142] Hypothermia reduces postinjury lethargy[29] but it does not diminish an already established brain damage.[37]

The spinal cord tolerates circulatory interruption about 6 times longer than the brain.

Negovskii and most Russian scientists are firmly convinced that the cause of death in posthypothermia (circulatory collapse) is induced during the cooling of the nervous system.

Hypothermia permits expansion of the short and unstable state observed just before death. This complicated state is the subject of many studies by the Russian physiologist Negovskii and his colleagues. Their goal is to study the mechanisms leading to death and the factors that help to postpone death. In other words, to study the basic differences between life and death, to understand their relationship, and to find effective methods for reanimation. The brain still remains at the forefront of their attention. Negovskii believes that the most characteristic features of the process of dying bear neurological character and that adaptation during dying takes place as a result of the nervous system.[102–105] The main probelm, he believes, is to prevent the brain from dying, and to maintain its functions during resuscitation. For this reason Russian scientists try to keep reinforced circulation to the brain during hypothermic open-heart surgery.[166]

Summary

Seldom is the protective role of hypothermia demonstrated better than during the cooling of nervous tissue, and especially the brain. The total permissible circulatory arrest of the brain is increased from 4 to 5 minutes to 1 or 2 hours when the brain is profoundly cooled, but a shallow cooling of the brain offers a much shorter, safe permissible circulatory arrest.

LOCALIZED BRAIN COOLING

Until recently in order to cool the brain of an organism or of a patient, the whole body had to be cooled. Cooling of the brain is useful only when the brain temperature is rather low. For this reason core-cooling techniques had to be used, but the core cooling is rather complex. Thus in order to use the protective effects of hypothermia during a brain intervention, two surgical teams had to be used, one of them involving neurosurgeons. Recently several new techniques have been developed for localized brain cooling. The body is kept only slightly hypothermic while the brain is profoundly cooled. There are several successful brain-cooling techniques used at the present time.

During the last 15 years a simple brain-cooling technique was developed[20,23,42,44,85,125,162,170–172,174] which induces fast and profound reduction in the brain temperature to 5 to 15 C[59] with only a small reduction in the core body temperature to 32 C. During this localized brain cooling, induced by carotid blood cooling through a heat exchanger, a rather long-lasting brain intervention can be performed. Some of them offer induction of 1-hour-long circulatory arrest.[59] If necessary, generalized body cooling, which is always brought forth by carotid blood cooling, can be prevented by concomitant gastric rewarming.[65] Infusion of small increments of catecholamines speeds the brain cooling. During the progressive lowering of the brain temperature the mean arterial pressure and cardiac rate decrease gradually.[168] At an intracerebral temperature of 15 C the mean arterial pressure is decreased to 50 percent of its normal value. The oxygen tension in the brain tissue of cooled animals stays at an unchanged value until a body temperature of 10 C is reached. With systemic warming of the brain, cardiovascular parameters rapidly return to basal levels.

White believes that his technique of preferential brain cooling offers the best protection to the higher centers of the CNS.[170] During preferential cooling of the brain, cerebral viability is maintained for several hours.[172,174]

Cooling changes the cerebral deposition of drugs[21] and profound cooling modifies the blood–brain barrier in experimental animals.[154]

Using the carotid perfusion technique of brain cooling in dogs we have shown that parts of the brain designated as "tumors" can be rewarmed by microwave energy to normothermic or slightly hyperthermic temperatures and that such rewarming increases the circulation through this part of the brain as well as the embedding of some anticancer drugs.

Microwave energy is used for brain tumor rewarming. However, much increased power of radiofrequency currents leads to localized thermal damage of brain in hypothermic animals.[155] In normothermic animals the secondary spread of necrosis is observed complicated with edema leading to unpredictable enlargement of lesions.[155] Small portions of the brain can be cooled—or rewarmed—by Peltier biothermodes also.[66]

Wolfson's washout cooling technique[19,20,55,159] consists of interruption of the circulation induced by ventricular fibrillation and of a cold saline infusion into carotid arteries. The technique is very promising and was used experimentally as well as clinically. Preferential brain cooling does not leave any neurological damage even after 60 minutes of circulatory arrest.[159] The preferential infusion cooling of the brain can be done with blood, though the use of ice-cold saline seems more beneficial.[74]

Other brain-cooling techniques encompass the intracranial (extravascular) perfusion for brain cooling in patients.[108–110,115] This technique is used for the surgical removal of neoplasms and in the management of cerebral aneurysms.[115] Craniocerebral hypothermia is beneficial also after injury of the brain,[176] even when applied several hours later. Russian scientists often use generalized hypothermia of a moderate degree with selective brain cooling of 7 to 10 C deeper for experimental or clinical work.[165,166]

Summary

Many organs or organ systems may be preferentially cooled to a very low temperature, leaving the rest of the organism normothermic or slightly hypothermic. In this way the complicated systemic perfusion of the body can be replaced by a more shallow surface cooling. Several successful brain-cooling techniques are described in the text of this chapter.

LOCALIZED SPINAL CORD COOLING

Spinal cord hypothermia has been introduced recently. Extravascular cold perfusion is used for fast cooling of the spinal cord.[3,5,71,78,81,107,109,113,114,145,148] This selective decrease in the temperature of the spinal cord can last 4 hours[4] without inducing any neurologic sequelae.

Spinal cord cooling is effective in arresting the development of severe neurological changes even if delayed for 3 to 4 hours after a severe spinal cord injury.[1,47] During this localized cooling the sensory blockade is observed at a temperature of 13 C.[3] The cardiovascular changes that are observed during localized spinal cord cooling are rather small.[5] Selective cooling of the spinal cord suppresses vasomotor activity and induces a decrease in the blood pressure and in the heart rate.[149] Spinal cord hypothermia activates the spinal vasomotor efferents and changes the blood pressure values.[147]

This technique proved to be useful in the treatment of impact injury to the spinal cord,[1,2,76] though there are reports that hypothermia does not help in experimental impact injury work done on rabbits.[115] Muscle spasticity in multiple sclerosis can also be decreased by this technique.[112] Local hypothermia of the spinal cord relieves spasticity and rigidity of cerebral palsy.[111] Spinal cord hypothermia has been used successfully for removal of spinal tumors in patients.[113]

Pain also can be controlled by cold subarachnoid saline injection.[76,86,135] The pain relief was very swift except in neoplastic patients where it lasted only temporarily.[135]

Localized spinal cooling appears to be more beneficial than steroid treatment.[47] However, there are a few reports indicating that steroids might be more effective than local spinal hypothermia in patients after traumatic injury.[26]

The technique of preferential cooling of segments of the spinal cord can be used to study the physiological processes of the part of the cord involved. Positive results will permit the eventual application of the knowledge acquired to the clinical problems of spinal cord trauma.

Summary

''Spinal cord hypothermia,'' localized spinal cord cooling, can be induced experimentally or clinically by nonvascular perfusion of parts of the spinal cord. This technique is used experimentally to study the physiological processes of a particular part of the spinal cord that is being cooled and then rewarmed. Clinically this technique is beneficial for treatment of impact injury, removal of spinal tumors, and suppression of pain.

CLINICAL APPLICATION

The usefulness of hypothermia as a means of protecting the brain threatened by anoxia during cerebrovascular surgery is well established. The most common complications in the case of postoperative situations after neurosurgery are brain hemorrhage, increased intracranial pressure, acute brain swelling, and a local cerebral hypoxia. All of these changes are ameliorated by hypothermia.

Hypothermia permits the surgeon to work in a bloodless field. Hypothermia is used as an adjunct to the therapy of head injury. It prevents brain damage due to anoxia by lowering the metabolic requirements of the brain and lowering the intracranial pressure at the same time. The generalized closed-chest core-cooling technique appears to be better than the open-chest method.[94] For this kind of treatment it might be useful to maintain the hypothermia for several days, not just several hours. A longer treatment would not be advisable because of pulmonary congestion, which is always a problem in a long-term generalized cooling.

Smith and Fay were the first to use shallow generalized hypothermia for treatment of pain.[52] In 1945 Fay showed that hypothermia decreases posttraumatic cerebral edema.[51]

Cerebral vascular insufficiency and injury are withstood much better and longer in hypothermia than in normothermia.[140] Furthermore, localized brain cooling is a valuable adjunct to microneurosurgical techniques for thromboendarterectomies of the small cerebral blood vessels. Local postoperative hypothermia of the brain reduces the ill effects after brain tumor removal.[115]

Hypothermia has been used successfully for treatment of intracranial aneurysms.[35,36,54,64,67,80,92–94,136,157,160,161,173] Resistance to surgical trauma is increased and surgical bleeding might be easier to control in hypothermia. Brain edema can be controlled by hypothermia.[124] A 50 percent reduction in epileptic seizures[150] was reported in patients whose brain was cooled to a temperature of 24 C. Even seriously ill patients such as those suffering from hypertension or recent cardiac infarction, can be safely cooled.[28] Furthermore, closed-chest generalized cooling protects the brain during intracerebral surgery and circulatory arrest.[63] Hypothermia is also beneficial in the management of cerebral anemia in children.[87]

However, the technique of hypothermia is used less commonly today in neurosurgery than a few years ago, especially in the United States, the reason being that the technique of surface cooling is time-consuming[30] and does not bring profound brain cooling. The technique of core cooling is complicated and requires a team of general surgeons as well as the neurosurgical team. Furthermore, relatively few clinical centers have accumulated sufficient experience with generalized core-cooling methods to permit the meaningful interpretation and comparison of the data obtained.[79] It appears also that even subtle differences in the perfusion techniques influence the clinical outcome.[123] In England, while some hospitals have interrupted use of hypothermia in neurosurgical practice on a broad basis, other hospitals use hypothermia in 30 percent of the cases for major intracranial operations.[36,88] In Continental Europe and in Russia,[15,33,176] hypothermia is still widely used as an adjunct to neurosurgery. One can hope that simple new localized brain-cooling techniques and localized spinal cord cooling will permit the use of the protective role of hypothermia in neurosurgery on a much broader scale in the near future.

Summary

Generalized surface cooling, though a rather slow process, protects an organism or a patient from brain damage if the body temperature is decreased to 28 to 30 C. A more profound core cooling protects the brain much better during neurosurgical operations, induced trauma, and so on, but requires two surgical teams, one for neurosurgery, another for core cooling. Recently developed simple selective brain-cooling techniques offer the same or better protection of the brain. Cooling of the brain is faster and more profound while the rest of the body stays normothermic or slightly hypothermic (above 30 C). It can be expected that these new techniques will find a more extensive use in the clinical and experimental work in the furture.

LEARNING AND BEHAVIOR IN HYPOTHERMIA

It is an accepted fact that animals trained before cooling perform well after rewarming.[126] Furthermore, experimental animals still display coordinated learned behavior even at a profoundly decreased body temperature,[13,100,128,139,169] though sometimes a short retrograde anmesia was observed induced by cooling.[138] Moreover, an organism in deep hypothermia can acquire a new behavior and learn or perform something new, a fact not known until recently. Previously it was thought that even a shallow hypothermia produced impairments in learning or in the performance abilities of experimental animals. The reason for this conclusion was the inappropriate choice of tests given to the hypothermic animals. It is clear now that motivation plays a more important role in the learning and performance of hypothermic organisms than it does in normothermic organisms. Bar pressing for food and solving maze problems for water or food acquisition are of less interest to hypothermic animals than to normothermic animals. This is why the test chosen is the deciding factor for establishing the presence or absence of learned behavior in animals at low body temperatures. Here are some of the examples that illustrate these facts.

Although it has been established that after cooling to a temperature of 30 C men are still able to vocalize,[52] experimental work failed to show the ability of the animals to learn during hypothermia. Thus cooling prevented mice from solving a water escape test,[49,153] acquiring a new conditioned avoidance response,[50] or learning at a body temperature of 25 C.[34] Furthermore, there were reports of the impairment of negative learning observed in even slightly hypothermic rats[34] and also a changed conditioned reflex activity in

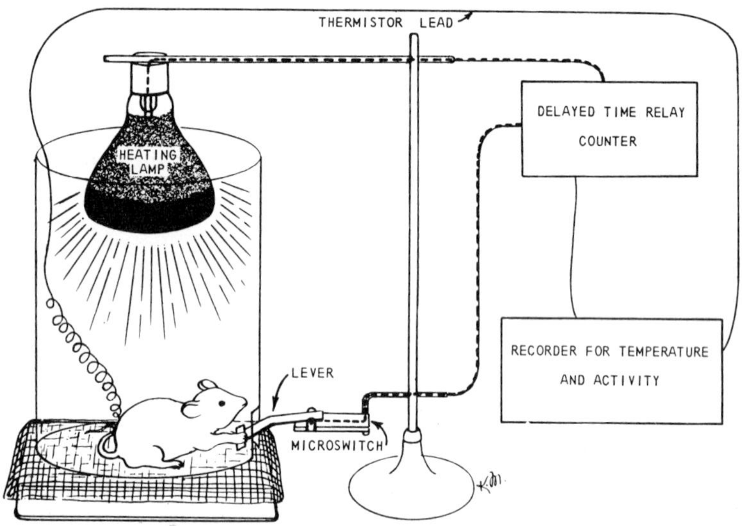

Fig. 6-1. Hypothermic "naive" rats are able to learn to press the lever to obtain the external heat from a lamp placed above the experimental chamber. They learn to press the lever and start to perform earlier than normothermic animals. The animals learn to perform this task even at a body temperature of 25 C.[118,119,121]

dogs[7,75] cooled to a body temperature of 30 C. However, when 30 C hypothermic rats were exposed to a critical situation in which they were strongly motivated, a situation in which they would die if they did not learn to rewarm themselves by accidental bar pressing for external heat, the rats quickly learned this task, 5 to 6 times faster than normothermic rats exposed to the same external cold. The criterion for learning and performance in the experiments was a sudden fourfold increase in bar pressing.[120] The animals were able to learn and perform the same task even at a lower body temperature of 24 to 25 C (Fig. 6-1).[118,119,121] At a somewhat lower body temperature the animals failed to perform. This critical temperature for instrumental acquisition was probably induced by motor incapability of the animals.[101] However, when the rats were "adapted" to hypothermia (several 2–3 hours cooling exposures), they were able to learn this task even at a body temperature of 23 C.[127,129,130] In another group of experiments, when pressing the bar for intracranial self-stimulation of the "pleasure center," the rats perform even at a body temperature of 21 to 22 C. This body temperature is the lowest critical temperature yet described for any acquired behavior.[132] During rewarming, however, the same rats did not press the lever for intracranial self-stimulation until their body temperature reached 35 C (Fig. 6-2).[132] The physiological basis for this striking difference in behavior is still unknown.

Another problem studied was the effect of cooling on behavior of pregnant or nursing rat mothers. The mothers reacted to their litters at a body temperature of 30 C, but not at lower temperatures.[17,18,163]

Summary

Hypothermia does not prevent animals from learning a new behavior or performing something they have learned before cooling. If the motivation is very strong, the animals learn even at a body temperature of 22 to 25 C. This body temperature is only 1 or 2 degrees higher than the critical temperature at which cessation of locomotion and "cold narcosis" are observed.

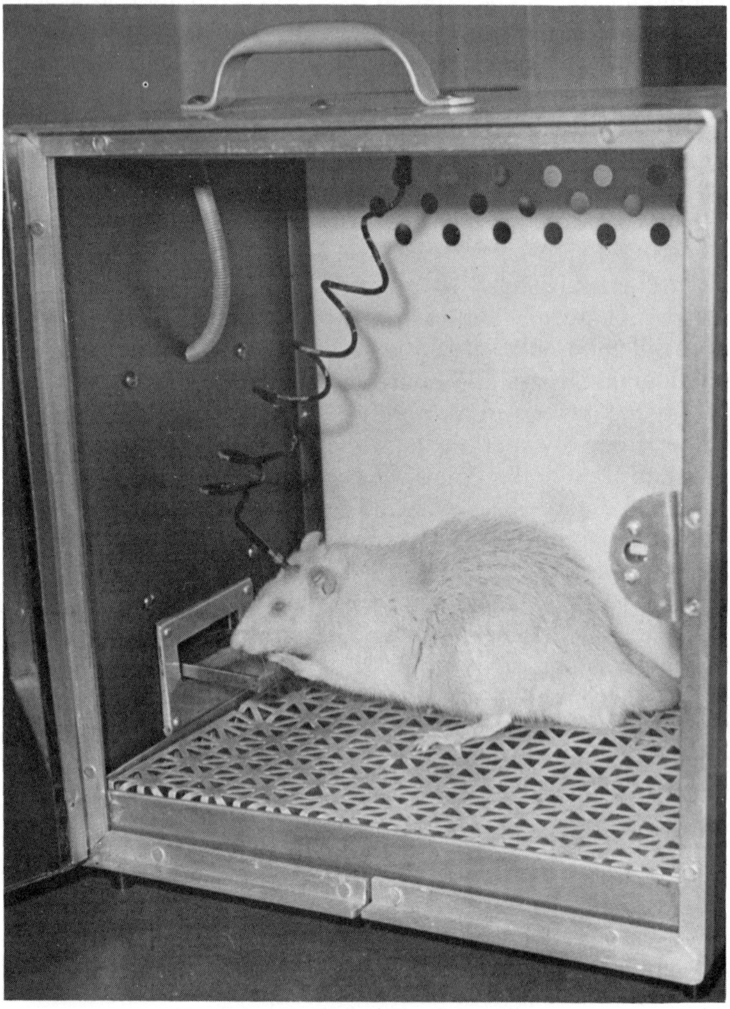

Fig. 6-2. Hypothermic rats press the lever for intracranial self-stimulation of the "pleasure center" even at a body temperature of 21 to 22 C. This body temperature is the lowest "critical temperature" (temperature of cessation) yet described for any acquired behavior.[132]

BIBLIOGRAPHY

1. Albin MS, White RJ, Acosta-Rua G, et al: Study of functional recovery produced by delayed localized cooling after spinal cord injury in primates. J Neurosurg 29:113–120, 1968
2. Albin MS, White RJ, Locke GE: Treatment of spinal cord trauma by selective hypothermic perfusion. Surg Forum 16:423–424, 1965
3. Albin MS, White RJ, Locke GS, et al: Localized spinal cord hypothermia: Anesthetic effects and application to spinal cord injury. Anesth Analg 46: 8–16, 1967
4. Albin MS, White RJ, MacCarty CS: Effects of sustained perfusion cooling of the subarachnoid space. Anesthesiology 24:72–80, 1963
5. Albin MS, White RJ, Yashon D, et al: Effects of localized cooling on spinal cord trauma. J Trauma 9:1000–1008, 1969
6. Aliukhin IS, Kalinina MK: Tissular respiration of the brain during hypothermia. Fiziol Zh (SSSR) 56:19–21, 1970
7. Altukhov GV, Khruleva LN, Gritsyik RI, et al: Reflex reactions and state of certain autonomic functions of white rats in hypothermia. Kosm Biol Med 3: 84–85, 1969
8. Altukhov GV, Kruleva LN, Gritsyik RI, et al: Influence of hypothermia of different degrees and durations on the higher nervous activity and vegetative functions of rats. Zh Vyssh Nerv Deiat 19:788–793, 1969
9. Anabtawi IN, Brockman SR: Protective effect of hypothermia on total occlusion of the cerebral circulation. Ann Surg 155:312–315, 1962
10. Andersen P, Gjerstad L, Pasztor E: Effects of cooling on sympathetic transmission through the cuneate nucleus. Acta Physiol Scand 84:433–447, 1972
11. Andersen P, Gjerstad L, Pasztor E: Effects of cooling on inhibitory processes in the cuneate nucleus. Acta Physiol Scand 84:448–461, 1972
12. Andjus RK, Cirkovic T, Genci R, et al: Brain metabolism and tolerance of hypothermic hibernators and nonhibernators to anoxia. Abstract, 4th Hibernation-Hypothermia Symposium, Aspen, 1971, pp 3–4
13. Andjus RK, Knopelmacher F, Russell RW, et al: Some effects of hypothermia on learning and retention. Q J Exp Psychol 8:15–23, 1956
14. Andrews PM, Panuska JA: Fractional distribution of cardiac output to the brains of hypothermic rats. The Physiologist 10:110, 1967
15. Arfel G: Variations in establishment of EEG after cardiac arrest. Symposium "On recovery period after resuscitation. Pathophysiology and treatment in experiment and clinics." Moskva, 1968, pp 8–12
16. Arfel G, duBouchet N: Repercussions electroencephalographiques de l'arret circulatoir sous hypothermie. Anesth Analg (Paris) 20:2–27, 1963
17. Arnovljevic-Brankovic J, Vidovic VL: Effet de l'hypothermie profonde sur le comportement maternel de la ratte. Arch Sci Physiol 13:161–157, 1959
18. Arnovljevic-Brankovic J, Vidovic VL: Changes in the performance of previously practised habits of albino rats under the influence of moderate hypothermia. Bull Inst Refrig Supply, Commission 6, Annexe 1961–64, 1961
19. Bacalzo LV, Wolfson SK: Resuscitation after unexpected circulatory arrest. Tolerance to total ischemia by cold carotid perfusion. Biomed Sci Instrum 5:75–79, 1969

20. Bacalzo LV, Wolfson SK: Preferential cerebral hypothermia. Tromethamine and dextran 40 and tolerance to circulatory arrest of 90–120 min. Arch Surg 103:393–397, 1971
21. Baldwin M, Farrier R, MacDonald F, et al: Cerebral deposition of drugs at low temperatures. J Neurosurg 20:637–646, 1963
22. Battista AF: Effect of cold on cortical potentials in the cat. Exp Neurol 19: 140–155, 1967
23. Bendandi G, Galleti G: Temperature distribution in the brain during profound selective cooling and anoxia of the central nervous system. J Cardiovasc Surg 4:65–71, 1963
24. Benjamin HB, Jochimsen P, Jochimsen W, et al: The effect of severe hypothermia on the central nervous system and on peripheral nerves. Rev Can Biol 22:433–436, 1963
25. Bjork VO, Hultquist G: Contraindications to profound hypothermia in open-heart surgery. J Thorac Cardiovasc Surg 44:1–13, 1962
26. Black P, Markowitz RS: Experimental spinal cord injury in monkeys: Comparison of steroids and local hypothermia. Surg Forum 22:409–411, 1971
27. Blozovski D, Blozovski M: Electrocorticogramme du jeune animal sous hypothermie et sous hyperthermie, J Physiol (Paris) 55:115–116, 1963
28. Boba A: Hypothermia: Appraisal of risk in 110 consecutive patients. J Neurosurg 19:924–933, 1962
29. Bouzarth WF, Kazi KH, Bubelis I, et al: Effect of temperature upon craniocerebral trauma. An experimental study in dogs. JAMA 199:567–569, 1967
30. Bouzarth WF, Madow L: A technique for immediate hypothermia and arteriography after cranial trauma. J Trauma 6:56–60, 1966
31. Boyd RJ, Connolly JE: The effect of hypothermia in experimental cerebral ischemia. Geriatrics 17:522–527, 1962
32. Brendel W, Reulen-Munchen J: Die Kalteschwellung des Gehirns. Langenbecks Arch Klin Chir 308:903–907, 1964
33. Bukov VA, Vinogradov VI: Cranio-cerebral hypothermia. How effective is possibility of removal of pathological consequences from cardiac arrest and clinical death. Symposium "On recovery period after resuscitation. Pathophysiology and treatment in experiments and clinics." Moscow, 1968, pp 28–32
34. Bureshova O, Buresh J, Hassamanova J, et al: The effect of decreased body temperature on conditioned reflex activity in the rat. Physiol Bohemosl 13:220–225, 1964
35. Campkin V: Moderate hypothermia and circulatory arrest for neurosurgical operations. Br J Anaesth 37:528–532, 1965
36. Campkin V, Dallas SH: Elective circulatory arrest in neurosurgical operations. Br J Anaesth 40:527–532, 1968
37. Cepki LP, Treshinski AI, Sviryakin VT, et al: Values of reestablished function of central nervous system after severe brain anoxia in sick patients treated by hypothermia. Symposium "On recovery period after resuscitation. Pathophysiology and treatment in experiment and clinics." Moscow, 1968, pp 122–124
38. Clasen RA, Pandolfi S. Hass GM: Interrupted hypothermia in experimental cerebral edema. Neurology 20:279–282, 1970

39. Collewijn H: Ionic Movements in the Cerebral Cortex. Amsterdam, Drukkerij, 1963, p 59
40. Collewijn H, Schade JP: Cerebral impedance changes in hypothermia. Arch Int Physiol Biochem 70:200–210, 1962
41. Collewijn H, Scade JP: Conductivity of the cerebral cortex after circulatory arrest at body temperatures from 37°C to 18°C. Arch Int Physiol Biochem 72:181–193, 1964
42. Connolly JE: Selective brain cooling for neurosurgery. Ann Chir Thorac Cardiovasc 1:1–2, 1962
43. Connolly JE, Boyd RJ, Calvin JW: The protective effect of hypothermia in cerebral ischemia: Experimental and clinical applications by selective brain cooling in the human. Surgery 52:15–24, 1962
44. Connolly JE, Harris EJ, Bruns DL, et al: An experimental study on the technique and effects of selective brain cooling. Surg Forum 11:405–407, 1960
45. Cushman A, Horn N, Rouhe S, et al: Diffuse head cooling as a method for producing a gradient of brain hypothermia and decreased blood volume. Surg Forum 22:418–419, 1971
46. deJong RH, Hershey WN, Wagman IH: Nerve conduction velocity during hypothermia in man. Anesthesiology 27:805–810, 1966
47. Ducker TB, Hamit HF: Experimental treatment of acute spinal injury. J Neurosurg 30:693–697, 1969
48. Dunn JM, Miller JA: Hypothermia combined with positive pressure ventilation in resuscitation of the asphyxiated neonate. Am J Obstet Gynecol 104:58–67, 1969
49. Essman WB, Sudak FN: Effect of body temperature reduction on response acquisition in mice. J Appl Physiol 17:113–116, 1962
50. Essman WB, Sudak FN: Effect of hypothermia on the establishment of a conditioned avoidance response in mice. J Comp Physiol Psychol 56:366–369, 1963
51. Fay T: Observations on generalized refrigeration in cases of severe cerebral trauma. Res Publ Assoc Neur Ment Dis 24:611–619, 1945
52. Fay T, Smith LW: Observations on reflex responses during prolonged periods of human refrigeration. Arch Neurol Psychiat 45:215–222, 1941
53. Fenstermacher JD, Li C, Levin VA: Extracellular space of the cerebral cortex of normothermic and hypothermic cats. Exp Neurol 27:101–114, 1970
54. Filatov IM: A method of extirpating arterio-venous aneurysms of the brain under conditions of controlled arterial hypotension and hypothermia. Vopr Neurokhir 34:8–12, 1970
55. Frank G, Tyers O, Wolfson SK: Automatic external cardiac massage. An adjunct to recovery from moderate hypothermia, profound preferential cerebral hypothermia and prolonged cardiopulmonary arrest. Arch Surg 98:771–775, 1969
56. Fukumura A: An experimental study of the cooling perfusion of the isolated brain utilizing an artificial solution, with special reference to the brain metabolism, blood-brain barrier and histopathological findings. J Kumamoto Med Soc 44:593–624, 1970
57. Gaevskaya MS: Biochemistry of Brain during Dying and Resuscitation of Organisms. Moscow, Medgiz, 1963, p 186

58. Galindo A, Baldwin M: Profound hypothermia and ventricular fibrillation during neurosurgery. Ann Surg 156:30–40, 1962
59. Galletti G, Mattioli G, Pagliani G, et al: Ipotermia profonda ed arresto circolatorio selettivi del sistema nervoso centrale. Gazz Int Med Chir 68:2892–2916, 1963
60. Gokhan N, Angelakos ET: Electroencephalographic activity after circulatory arrest in the hypothermic dog. J Appl Physiol 18:69–72, 1963
61. Goldman SS, Willis JS: Cold resistance of the brain during hibernation. I. K^+ transport in cerebral cortex slices. Cryobiology 10:212–217, 1973
62. Goldman SS, Willis JS: Cold resistance of the brain during hibernation. II. Na-K-activated ATPase. Cryobiology 10:218–224, 1973
63. Gonski A, Johnston JB, Hercus VM, et al: Profound hypothermia for intracranial surgery. Med J Aust 1:318–320, 1964
64. Hale DE, Collis JS Jr, King MH: Intracranial aneurysmal surgery with and without hypothermia. Surgery 52:338–341, 1962
65. Hansebout RR, Peterson EW, Ringer TR, et al: Experiences with core temperature maintenance during the course of regional profound brain hypothermia. Med Res Eng 9:9–13, 1970
66. Hayward JN, Ott LH, Stuart DG, et al: Peltier biothermodes. Am J Med Electron 24:11–19, 1965
67. Henre FW: Hypothermia for operations during pregnancy. Anesth Analg 44:424–428, 1965
68. Herrmann HD, Dittmann J: Examination of the metabolism of oedematous brain tissue. I. Alterations of the metabolism in the cold-induced oedema of the rabbit brain measured manometrically in vitro. Acta Neurochir 22:167–175, 1970
69. Hirsch H, Breuer M, v Buch KG, et al: Uber Krampfpotentiale in Hypothermie. Pfluegers Arch 277:251–269, 1963
70. Horecky J, Pivkova A: Blood flow changes during hypothermic brain perfusion. Med J Bratislava 34:259–270, 1963
71. Howitt WM, Turnbull IM: Effects of hypothermia and methysergide on recovery from experimental paraplegia. Can J Surg 15:179–186, 1972
72. Hurwitz BS, Wolfson SK: Brain lactate in anoxia and hypothermia: Relationship to brain viability. Exp Neurol 23:426–434, 1969
73. Ichiyanagi K, Matsuki M, Masuko K, et al: Effect of altered arterial carbon dioxide tensions on the electroencephalogram during hypothermia. Acta Anaesth Scand 13:173–183, 1969
74. Icoz MV, Wolfson SK: Tolerance to total ischemia in dogs after cold blood or cold physiologic saline perfusion of the brain. Surg Forum 17:403–405, 1966
75. Karpovich OA: Changes in the motor conditioned reflex in dogs as the result of excessive cooling and subsequent warming, in Starkov PM (ed): Problem of Acute Hypothermia. New York, Pergamon Press, 1960, pp 32–43
76. Kelly DL Jr, Lassiter KRL, Calogero JA, et al: Effects of local hypothermia and tissue oxygen studies in experimental paraplegia. J Neurosurg 33: 554–563, 1970
77. Klatzo I, Li CL, Long DM, et al: The effect of hypothermia on electric impedance and penetration of substances from the CSF into the periventricular brain tissue. Prog Brain Res 29:385–396, 1967

78. Klussmann FW: Der Einflus der Temperatur auf die afferente und efferente motorische Innervation des Ruckenmarks. I. Temperatur Abhangingkeit der afferenten und efferenten Spontantatigkeit. Pfluegers Arch 305:295–315, 1969
79. Kramer RS, Sanders AP, Lesage AM, et al: The effect of profound hypothermia on preservation of cerebral ATP content during circulatory arrest. J Thorac Cardiovasc Surg 56:699–709, 1968
80. Leblanc G, Bertho E: Resection d'un anevrisme cerebral a l'aide de l'hypothermie profonde. L'arret circulatoire total et l'exsanguination. Laval Med 33:414–418, 1962
81. Lumb WV, Brasmer TH: Improved spinal plates and hypothermia as adjuncts to spinal surgery. J Am Vet Med Assoc 157:338–342, 1970
82. Malmejac J, Chardon G, Bonnet D: Hyperexcitabilite transitoire des neurones postganglionnaires en hypothermie controlee. C R Soc Biol (Paris) 155: 1633–1634, 1965
83. Marco P, Horecky J, Pechan J: Effect of deep hypothermia on the free nucleotides of the dog brain during anoxia. Vnitr Lek 10:105–110, 1964
84. Massopust LC Jr, Albin MS, Barnes HW, et al: Cortical and subcortical responses to hypothermia. Exp Neurol 9:249–261, 1964
85. Massopust LC, Wolin LR, White RJ, et al: Electroencephalographic characteristics of brain cooling and rewarming in monkey. Exp Neurol 26:518–526, 1970
86. Mathews GJ, Pace-Florida A: Intrathecal cold saline for the relief of intractable pain. Can Med Assoc J 103:1143–1146, 1970
87. McCredie DA: The use of hypothermia in pediatric emergencies. J Pediatr 61:653–659, 1962
88. Mc Dowall DG: The current usage of hypothermia in British neurosurgery. Br J Anaesth 43:1084–1087, 1971
89. McQueen JD, Jeanes LD: Influence of hypothermia on intracranial hypertension. J Neurosurg 19:277–288, 1962
90. Mendler N: Electrolyte and metabolite alterations in the rat brain after cooling to 4–2°C with a heart-lung machine. Z Ges Exp Med 146:206–225, 1968
91. Messmer K, Brendel W, Reulen HJ, et al: Elektrolytveranderungen in tiefer Hypothermie: III. Beziehunger zur biologischen Uberlebenszeit bei Kunstlichem Kreislauf. Pfluegers Arch 288:240–261, 1966
92. Mickenfelder JD, Kirklin JW, Uihlein A: Clinical experience with a closed-chest method of producing profound hypothermia and total circulatory arrest in neurosurgery. Ann Surg 159:125–131, 1964
93. Michenfelder JD, MacCarty CS, Theye RA: Physiologic studies following closed-chest technique of profound hypothermia in neurosurgery. Anesthesiology 25:131–136, 1964
94. Mickenfelder JD, Terry HR, Daw EF, et al: Profound hypothermia in neurosurgery. Open-chest versus closed-chest techniques. Anesthesiology 24:177–184, 1963
95. Mickenfelder JD, Theye RA: Hypothermia: Effect on canine brain and whole-body metabolism. Anesthesiology 27:1107–1112, 1968
96. Miller JA: New approaches to preventing brain damage during asphyxia. Am J Obstet Gynecol 110:1125–1133, 1971

97. Miller JA, Miller FS: Studies on prevention of brain damage in asphyxia. Dev Med Child Neurol 7:607–619, 1965
98. Miller JA, Miller FS: Interactions between hypothermia and hypoxia-hypercapnia in neonates. Fed Proc 25:1338–1341, 1966
99. Millet R, Viale-Millet D: A propos de 42 cas d'hypothermie moyenne en neuro-chirurgie. Anesth Analg (Paris) 19:463–473, 1962
100. Mrosovsky N: Retention and reversal of conditioned avoidance following severe hypothermia. J Comp Physiol Psychol 56:811–813, 1963
101. Mrosovsky N: Lowered body temperature, learning and behavior, in Fisher KC, Dawe AR, Lyman CP, Schonbaum E, South FE (eds): Mammalian Hibernation, Vol III. New York, Am Elsevier, 1967, pp 152–174
102. Negovskii VA: Some physiopathologic regularities in the process of dying and resuscitation. Circulation 23:452–457, 1961
103. Negovskii VA: Resuscitation and Artificial Hypothermia. Russian publ Medgiz, Moscow. Translated into English by Consultants Bureau, New York, 1962, p 314
104. Negovskii VA: Contributions to Reanimation and Hypothermia. Moskva, Medicina, 1964, p 142
105. Negovskii VA: Aspects metabolique et toxemiques de l'irreversibilite de la mort clinique. Agressologie 9:393–399, 1968
106. Negovskii VA, Soboleva VJ, Gurvich NL, et al: Deep hypothermia as a method of prolonging the clinical death periods. Bull Exp Biol Med 11:39–43, 1963
107. Negrin J: Prevention des lesions ischemique de la moelle epiniere par l'hypothermie regionale extravasculaire. Rev Neurol (Paris) 106: 725–729, 1962
108. Negrin J: Hypothermie regionale directe du cerveau par perfusion intracranienne extravasculaire. Rev Neurol (Paris) 108:923–927, 1963
109. Negrin J: Extravascular perfusion for selective regional hypothermia of the central nervous system (brain or spinal cord). Acta Neurochir 12:88–95, 1964
110. Negrin J: Regional cooling of central nervous system by extravascular perfusion hypothermia. NY State J Med 65:2908–2913, 1965
111. Negrin J: Local hypothermia of the spinal cord for relief of spasticity and rigidity: Preliminary observations. Arch Phys Med Rehabil 47:169–173, 1966
112. Negrin J: Spinal cord hypothermia to relieve muscle spasticity in multiple sclerosis: Preliminary observations. J Nerv Ment Dis 144:430–434, 1967
113. Negrin J: Spinal cord hypothermia in neurological surgery. Int Surg 52:264–267, 1969
114. Negrin J: The hypothermostat. An instrument to obtain local hypothermia of the brain or spinal cord. Int Surg 54:93–106, 1970
115. Negrin J: Hypothermia of the central nervous system. Trans NY Acad Sci 33:557–563, 1971
116. Oja SS, Oja H, Sarajas HSS: Cerebral free amino acids in rats undergoing varying periods of anesthesia and hypothermia. Ann Acad Sci Fenn (Biol) 142:1–14, 1968
117. Ookawa T, Tateishi T: Relation between the chick electroretinogram and body temperature. Experientia 26:277–278, 1970

118. Panuska JA: Instrumental shock escape performance during hypothermia. Cryobiology 2:23–24, 1965
119. Panuska JA: The non-linear suppression of animal performance during progressive hypothermia. Broteria (Sci Nat) 36:47–62, 1967
120. Panuska JA, Popovic V: Learning in hypothermic rats. J Appl Physiol 18: 1016–1018, 1963
121. Panuska JA, Popovic V: Critical temperature for instrumental response acquisition in hypothermic rats. J Appl Physiol 20:1275–1277, 1965
122. Patterson RH, McSherry CK, Schwartz MS: Hyperbaric oxygen, hypothermia, and cerebral ischemia in the dog. Int Surg Res 8:279–285, 1968
123. Patterson RH, Ray BS: Profound hypothermia for intracranial surgery: Laboratory and clinical experiences with extracorporeal circulation by peripheral cannulation. Ann Surg 156:377–391, 1968
124. Paul B: Significance of controlled hypothermia in the treatment of brain edema (experimental studies in the dog). Zentralbl Chir 96:697–714, 1971
125. Peterson EW, Ringer TR: Refroidissement du cerveau au moyen d'un echangeur de chaleur place en continuite avec la circulation carotidienne. Neurochirurgie 10:651–658, 1964
126. Popovic P: Effet de l'hypothermie profonde prolongee sur l'activite nerveuse superieure. C R Soc Biol (Paris) 151:1001–1003, 1957
127. Popovic P: Conditionnement instrumental du rat en hypothermie. These du doctorat, 1966, Toulouse, France
128. Popovic P, Horecky J, Popovic V: Instrumental responses in rats after hypothermic cardiopulmonary by-pass. Proc Soc Exp Biol Med 126:225–228, 1967
129. Popovic P, Panuska JA, Popovic V: Instrumental acquisition in rats after twelve exposures to deep hypothermia. Proc Soc Exp Biol Med 122:337–341, 1966
130. Popovic P, Panuska JA, Popovic V: Adaptation to hypothermia, in Biometeorology, Vol II. New York, Pergamon Press, 1966, pp 276–282
131. Popovic P, Popovic V: Survival of newborn ground squirrels after supercooling or freezing. Am J Physiol 204:949–952, 1963
132. Popovic P, Silver AB, Popovic V: Critical temperature for intracranial self-stimulation in white rats. Am J Physiol 214:801–803, 1968
133. Prusiner S, Wolfson SK: Hypothermic protection against cerebral edema of ischemia. Prevention of cerebral edema in the rat after prolonged circulatory arrest. Arch Neurol 19:623–627, 1968
134. Putkonen PTS, Sarajas HSS: Central nervous function in hypothermic rabbits. Scand J Clin Lab Invest 21:65–66, 1968
135. Raskind R, Weiss SR, Huertas J: Hypothermic subarachnoid saline injection as a method of pain control. Am Surg 38:142–144, 1972
136. Rehder K, Kirklin JW, MacCarty CS, et al: Physiologic studies following profound hypothermia and circulatory arrest for treatment of intracranial aneurysm. Ann Surg 156:882–889, 1962
137. Reulen HJ, Aigner P, Brendel W, et al: Electrolytveranderungen in tiefer Hypothermie. Pfluegers Arch 288:197–219, 1966
138. Riccio D, Stikes ER: Persistent but modifiable retrograde amnesia produced by hypothermia. Physiol Behav 4:649–652, 1969

139. Richman CL, Parrett G, Black-Schaffer B, et al: The effect of deep hypothermia on retention and motivation in the rat. Psychonal Sci 9:275–276, 1967
140. Rosomoff HL: Pathophysiology of the central nervous system during hypothermia. Acta Neurochir 13:11–12, 1964
141. Rosomoff HL, Gilbert R: Brain volume and cerebrospinal fluid pressure during hypothermia. Am J Physiol 183:19–22, 1955
142. Rosomoff HL, Shulman K, Raynor R, et al: Experimental brain injury and delayed hypothermia. Surg Gynecol Obstet 110:27–32, 1960
143. Sarajas HSS, Oja H, Oja SS: Variables influencing the energy metabolism of the brain in normo- and hypothermia. Ann Med Exp Fenn 46:547–551, 1968
144. Sarajas HSS, Putkonen PTS: Central nervous and visceral reaction patterns in rabbits warming up from deep hypothermia. Ann Acad Sci Fenn 144:1–22, 1968
145. Selker RG: Icewater irrigation of the spinal cord. Surg Forum 22:411–413, 1971
146. Silverstone JT, Taunahill MM, Treland JA: Psychiatric aspects of profound hypothermia in open-heart surgery. J Thorac Cardiovasc Surg 59:193–200, 1970
147. Simon E: Kreislaufwirkungen der spinalen Hypothermie. J Neurovisc Relat 31:223–259, 1969
148. Simon E: Aktivitatsanderungen im cervikalen Sympathikus wahrend spinaler Hypothermie. J Neurovisc Relat 31:260–274, 1969
149. Simon E, Rautenberg W, Usinger W, et al. Der Einflus der spinalen Hypothermie auf die spinalen vasomotorischen Zentren. J Neurovisc Relat 31: 350–372, 1970
150. Sourek K, Travnicek V: General and local hypothermia of the brain in the treatment of intractible epilepsy. J Neurosurg 33:253–259, 1970
151. Stephenson FM, Du JN, Oliver TK: The effect of cooling on blood gas tensions in newborn infants. J Pediatr 76:848–852, 1970
152. Suda I, Kito K, Adachi C: The viability of long-term frozen cat brain in vitro. Nature 212:268–270, 1966
153. Sudak FN, Essman WB: Maze acquisition and retention in hypothermic mice. J Appl Physiol 17:747–750, 1962
154. Sutton CH, Nunnally RL, Carrol FB: Protection of the microwave-irradiated brain with body-core hypothermia. Annual Meeting of the Society of Cryobiology, Key Biscayne, Florida, 1973
155. Sutton CH, Soriano DB, Tiell ML: Modification of secondary spread of thermal injury in the central nervous system with systemic hypothermia. Trans Am Neurol Assoc 95:316–317, 1970
156. Svanes K: The effect of barbiturate anesthesia and hypothermia on the edema formation caused by subcutaneous injection of 5-hydroxytryptamine in mice. Acta Physiol Scand 72:378–382, 1968
157. Terry HR, Daw EF, Michenfelder JD: Hypothermia by extracorporeal circulation for neurosurgery. An anesthetic technic. Anesth Analg 41:241–248, 1962
158. Turinsky J, Mukherji B, Sloviter HA: Effects of induced hypothermia on amino acids and glycogen in rat brain. J Neurochem 18:233–235, 1971
159. Tyers GFO, Wolfson SK: Automatic external cardiac massage: An adjunct to recovery from moderate general hypothermia, profound preferential cerebral

hypothermia and prolonged cardiopulmonary arrest. Arch Surg 98:771–775, 1969
160. Uihlein A, MacCarty CS, Mickenfelder JD, et al: Deep hypothermia and surgical treatment of intracranial aneurysms. JAMA 195:639–641, 1966
161. Uihlein A, MacCarty CS, Svien HJ, et al: Hypothermia for operations on intracranial aneurysm with the aid of open and closed thoracic perfusions. Minn Med 46:255–258, 1963
162. Verdura J, White RJ, Albin MS: Profound selective hypothermia and arrest of arterial circulation to the dog brain. J Neurosurg 24:1002–1006, 1966
163. Vidovic VL, Arnovljevic-Brankovic J: Effet de l'hypothermie moderee sur le comportement maternel de la rate. Experientia 16:558–562, 1960
164. Vindyuk VP, Schegolkova GG: Blood filling of the brain in craniocerebral hypothermia. J Pathol Physiol Gen Pathol 33:33–35, 1968
165. Vindyuk VP, Schegolkova GG: Hyperemia of the cerebrum during craniocerebral hypothermia. Biull Eksp Biol Med 68:33–35, 1969
166. Vishnevsky AA, Darbinian TM, Portnoy VF, et al: A new method of open heart surgery—Isolated artificial cerebral circulation combined with general moderate hypothermia. J Cardiovasc Surg 5:58–66, 1964
167. Vladimirov GY: The effect of interruption of the circulation of the brain during hypothermia on cerebral metabolism, in Palladin AV (ed): Problems of the Biochemistry of the N. S. Oxford, Pergamon Press 1964, p 207
168. Walker RL, Schlobohm RM, Cooke FN, et al: Bradycardia with carotid system infusions of cold blood during endarterectomy. Can Anaesth Soc J 17:221–226, 1970
169. Westin B, Miller JA, Boles A: Hypothermia induced during asphyxiation. Its effects on survival rate, learning and maintenance of the conditioned response in rats. Acta Paediatr 52:49–60, 1963
170. White RJ: Preservation of cerebral function during circulatory arrest and resuscitation: Hypothermic protective considerations. Resuscitation 1:107–115, 1972
171. White RJ, Massopust LA, Wolin LR, et al: Profound selective cooling and ischemia of primate brain without pump or oxygenator. Surgery 66:224–232, 1969
172. White RJ, Wolin LR, Massopust LC, et al: Extracorporeal perfusion of dog and monkey brain during circulatory arrest. Resuscitation 1:275–284, 1973
173. Willi MD: Kunstliche Hypotonie und Hypothermie mit Halothan. Der Anaesthesist 9:107–108, 1960
174. Wolin LR, Massopust LC, White RJ, et al: Arrest of cerebral blood flow and reperfusion of the brain in the rhesus monkey. Resuscitation 1:39–44, 1973
175. Zakhary R, Miller JA, Miller FS: Hypothermia, asphyxia and brain carbohydrates in newborn puppies. Biol Neonat (Basel) 11:36–49, 1967
176. Zhmurko SF: Cranio-cerebral hypothermia in patients with acute craniocerebral injury. Khirurgia 47:40–43, 1971

7

Protective Effects of Hypothermia, Organ Preservation, and Effect of Drugs

"All this has been told before
But since nobody listened
It must be said again."

Andre Gide

PROTECTIVE ROLE OF HYPOTHERMIA

In most physiologically detrimental situations (ischemia, anoxia, shock, intoxication) a homeothermic organism spontaneously leaves normothermia for a hypothermic body temperature. It is clear that under these conditions hypothermia appreciably extends the survival of the organism. Normothermia returns spontaneously after removal of the detrimental conditions if the body temperature of the homeotherm is not already too low. Under some conditions hypothermia might even potentiate the detrimental conditions such as barbiturate poisoning.[103] In hypothermia the lethal concentration of barbiturates is lower than under normothermic conditions. This and similar cases of increased toxicity or the increased impairment of a function in hypothermia are exceptions to the rule.

Since the protective role of hypothermia is mentioned throughout the entire book this chapter is mostly a summary of the major work done in this field.

Today hypothermia is used in many detrimental situations. Hypothermia has proved to be protective in many cases, such as oxygen poisoning,[104] hypoxia,[1,5,36,64,85,92] ischemia,[94] asphyxia in infants,[84,86,101,102,136] high-altitude effects,[133] hemorrhagic shock,[31,91,93,116] traumatic shock,[19,107] peptone shock,[83] endotoxin shock,[139] and bacteremic and septic shock.[17,18,115]

Hypothermic protection has been proved effective in circulatory and cardiac arrest surgery of heart and blood vessels (Chapter 3). Hypothermia exerts a protective role against complete depletion of the red blood cell volume (''asanguineous'' organisms) and extreme acute anemic anoxia.[34,35,55,56,90,98] The protective effect of hypothermia was established in trauma or ischemia of the central nervous system,[92,137] electrically induced seizures,[99] and the alleviation of pain. Hypothermia has been used successfully for amputation of organs,[28] in severe intoxications,[112–114,128] alloxan intoxication,[63,110] edema formation after administration of some drugs,[126] bacterial infection,[24] second- and third- degree burns,[97,106,119,144] liver damage,[81] and malignant hyperthermia.

The protective role of hypothermia has also been shown effective in drowning,[76] x-irradiation,[7,9,10,12,20,21,38,39,48,66,87,88,105,123] and increased G forces.[15,16,130] Hypothermia has been proposed for long-term interplanetary space flights.[37] It has been suggested that a state of suspended animation would eliminate many problems such as the amount of food and oxygen to be used, as well as the problem of isolation.

Use of hypothermia in cancer chemotherapy was tried with the hope of protecting healthy cold tissues from drug toxicity. Hypothermia, induced by external thoracic cage cooling, protects bone marrow from the effects of nitrogen mustard.[120,121] Hypothermia was found to be protective in the treatment of advanced head and neck cancers in patients with ethoglucid[23] or with other anticancer agents.[42,61,108,117,143] Cooling and rewarming show striking temperature differences of effect on the action of anticancer drugs sometimes permitting synchronization of cell cultures.[41,77]

Binding of antitumor agents to the cells is appreciably decreased during cooling of tumor cells,[32,33,109] though there are some investigators who did not find temperature dependency for drug binding.[29]

It is generally accepted that only profound hypothermia can fully exert its protective role. Fortunately, recent advances in cooling techniques have decreased the lethal limits of hypothermia to much lower levels than was thought possible in the past. Thus, it has been established that adult homeothermic animals can survive a body temperature close to the freezing point,[4,85] while newborn homeothermic mammals survive supercooling to a temperature of −8 C.[101,102] Man can survive for 1 to 2 hours a body temperature of only 4 C above the freezing point.[95] Homeothermic animals can survive hypothermic exposure to 2 C for several hours when their circulation has been extracorporeally supported. Since it is possible to safely cool animals and human patients deeper today than several years ago, it is now possible to obtain better hypothermic protection.

Summary

Spontaneous hypothermia develops in almost every situation that is harmful to a homeothermic organism. Spontaneous or induced hypothermia protects organisms from hypoxia, shock, intoxication, and x-irradiation, and permits a much longer treatment time than would be possible at a normal body temperature. But hypothermia per se does not remove harmful conditions or treat an endangered organism or a sick patient.

ORGAN PRESERVATION

Recently new techniques have been developed for the long-term preservation of tissues and organs. Generally these techniques are combined with profound cooling of the isolated organs. The term "hypothermic" should not be used for an isolated organ. The terms hypothermia, normothermia, and hyperthermia are to be used when the temperature-regulative processes of a whole homeothermic organism are involved, not for poikilothermia or for parts of the body. The term hypothermia is still used in the field of organ preservation. In order to preserve the functional viability of an extirpated organ, an intravascular perfusion of a cold electrolyte solution or a cold plasma is used. The organ is cooled very quickly. Each decrease of 10 C (van't Hoff's law) decreases the metabolic rate of the cooled organ by two- or threefold. Ideally the long-term preservation of organs for clinical use would be by freezing, and would involve organ storage and tissue typing. Currently, the only completely successful freezing undertakings have been the commercial use of frozen sperm and the clinical use of frozen plasma, frozen red cells, and frozen skin. The specific problems of organ freezing and thawing are associated mainly with organ size and with the process of rewarming. It is hoped that controlled and uniform rewarming with microwave energy will solve these problems in the near future (Chapter 1). Presently localized hypothermia, simple cooling of the organs, is the only means to extend the survival of isolated organs appreciably.

Hypothermia extends the functional viability of most of the isolated organs that are used either experimentally or clinically for transplantation. This applies to the heart,[54,100,124,127,131,134,140] lung,[30,129,138] kidney,[11,46,47,58,78,125] liver,[22,25,40,59,65] pancreatic islets.[8,57]

Summary

Hypothermia extends the functional viability of harvested organs from several hours to 3 days. Until adequate techniques are developed for the successful freezing and thawing of organs for transplantation, hypothermia (in combination with perfusion) remains the only tool that prolongs the survivability of isolated organs.

DRUGS IN HYPOTHERMIA

Effect on Body Temperature

The action of drugs is often modified by a rise or a fall in body temperature. The effect of temperature on drug action is not always identical in vitro and in vivo.[142] There are drugs that induce hypothermia, such as Thorazine (chlorpromazine), large amounts of epinephrine, propanol, or eserine.[6,44,49,62,82,132] Many drugs that act as general depressants or excitants of CNS cause nonspecific changes in body temperature. During general anesthesia one observes a decrease in thermoregulatory control mechanisms and a subsequent decrease (or increase) of body temperature. Azotemia leads to hypothermia.[27] Even cholesterinase inhibitors that pass through the blood–brain barrier induce hypothermia.[80]

One of the drugs that depresses thermoregulation and decreases body temperature of normothermic animals is pentobarbital.[68] The degree of hypothermia depends on the amount of the barbiturate administered. Severe hypothermia occurs after intoxication with barbiturates.[26,60,67] The depth of hypothermia will depend on the environmental temperature as well as the duration of exposure. Marihuana[70,71] and 6-hydroxydopamine[89,122] lead to spontaneous hypothermia, as does morphine.[69,72–75] Some anticancer agents lead to spontaneous hypothermia also.[3]

In diabetic acidosis[79] and even more so in diabetic coma, the body temperature of patients might be decreased to astonishingly low levels.[118]

Drug Metabolism

Drug metabolism is altered in hypothermia, mainly by the depth of the hypothermia. However, the distribution of drugs appears to be unchanged, as in the case of barbiturates.[96]

Hypothermia induces changes in drug action, and sometimes decreases the toxicity or even the effectiveness of some drugs. The effect of other drugs remains unchanged and for some the lowering of the body temperature means an increased toxicity. Thus a new pharmacology of hypothermia is born. The picture of drug action is further complicated by a decreased absorption of some and a decreased excretion of others, especially through the kidney. The decreased metabolism of drugs, especially those associated with liver function, increases the duration of their effects.

The uptake of ^{14}C-atropine is decreased 3 times in profound hypothermia.[52]

The average lethal dose of digitalis (Digoxin) in hypothermia is twice as large as compared to normothermic conditions.[14] Hypothermia gives more time for removal of the effects of digitalis toxicity as well.[2] In hypothermia therapeutic as well as lethal doses of G-strophantin (ouabain) are doubled as compared to normothermic conditions.[43] The neurovascular blocking effect of suxamethonium[141] is doubled even in shallow hypothermia while the lethal concentration of potassium in serum is decreased.[45]

The heart stops at a lower body temperature after alcohol administration.[13,135]

^{14}C-atropine is metabolized in liver in hypothermic rats.[51] The effect of deep hypothermia is much greater on renal excretion of atropine than on hepatic excretion. Even at body temperature of 17 C the liver is still capable of completely altering the drug that will be excreted into the bile.[51] Degenerative changes of the liver cells after poisoning with carbon tetrachloride are smaller if the experimental animals (rats) are cooled 1 hour after poisoning and if the cooling was rather prolonged.[111] Liver metabolism of procaine[50] and acetylation[53] are present in hypothermia although appreciably decreased in accordance with van't Hoff's law.

Summary

Drug metabolism is decreased in hypothermia. The toxicity of some drugs is decreased and that of others is increased in hypothermia. Some drugs decrease the body temperature of an experimental animal or a patient, either increasing or decreasing their toxicity. The picture of drug action is further complicated by a decreased absorption and a decreased excretion of drugs. In clinically induced hypothermia the rule of thumb is still—until we learn more about drugs in hypothermia—as few and as little drugs as possible.

BIBLIOGRAPHY

1. Adolph EF, Goldstein J: Survival of rats and mice without oxygen in deep hypothermia. J Appl Physiol 14:599–604, 1959
2. Akhtar M, Chakravarti RN, Sarkar AK, et al: Effect of hypothermia on digitalis toxicity: An experimental study. Indian J Med Res 59:58–63, 1971
3. Amblard P, Dugois P, Imbert R, et al: Apropos of 2 accidents during general treatments with methotrexate. Bull Soc Fr Dermatol Syphillgr 78:85–87, 1971
4. Andjus RK: Suspended animation in cooled, supercooled and frozen rats. J Physiol 128:547–556, 1955
5. Andjus RK, Cirkovic T, Cuperlovic N, et al: Brain metabolism and resistance of a hibernator (*Citellus citellus*) and the rat to different anoxic conditions, including cardiac arrest in deep hypothermia. Ann Acad Sci Fenn A.4 71/1, Helsinki, 1964, pp 11–23

6. Arkenau C, Bosse AJ, Schaum E: Comparative studies on the effect of propranolol and oxyfedrine on body temperature in hypothermia. Arzneimittelforschung 19:1828–1829, 1969
7. Ashwood-Smith MJ, Leong GF: The protective effect of deep body hypothermia on X-ray induced mitotic aberrations of regenerating rat liver. U S Naval Radiological Defense Laboratory, USNRDL-TR-666, 1963, pp 1–19
8. Ballinger WF, Lacy PE: Transplantation of intact pancreatic islets in rats. Surgery 72:175–186, 1972
9. Barr RE, Musacchia XJ: Radiation sensitivity of the hibernating ground squirrel, *Citellus tridecemlineatus*. Proc Soc Exp Biol Med 124:1204–1207, 1967
10. Barr RE, Musacchia XJ: Postirradiation hibernation and radiation response of ground squirrels: Telemetry surveillance. Radiat Res 51:631–637, 1972
11. Belzer FO: Current methods of kidney storage. Cryobiology 5:444–446, 1969
12. Bernshtein VA: Radiosensitivity under hypothermic conditions. Med Radiol 16:80–90, 1971
13. Bertho E, deAranguren V, Perez AP: Etude experimentale de l'hypothermie profonde a l'aide de l'alcool intraveineux et de l'adrenaline. Can J Surg 7: 443–453, 1964
14. Beyda EJ, Jung M, Bellet S: Effect of hypothermia on the tolerance of dogs to digitalis. Circ Res 9:129–135, 1961
15. Black-Schaffer B: Protection by deep hypothermia and immersion against 2300 G acceleration of a non-hibernator (rat) and a hibernator (hamster). Aerospace Med 33:286–296, 1962
16. Black-Schaffer B, Hensley JT, Simson LR: Protection of the adult mouse against 1,800 G acceleration by hypothermic immersion. Aerospace Med 32:1119–1126, 1961
17. Blair E, Cowley A, Mansberger AR, et al: Physiologic rationale for hypothermia in septic shock. Surg Forum 13:20–22, 1962
18. Blair E, Henning G, Hornick R, et al: Hypothermia in bacteremic shock. Arch Surg 89:619–629, 1964
19. Bliumin IS, Vilensky IT: Potentiated anesthesia and hypothermia in the treatment of traumatic shock. Exp Surg 6:46–48, 1960
20. Brehm R, Brunner J, Domanig E, et al: Problematik und Klinik der Bestrahlung in Hypothermie. Wien Klin Wochenschr 81:743–744, 1969
21. Brunner J, Domanig E, Fochem K, et al: Zur Methodik der einzeitigen Rontgenbestrahlung in Hypothermie. Strahlentherapie 139:431–434, 1970
22. Clot JP, et al: Experimental study of the possibilities of liver preservation for 24 hours and longer under hypothermia, hyperbaric oxygen and perfusion. II. Biochemical results. Ann Chir 25:181–192, 1971
23. Condon HA: Protective hypothermia for cancer chemotherapy. Br J Anaesth 39:806–811, 1967
24. Eiseman B, Wotkyns RS, Hirose H: Hypothermia and infection. Three mechanisms of host infection in type III pneumococcal peritonitis. Ann Surg 160:994–1006, 1964
25. Elmslie RG, Pirola RC, Coroneos N, et al: Function of the liver after isolated cold perfusion. Surg Gynecol Obstet 131:694–696, 1970

26. Fell RH, Gunning AJ, Bardhan KD, et al: Severe hypothermia as a result of barbiturate overdose complicated by cardiac arrest. Lancet 1:392–394, 1968
27. Freeman RM: The role of magnesium in the pathogenesis of azotemic hypothermia. Proc Soc Exp Biol Med 137:1069–1072, 1971
28. Fuson RL: Hypothermia prior to amputation. Arch Surg 85:1008–1010, 1962
29. Gale GR, Morris CR, Atkins LM, et al: Binding of an antitumor platinum compound to cells as influenced by physical factors and pharmacologically active agents. Cancer Res 33:813–818, 1973
30. Garzon AA, Cheng C, Pangan J, et al: Hypothermic hyperbaric lung preservation for twenty-four hours with replantation. J Thorac Cardiovasc Surg 55: 546–554, 1968
31. Giaja I: Hypothermia. J Biol Med 42:545, 1953
32. Goldenberg GJ, Lyons RM, Lepp JA, et al: Sensitivity to nitrogen mustard as a function of transport activity and proliferative rate in L5178/Y lymphoblasts. Cancer Res 31:1616–1619, 1971
33. Goldenberg GJ, Vanstone CL, Israels LG, et al: Evidence for a transport carrier of nitrogen mustard in nitrogen mustard-sensitive and -resistant L5178/Y lymphoblasts. Cancer Res 30:2285–2286, 1970
34. Gollan F, Aono M: The effect of temperature on asanguineous rabbits. Cryobiology 10:321–327, 1973
35. Gollan F, Hoffman JE, Jones RM: Maintenance of life of dogs below 10°C without hemoglobin. Am J Physiol 179:640, 1954
36. Gollan F, Nelson IA: Anoxic tolerance of beating and resting heart during perfusion at various temperatures. Proc Soc Exp Biol Med 95:485–487, 1957
37. Gooden BA: Hibernation, hypothermia and interplanetary flight. Spaceflight 12:167–169, 173, 1970
38. Hajdukovic S: Hypothermia and irradiation. Voj San Pregled 14:348–353, 1957
39. Hajdukovic S, Herve A, Vidovic V: Diminution de radiosensibilite du rat adult en hypothermie profonde. Experientia 10:343–344, 1954
40. Ham JM, Rose M, Kerne I: Liver function after cooling with two types of electrolyte solution. Aust NZ J Surg 40:89–91, 1970
41. Hara T: Temperature dependency of anti-cancer chemotherapeutic effect. Kumamoto Med J 22:140–149, 1969
42. Harrison DFN: The use of hypothermia in intra-arterial chemotherapy for head and neck cancer. J Laryngol 81:173–185, 1967
43. Hausler HF, Wieland M: Die Wirkung von g-Strophanthin am Herz-Lungenpreparat des Meerschweinchens bei Hypothermie, Normaltemperatur und Hyperthermie. Naunyn-Schmiedeberg's Arch Exp Pathol Pharmak 242: 403–408, 1962
44. Higgins EA, Iampietro PF, Adams T, et al: Effects of a tranquilizer on body temperature. Soc Exp Biol Med 115:1017–1019, 1964
45. Hoff HE, Deavers S, Huggins RA: Potassium distribution and toxicity in hypothermia. J Appl Physiol 16:250–252, 1961
46. Humphries AL: Problems with various perfusates for kidney preservation. Cryobiology 5:447–453, 1969
47. Humphries AL, Russell R, Gregory J, et al: Hypothermic perfusion of the canine kidney for 48 hours followed by reimplantation. Am Surg 30:748–752, 1964

48. Jaroslow BJ, Smith DE, Williams M, et al: Survival of hibernating ground squirrel (*Citellus tridecemlineatus*) after single and fractionated doses of cobalt-60 gamma radiation. Radiat Res 38:379–388, 1969
49. Johnson GE, Sellers EA, Schonbaum E: Interrelationship of temperature on action of drugs. Fed Proc 22:745–749, 1963
50. Kalser SC, Kelvington EJ, Kunig R, et al: Drug metabolism in hypothermia, uptake, metabolism, and excretion of C^{14}-procaine by the isolated, perfused rat liver. J Pharmacol Exp Ther 164:396–404, 1968
51. Kalser SC, Kelvington EJ, Randolph MM, et al: Drug metabolism in hypothermia. I. Biliary excretion of C^{14}-atropine metabolites in the intact and nephrectomized rat. J Pharmacol Exp Ther 147:252–259, 1965
52. Kalser SC, Kelvington EJ, Randolph MM: Drug metabolism in hypothermia. II. C^{14}-atropine uptake metabolism and excretion by the isolated perfused rat liver. J Pharmacol Exp Ther 147:260–269, 1965
53. Kalser SC, Kelvington EJ, Randolph MM: Drug metabolism in hypothermia. Uptake, metabolism and excretion of S^{35}-sulfanilamide by the isolated, perfused rat liver. J Pharmacol Exp Ther 159:389–398, 1968
54. Kamiyama TM, Webb WR, Ecker RR: Preservation of the anoxic heart with a metabolic inhibitor and hypothermia. Arch Surg 100:596–598, 1970
55. Klebanoff G: Infectious hepatitis complicated by coma. Principles of management including the adjunctive use of asanguineous hypothermic total body perfusion. Resuscitation 1:327–333, 1972
56. Klebanoff G, Hollander D, Cosima LB, et al: Asanguineous hypothermic total body perfusion in the treatment of stage IV in hepatic coma. J Surg Res 12:1–7, 1972
57. Knight MJ, Scharp DW, Kemp CB, et al: Effects of cold storage on the function of isolated pancreatic islets. Cryobiology 10:89–90, 1973
58. Ladaga LG, Nabseth DC, Besznyak I, et al: Preservation of canine kidney by hypothermia and hyperbaric oxygen. Long-term survival of autografts following 24-hour storage. Ann Surg 163:553–558, 1966
59. Lambotte L: Influence of temperature on sodium-potassium exchange produced by ouabain in the perfused dog liver. Arch Int Physiol Biochem 77: 331–333, 1969
60. Lash RF, Burdette JA, Ozdil T: Accidental profound hypothermia and barbiturate intoxication: A report of rapid core rewarming by peritoneal dialysis. JAMA 201:123–124, 1967
61. Lawton RL, Llewellyn NL, Stanford W: General hypothermia and survival following use of alkylating agent. J Surg Res 3:159–161, 1963
62. Lettau HF, Sellers EA, Schonbaum E: Modification of drug-induced hypothermia. Can J Physiol Pharmacol 42:745–755, 1964
63. Levet E, Cier A, Girod C: Inhibition of the diabetogenic effects of alloxan in rats in deep hypothermia. C R Soc Biol (Paris) 164:2298–2301, 1970
64. Levy JV, Richards V: Effect of oxygen at high pressure (OHP) on asphyxial survival time of rats. Proc Soc Biol Med 109:941–944, 1962
65. Lie TS, Yamamoto T, Bohmer F: Preservation of pig liver for transplantation. Initial perfusion and simple hypothermia. Zentralbl Chir 96:430–436, 1971
66. Liebecq-Hutter S, Mewissen DJ, Bacq ZM: Action de la chlorpromazine sur la survie des souris irradiees en relation avec l'hypothermie quelle provoque. Arch Int Physiol Biochem 66:546–551, 1958

67. Linton AL, Ledingham I McA: Severe hypothermia with barbiturate intoxication. Lancet 1:24–26, 1966
68. Lomax P: The hypothermic effect of pentobarbitol in the rat: Sites and mechanisms of action. Brain Res 1:296–302, 1966
69. Lomax P: Investigations on the central effects of morphine on body temperature. Arch Biol Med Exp 4:119–124, 1967
70. Lomax P: Acute tolerance to the hypothermic effect of marihuana in the rat. Res Commun Chem Pathol Pharmacol 2:159–167, 1971
71. Lomax P, Campbell C: Phenitrone and marihuana induced hypothermia. Experientia 27:1191–1192, 1971
72. Lotti VJ, George R, Lomax P: Hypothermia following intracerebral injection of morphine. Proc West Pharmacol Soc 8:33–35, 1965
73. Lotti VJ, Lomax P, George R: Temperature responses in rat following intracerebral microinjection of morphine. J Pharmacol Exp Ther 150:135–139, 1965
74. Lotti VJ, Lomax P, George R: *N*-allylnormorphine antagonism of the hypothermic effect of morphine in the rat following intracerebral and systemic administration. J Pharmacol Exp Ther 150:420–425, 1965
75. Lotti VJ, Lomax P, George R: Heat production and heat loss in the rat following intracerebral and systemic administration of morphine. Int J Neuropharmacol 5:75–83, 1966
76. Madden FR, Stemler FW, Hiestand WA: Effect of certain chemical agents and physical conditions on the body temperature of mice and the relationship of temperature to drowning survival. Am J Physiol 180:121–123, 1955
77. Mahaley MS, Woodhall B: Effect of temperataure in the vitro action of anticancer agents on VX_2 carcinoma. J Neurosurg 18:269–272, 1961
78. Manax WG, Bloch JH, Largiader F, et al: Organ perfusion before transplantation with particular reference to the kidney. Surgery 57:528–534, 1965
79. Matz R: Hypothermia in diabetic acidosis. Hormones 3:36–41, 1972
80. Meeter E, Wolthuis OL, Van Benthem MJ: The anticholinesterase hypothermia in the rat: Its practical application in the study of the central effectiveness of oximes. Bull WHO 44:251–257, 1971
81. Melnak Z, Varga F: The effect of hypothermia on thioacetamide induced hepatic damage. Acta Physiol Acad Sci Hung 34:951–958, 1968
82. Meltzer H: Chlorpromazine-induced hypothermia and increased plasma creatine phosphokinase activity. Biochem Pharmacol 20:1739–1748, 1971
83. Mietkiewski E, Gracki H, Szczepanski B: Verlauf des Peptonschocks bei kunstlich unterkuhlten Hunden. Arch Int Pharmacodyn 117:328–340, 1958
84. Miller JA: Some unconventional approaches to the problem of asphyxia of the newborn. Acta Paediatr 52:198–199, 1962
85. Miller JA, Miller FS: Factors contributing to successful reanimation of mice cooled to less than 1°C. Am J Physiol 196:1218–1223, 1959
86. Miller JA, Miller FS, Westin B: Hypothermia in the treatment of asphyxia. Biol Neonatorum 6:148–163, 1965
87. Musacchia XJ, Barr RE: Survival of whole-body-irradiated hibernating and active ground squirrels, *Citellus tridecemlineatus*. Radiat Res 33:348–356, 1968
88. Musacchia XJ, Barr RE: Postirradiation hibernation and radiation response of ground squirrels: Telemetry surveillance. Radiat Res 51:631–637, 1972

89. Nakamura K, Thoenen H: Hypothermia induced by intraventricular administration of 6-hydroxydopamine in rats. Eur J Pharmacol 16:46–54, 1971
90. Neely WA, Turner MD, Haining JL: Asanguineous total body perfusion. JAMA 184:718–721, 1963
91. Negovskii VA: Some physiopathologic regularities in the process of dying and resuscitation. Circulation 23:452–457, 1961
92. Negovskii VA: Resuscitation and Artificial Hypothermia. New York, Consultants Bureau, 1962, 314 pp
93. Negovskii VA: Aspects metaboliques et toxemiques de l'irreversibilite de la mort clinique. Agressologie 9:393–399, 1968
94. Negovskii VA, Sobolef VI: Reanimation des fonctions vitales de l'organisme apres des delais prolonges de la mort clinique dans des conditions d'hypothermie. Inst Int Froid 6:75–79, 1959
95. Niazi SA, Lewis FY: Profound hypothermia in man. Ann Surg 147:264–266, 1958
96. Nurmand LB, Pervik CG, Parna RA: Distribution of barbiturates in a hypothermic organism. Farmarkol Toksikol 28:534–535, 1965
97. Ofeigsson OJ: Observations and experiments on immediate cold water treatment for burns and scalds. Br J Plast Surg 12:104–119, 1959
98. Osteen RT, Klebanoff G: The effects of hemodilution, hypothermia, and hyperbaric oxygenation of intact dogs. Cryobiology 7:263–264, 1971
99. Owens G: Effect of hypothermia on seizures induced by physical and chemical means. Am J Physiol 193:560–562, 1958
100. Pitzele S, Sze S, Dobell ARC: Functional evaluation of the heart after storage under hypothermic coronary perfusion. Surgery 70:569–577, 1971
101. Popovic P, Popovic V: Survival of newborn ground squirrels after supercooling or freezing. Am J Physiol 204:949–952, 1963
102. Popovic P, Popovic V: Survival of young rats after supercooling to −3°C. Cryobiology 2:23, 1965
103. Popovic V: Survival time of hypothermic white rats (15°C) and ground squirrels (10°C). Am J Physiol 199:463–466, 1960
104. Popovic V, Gerschman R, Gilbert DL: Effect of high oxygen pressure on ground squirrels in hypothermia and hibernation. Am J Physiol 206:49–50, 1964
105. Praslicka M, Marko L, Horak J: Modification of radiation injury in blood, bone marrow, and spleen by long-term postirradiation hypoxic hypothermia. Radiat Res 40:490–502, 1969
106. Reynolds LE, Brown CR, Price PB: Effects of local chilling in treatment of burns. Surg Forum 6:85–87, 1955
107. Ricca RA, Fink K, Katzin LI, et al: Effect of environmental temperatures on experimental traumatic shock in dogs. J Clin Invest 24:127–139, 1945
108. Rioux P, Durand H, Masson V: Contribution de l'anesthesie hypothermisante dans 24 cas de perfusion anticancereuse. Laval Med 36:573–577, 1965
109. Rochlin DB, Thaxter TH, Dickerson AG, et al: The effect of tissue temperature on the binding of alkylating agents in the isolation perfusion treatment of cancer. Surg Gynecol Obstet 113:555–561, 1961
110. Sahovic X, Armovljevic V, Popovic V: Le pouvoir thermogenetique dans le diabete alloxanique experimental. Glas Acad Serbe Sci 205:51–59, 1952

111. Schlicht I: Der Einfluss der Hypothermie auf die Leber bei experimenteller Tetrachlorkohlenstoff Vergiftung. Klin Wochenschr 42:806–812, 1964
112. Schlicht I: Die experimentelle Leberdystrophie in protrahierter Hypothermie. Untersuchungen mit Tetrachlorkohlenstoff und Thioacetamid. Z Ges Exp Med 156:183–194, 1971
113. Schlicht I, Scholz A: Die Schutzwirkung der Hypothermie auf die Leberfunction bei Tetrachlorkohlenstoffvergiftung. Verh Dtsch Ges Inn Med 135:775–778, 1965
114. Scholz A, Schlicht I, Daugs J, et al: Die Schutzwirkung der Hypothermie auf die Niere bei Sublimatvergiftung. Verh Dtsch Ges Inn Med 156:935–938, 1965
115. Schumer W: Hypothermia in septic shock. Am J Surg 103:432–436, 1962
116. Schumer W: Moderate hypothermia in controlled hemorrhage in dogs. Physiologic response of the microcirculation. Am Surg 32:347–354, 1966
117. Shingleton WW, Smith AG: Hypothermia against lethal dose of mechlorethamine. Arch Surg 82:400–404, 1961
118. Shirriffs GG, Bewsher PD: Hypothermia, abdominal pain and lactic acidosis in phenformine treated diabetic. Br Med J 3:506, 1970
119. Shulman AG: Ice water as primary treatment of burns. JAMA 173:1916–1919, 1960
120. Silberman R: The marrow protective effect of external thoracic cage cooling. Following parenteral nitrogen mustard in large doses. S Afr Cancer Bull 1: 4–13, 1967
121. Silberman R, Hofmeyer JJC: Protection of thoracic bone marrow by external hypothermia during administration of nitrogen mustard in dogs. Ann Surg 163:60–66, 1966
122. Simmonds MA, Uretsky NJ: Acute hypothermic response of the rat to intraventricular injection of 6-hydroxydopamine. Br J Pharmacol 40:564P–565P, 1970
123. Smith DE: The influence of X-irradiation upon dormancy in vertebrates. J Exp Zool 139:85–94, 1958
124. Smith NT, Gershwin ME, Hurley EJ: Hemodynamic effect of ouabain on the surgically denervated autotransplanted dog heart. Arch Int Pharmacodyn 173:95–114, 1968
125. Stevens LE, Swenson FC, Freeman JS: Preservation of kidneys in vitro: Value of hypothermia. Am J Surg 112:728–732, 1966
126. Svanes K: Effect of barbiturate anesthesia and hypothermia on edema formation caused by subcutaneous injection of 5-hydroxytryptamine in mice. Acta Physiol Scand 72:378–382, 1968
127. Tamai T: Studies of cat heart muscle during recovery from prolonged hypothermia. Automatic activity, excitability and refractoriness. 44th General Meeting, Section III, 17th General Assembly, Japanese Medical Society, 1967
128. Thom R, Schlict I: Die Ultrastruktur der Rattenleber bei Tetrachlorkohlenstoffvergiftung und protrahierter Hypothermie. Virchows Arch Abt A Pathol Anat 349:115–123, 1970
129. Thomas PA, Buchman RJ: Successful 20 hour preservation of ischemic canine lung by hypothermia combined with minimal ventilation. J Thorac Cardiovasc Surg 62:176–182, 1971

130. Tillman FC, Miller JA: Hypothermia and resistance of mice to lethal exposures to high gravitational forces. Aerospace Med 43:860–866, 1972
131. Trunkey D, Degenhardt T, Chartrand C, et al: Preservation of canine hearts. Cryobiology 6:515–521, 1970
132. Varagic VM, Zugic M, Kazic T: The hypothermic effect of eserine in the rat. Naunyn Schmiedebergs Arch Pharmakol 270:407–418, 1971
133. Voinova II: Use of hypothermia for preventing the negative effect of oxygen inadequacy on vestibular reflexes. Space Biol Med 4:120–123, 1970
134. Webb WR: Cardiac preservation. Cryobiology 5:423–428, 1969
135. Webb WR, Harrison N, Dodds R, et al: Protective effect of ethyl alcohol in profound hypothermia. Cryobiology 4:290–294, 1968
136. Westin B, Nyberg R, Miller JA, et al: Hypothermia and transfusion with oxygenated blood in the treatment of asphyxia neonatorum. Acta Paediatr Suppl 139:1–80, 1962
137. White RJ: Modifications in primate cerebral circulation and electrical activity with profound hypothermia. Cryobiology 9:383–392, 1972
138. William LJ, Morton DL: Influence of ischemia and hypothermia on the ability of the transplanted primate lung to provide immediate and total respiratory support. J Thorac Cardiovasc Surg 62:752–762, 1971
139. Williams TB, Cavanagh D: Experimental endotoxin shock. The effect of hypothermia on outcome. Am J Obstet Gynecol 108:1171–1174, 1970
140. Willman VL, Barner HB: Anatomical and physiological considerations in cardiac preservation. Cryobiology 5:413–422, 1969
141. Wislicki L: Effects of hypothermia and hyperthermia on the action of neuromuscular blocking agents. I. Suxamethonium. Arch Int Pharmacodyn 126: 68–78, 1960
142. Wislicki L: Drugs and body temperature. Georgetown Med Bull 15:137–141, 1961
143. Woodhall B, Hall K, Mahaley S, et al: Chemotherapy of brain cancer. Ann Surg 150:640–652, 1959
144. Zitowitz L, Hardy JD: Influence of cold exposure on thermal burns in rats. J Appl Physiol 12:147–154, 1958

8

Spontaneous, Accidental, and Prolonged Hypothermia

Spontaneous hypothermia develops whenever the temperature-regulating mechanisms of a homeotherm fail. This can happen after the administration of a general anesthetic, a muscle relaxant, or other drugs.[5,12] The hypothermia that develops in anesthetized patients[25] is often so profound that some clinicians call it partial or total poikilothermia. Of course, this is not a correct description of what is really happening. Anesthetized patients can enter hypothermia or hyperthermia, depending mainly on the amount of anesthetic administered and on the temperature of the operating room. Other physiologically detrimental situations may induce decreases in the body temperature, leading to development of spontaneous hypothermia. This occurs in hypothyroidism, after x-irradiation, in prostatic hyperplasia,[27] in chronic diabetes,[36] in uremic conditions,[7,23] after alcohol intoxication,[18] in hypoglycemia,[40] or in hypnosis.[15] Spontaneous hypothermia could be lethal,[1,28] especially in elderly persons[20] and in undernourished people or infants.[13,14,26,35,44] Another unusual type of spontaneous hypothermia, called "episodic hypothermia," is characterized by a shallow decrease of body temperature which might last for several weeks.[41]

ACCIDENTAL HYPOTHERMIA

Accidental hypothermia appears whenever the heat production of a homeotherm is not large enough to meet the heat loss.[22,45] In this situation the person becomes hypothermic in time due to the external cold. Often, this condition was reported to happen in aged people,[6,43] in newborn,[13,14] during shipwrecks in cold seas,[16] in ill-prepared mountain climbers,[34] or in persons lost in cold caverns.[17] People who live in severely cold climates without adequate heat or shelter, or who are not protected during snowstorms, are sometimes victims of accidental hypothermia.[9]

What can be done in the case of spontaneous or accidental hypothermia in order to save the patient's life? In the case of spontaneous hypothermia the first and most important thing is to find the main cause that led to the hypothermia and to remove the dangerous condition immediately. Almost any rewarming technique (surface rewarming with warm blankets, a warm bath, extracorporeal blood warming, or microwave warming) should be helpful[42] if the duration of hypothermia was not very long. Fast rewarming appears to be beneficial,[3,24] though some investigators believe that slow rewarming is better.[46] Intravenous administration of large amounts of fluids is probably beneficial.[33] Unfortunately after an extended hypothermic episode, the patient cannot be saved by any presently known technique and will usually die during rewarming or a few hours later. Similarly, deeply cooled animals can be successfully rewarmed during the first 5 to 6 hours of hypothermia (biological survival) but not later (clinical survival).[29–32]

PROLONGED HYPOTHERMIA

Prolonged hypothermia was first used by Smith and Fay in 1939[37] and applied to the treatment of cancer in human patients. Two years later prolonged hypothermia was used for treatment of schizophrenic patients.[4,39] Chronic hypothermia develops in patients with intracranial hypothalamic lesions.[10] Long-lasting extracorporeal hypothermia represented a problem several years ago[19] but not any more. Patients can be core cooled and kept hypothermic for many hours.

Experimental animals (dog) can be kept hypothermic for 72

hours when their body temperature is decreased to 26 to 30 C.[8,21] Cooling to 24 to 25 C decreases survival to 20 to 24 hours.[2,11,38] Safe survival time is limited to 5 to 6 hours at a body temperature of 15 C[29–32] and only to 2 hours at a body temperature of 4 C.[33]

Summary

When the heat loss of a homeotherm exceeds the heat production, hypothermia develops. This can happen in regions of cold climate, in very old or in very young persons, or in physiologically detrimental situations as the result of irradiation, uremia, and so on. Fast rewarming and the administration of intravenous fluid appear to be beneficial for the successful rewarming from spontaneous hypothermia.

BIBLIOGRAPHY

1. Adelstein AM: Certification of hypothermia deaths. Br Med J 1:482, 1973
2. Connaughton PJ, Holt G, Lewis FJ: Prolonged hypothermia below 25°C for periods over 20 hours: Influence of therapy and technique on survival. Surgery 50:372–381, 1961
3. D'Amato HE, Covino BG: Relative merits of slow versus rapid rewarming and internal versus external rewarming following acute general and local hypothermia. Arctic Aeromed Lab Tech Note AAL-TIV-59-4, 1958
4. Dill DB, Forbes WH: Respiratory and metabolic effects of hypothermia. Am J Physiol 132:685–697, 1941
5. Dripps RD: The physiology of induced hypothermia, in Dripps RD (ed): Proceedings of a Symposium. Washington, D.C., National Academy of Sciences, 1956
6. Fox RH, MacGibbon R, Davies L, et al: Problem of the old and the cold. Br Med J 1:21–24, 1973
7. Freeman RM: The role of magnesium in the pathogenesis of uremic hypothermia. Clin Res 17:52, 1969
8. Gray TC: Reflections in circulatory control. Lancet 1:383–389, 1957
9. Gregory RT: Accidental hypothermia. I. An Alaskan problem. Alaska Med 13:134–136, 1971
10. Hockaday TDR, Cranston WI, Cooper KE, et al: Temperature regulation in chronic hypothermia. Lancet 1:428–432, 1962
11. Horvath SM, Hutt BK, Spurr GB, et al: Some metabolic responses of dogs having low body temperatures. Science 118:100–101, 1953
12. Karger S: The pharmacology of thermoregulation, in Schonbaum E, Lomax P (eds): Proceedings of Satellite Symposium, San Francisco, 1972.

13. Kintzel HW: Der Energiestoffwechsel Fruhgeborener bei langehaltender Hypothermie. Monatsschr Kinderheilkd 114:544–550, 1966
14. Kintzel HW: Die Blutzucker-regulation und der Saurebasenhaushalt Frugeborener wahrend langehaltender Hypothermie. Monatsschr Kinderheilkd 115: 477–479, 1967
15. Kissen AT, Reifler CB, Thaler VH: Modification of thermoregulatory responses to cold by hypnosis. J Appl Physiol 19:1043–1050, 1964
16. Klintsevich GN: Cold injury in shipwreck. Voen Med Zh 1:64–65, 1970
17. Kreider MB: Physical and physiological factors in fatal exposures to cold. Natl Speleol Soc Bull 29:1–12, 1967
18. Laufman H: Profound accidental hypothermia. JAMA 147:1201–1212, 1951
19. Lesage MA, Young WG, Sealy WC: Studies on tolerance to prolonged deep hypothermia. Technical Documentary Report AAA-TDR 63-20 of Arctic Aeromed Lab, 1963, p 14
20. Lloyd EL: Diagnositic problems and hypothermia. Br Med J 3:417, 1972
21. MacPhee I, Gray CT, Davis S: Effects of hypothermia on adrenocoritcal response to operation. Lancet 2:1196–1199, 1958
22. Mant AK: Autopsy diagnosis of accidental hypothermia. J Forensic Med 16: 126–129, 1969
23. McKean W: Renal failure after accidental hypothermia. Br Med J 1:463–464, 1970
24. Meriwether WD, Goodman RM: Severe accidental hypothermia with survival after rapid warming. Case report, pathophysiology and review of the literature. Am J Med 53:505–510, 1972
25. Morris RH: Influence of ambient temperature on patient temperature during intraabdominal surgery. Ann Surg 173:230–233, 1971
26. Mulber H: Clinical aspects and pathology of hypothermic lesions of young infants. Munch Med Wochenschr 113:1678–1685, 1971
27. Patton RD: Hypothermia and profound acidosis due to benign prostatic hyperplasia. J Urol 105:547–548, 1971
28. Popovic P: Effet de l'hyperthermie ou de l'hypothermie precedentes sur les temperatures lethales limits. C R Soc Biol (Paris) 151:1003–1005, 1957
29. Popovic V: De l'hypothermie lethargique prolongee. Arch Sci Physiol (Paris) 9:219–229, 1955
30. Popovic V: Lethargic hypothermia in hibernators and nonhibernators. Ann NY Acad Sci 80:320–331, 1959
31. Popovic V: Physiological characteristics of rats and ground squirrels during prolonged lethargic hypothermia. Am J Physiol 199:467–471, 1960
32. Popovic V: Survival time of hypothermic white rats (15°C) and ground squirrels (10°C). Am J Physiol 199:463–466, 1960
33. Popovic V, Kostolny I, Pass K, et al: Survival of extracorporeally cooled dogs after one hour circulatory arrest. Cryobiology 8:390, 1971
34. Pugh LGCE: Accidental hypothermia in walkers, climbers, and campers: Report to the Medical Commission on Accident Prevention. Br Med J 1:123–129, 1966
35. Schmidt G, Kintzel HW, Eysold R: Elektroencephalographische Untersuchungen Fruhgeborener wahrend langehaltenden Hypothermie. Z Kinderheilkd 98:246–253, 1967

36. Shirriffs GG, Bewsher PD: Hypothermia, abdominal pain and lactic acidosis in phenformine-treated diabetic. Br Med J 3:506, 1970
37. Smith LW, Fay T: Temperature factors in cancer and embryonal cell growth. JAMA 113:653–660, 1939
38. Spurr GB, Hutt BK, Horvath SM: Prolonged hypothermia in the dog. Am J Physiol 178:275–282, 1954
39. Talbott JH, Consalazio WV, Pecora LJ: Hypothermia. Arch Int Med 68:1120–1132, 1941
40. Tashima CK: Hypoglycemia in hypothermia. N Engl J Med 289:920–921, 1973
41. Thomas DJ: Episodic hypothermia. Lancet 2:449, 1973
42. Truscott DG: Accidental profound hypothermia. Successful resuscitation by core rewarming and assisted circulation. Arch Surg 106:216–218, 1973
43. Watts AJ: Hypothermia in the aged: A study of the role of cold sensitivity. Environ Res 5:119–126, 1972
44. Wigglesworth R: Hypothermia. Br Med J 1:482, 1973
45. Zingg W: Accidental hypothermia. Med Serv J Can 22:399–410, 1966
46. Zingg W: Fast and slow rewarming after acute and prolonged hypothermia in rabbits. J Trauma 9:250–256, 1969

9

Differential Hypothermia

(H. A. Sybers collaborated in the writing of this chapter.)

Cooling or warming of a small segment or group of tissues of intact organisms can have a striking effect on their physiology. The cooling or heating of a small area in the hypothalamus by implanted thermodes will lead to a pronounced hyperthermia or hypothermia, respectively.[6] In most cases the localized cooling has to be profound to induce changes: the electroretinogram of a selectively cooled eye is changed only when the eye is preferentially cooled below a temperature of 27 C.[62] Preferential brain, lung, gastric, colonic, kidney, or extremity cooling and their physiological applications and the protective effects of hypothermia have been discussed in other chapters. The technique of localized liver[21] or vaginal[12] cooling has also been described in the literature. It was also demonstrated that a decrease in the temperature of a tissue will protect the cold cells from the lethal effects of total body irradiation.[61]

Drug response is affected by the level of the body temperature following van't Hoff's law. The protective effect of cooling is manifested in cancer chemotherapy.[5,9,19] Cooling protects the bone marrow from anticancer agents administered to experimental animals[13,49,64] or human patients.[13,53,54,55] The induced leukocytopenia is appreciably smaller if the anticancer drugs are administered in hypothermia. The toxicity of nitrogen mustard is decreased in hypothermia, in both animals[57] and patients.[56]

Embedding of anticancer drugs is greater in the warm tissues than in the cold. After diathermic heating of tissues in dogs or rabbits, ^{14}C-labeled nitrogen mustard is found in significantly greater amounts in the warm muscle or in the warm tumor tissue.[50]

Even simple warming of a group of cells leads to their destruction. This sensitivity of tumor cells to heat has been known for a long time. In 1874 an article was published dealing with a growing cheek tumor which was eventually "healed by hot water baths."[3] Besides the temperature, the time (duration of exposure) plays an important role. Warming of HeLa cells to 42 C for 30 minutes leads to pronounced changes. A temperature of 44 C destroys the HeLa cells if the exposure is prolonged.[11] Nuclear DNA and nucleolinear material disappear after an exposure of growing cells to a temperature of 45 C lasting at least 1 hour.[16] In a cell culture the heat might preferentially affect some cells but not others. Furthermore, there is a differential temperature sensitivity between the normal and the cancer cells.[2,10,15,60] A temperature of 42 C, which lasts 24 hours, affects cancer cells in vitro. Temperatures above 42 C induce lethal changes in cancer cells while leaving many normal cells unaffected. This high temperature causes irreversible damage.[58]

A new approach based on temperature differential (warm versus cold effect) was developed for cancer chemotherapy and for the embedding of biologically important pharmaceuticals in various tissues. Differential hypothermia has been initiated in experimental and clinical situations during the past decade. The use of generalized body or organ system cooling combined with localized tissue warming was undertaken to increase the metabolism and the circulation of selected warm tissues while keeping metabolic requirements of the cooled tissues at a very low level. This technique was developed and applied for tumor treatment in experimental animals, with or without chemotherapy. It was hypothesized that the metabolism of fast reproducing malignant tumor cells might be higher than that of normal tissues. Therefore, if the withdrawal of metabolic support for normothermically kept tumor cells is induced through generalized body cooling, this may lead to tumor damage due to an insufficient nutrient supply and an insufficient metabolite irrigation.

In order to achieve this goal hamsters were cooled to a temperature of 4 C during 10 hours, while transplanted cheek-pouch tumors remained at 37 C. The result of this experiment was the eradication of tumors (Fig. 9-1).[37] While tumor cells shrink and die, the muscle cells of the cheek pouch after the treatment undergo chronic inflammation and degenerative changes. Several weeks later, however, the recuperation of the cheek pouch is fully completed. When hypothermia lasted 2 or 4 hours the tumor regressed somewhat, but after several days continued to grow as in the control animals.[37] Generalized cooling of the body to only 28 to 30 C while the tumors are kept normothermic, results in tumor disappearance, provided that the cooling–warming treatment is extended to 24 hours (Fig. 9-2).[40,41] Similar results after 10 hours differential hypothermia treatment were obtained on hamsters with cheek-pouch adenovirus type-12 transplanted tumors or on hamsters with brain transplanted tumors.[23] The most striking feature of this treatment is destruction of nuclei of tumor cells.[59] Electron microscopy of adenovirus type-12 induced tumors inoculated into the cheek pouches of Syrian hamsters clearly suggests the possibility of selective destruction of tumor cells by differential hypothermia. If the tumor was implanted in both cheek pouches and only one side was warmed, a 24-hour hypothermia of 30 C had no effect on the growth rate of the cold tumor while the warm tumor disappeared.[40,41] When generalized cooling of tumor-bearing animals was employed, the tumors continued to grow as in control animals.[1,8,44] There are reports that hypothermia itself might be beneficial for treatment of tumors.[4,7,22,24,63,65] Observations made on hibernating animals show that tumors resume normal growth after arousal from hibernation.[17]

Nonhibernators cannot tolerate as profound and extended a cooling as artificially cooled hibernators.[27–29,33] In order to decrease the duration of hypothermia, 5-fluorouracil (FU), an anticancer drug, was combined with differential hypothermia. One hour of differential hypothermia in hamsters (body 4 C, tumor 37 C) and FU 50 mg/kg led to regression and complete disappearance of tumors within 4 weeks. When the same amount of FU was injected into normothermic tumor-bearing animals or hypothermic animals with hypothermic tumors, neither tumor size nor body weight of the animals was affected. It was concluded that chemotherapeutic action of 5-flourouracil was greatly enhanced when this anticancer drug was used in combination with 1-hour-long differential hypothermia (Fig. 9-3).[38,39,42] Similar results were obtained with 7,12-dimethylbenz-(α)-anthracene (DMBA)-induced tumors in

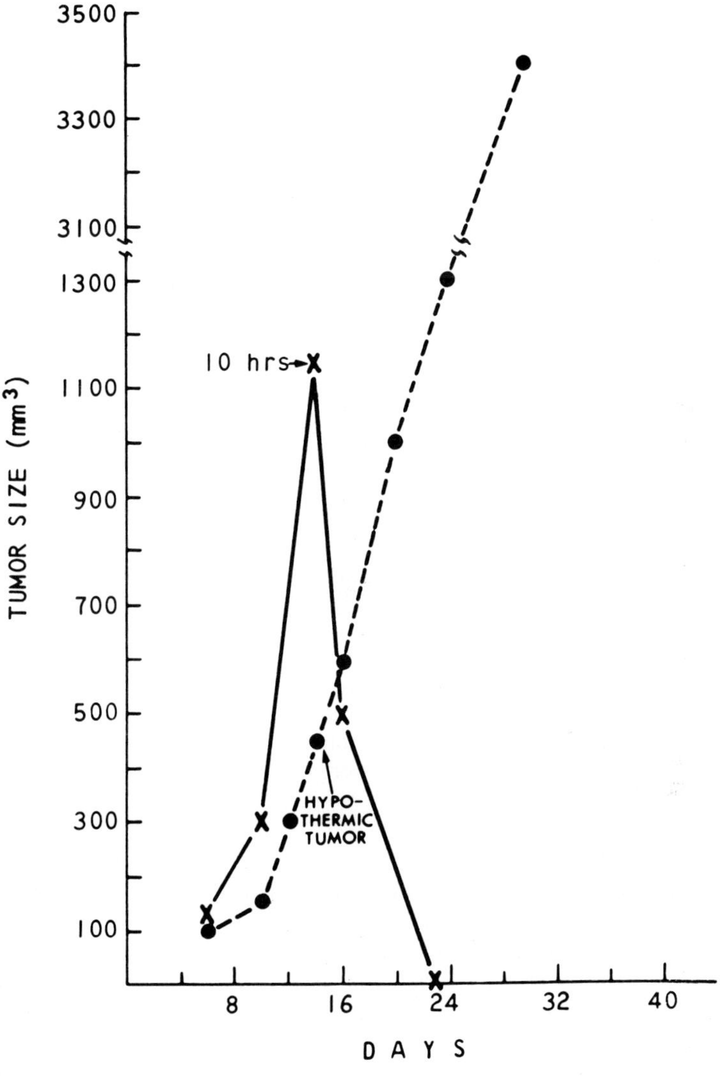

Fig. 9-1. Differential effect of local temperature of hypothermic animals on growth of tumors. The body of an animal with two tumors was cooled to a temperature of 4 C for 10 hours. The larger tumor was kept at 37 C (solid line), while the other tumor (dashed line) was kept at 4 C. The former disappeared while the latter continued to grow.[37]

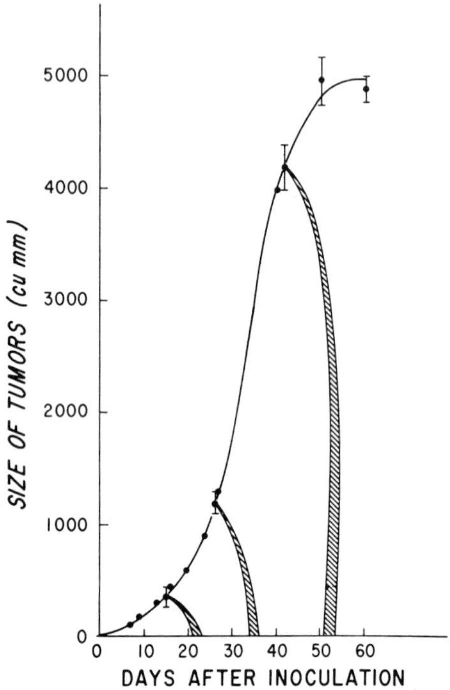

Fig. 9-2. Tumor growth (solid line) and tumor disappearance after exposure of golden hamsters for 24 hours to 30 C hypothermia while the tumors were kept normothermic.[40,41]

rats,[32] Yoshida sarcoma in rats,[18] or spontaneous mammary tumors in cannulated C_3H mice[26] when used in differential hypothermia experiments.[46,47]

In order to study possible mechanisms causing tumors to disappear after differential hypothermia and 5-fluorouracil, distribution and concentration of ^{14}C-labeled fluorouracil in the tissues of differentially cooled hamsters were studied and compared to the distribution of ^{14}C-labeled fluorouracil in normothermic and hypothermic animals. The results show that FU administered to normothermic animals is speedily utilized and excreted. On the other hand, the radioactivity of the blood remained high during the hypothermic state, indicating a high concentration of FU in the blood (Fig. 9-4).[42] This could be caused either by a decreased utilization of FU, a

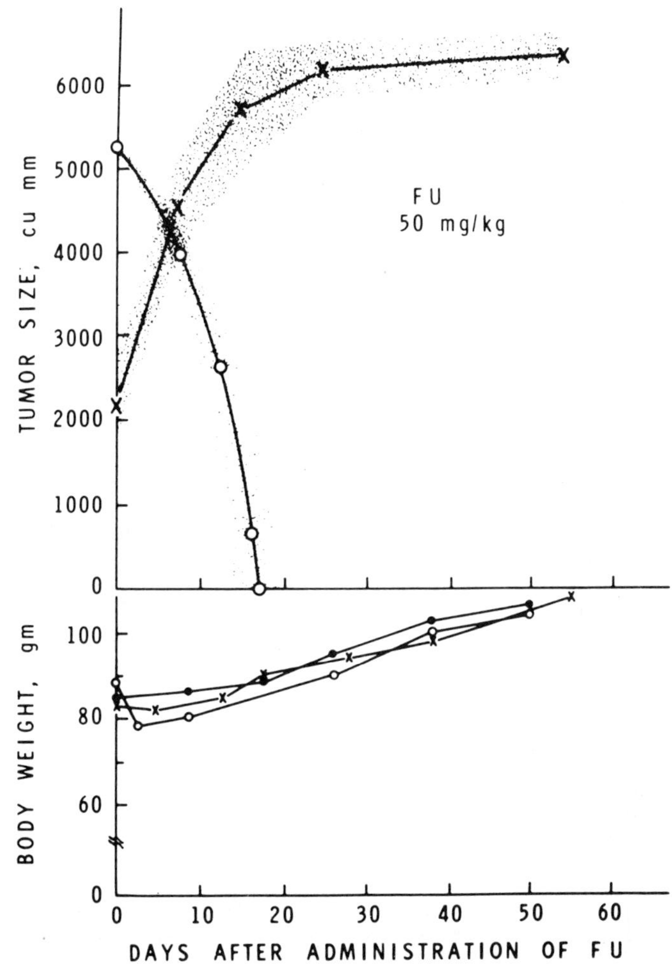

Fig. 9-3. Upper: Recession of normothermic tumors in hypothermic animals (open circles) after single injection of 50 mg/kg of 5-fluorouracil (FU). The same amount of FU when injected in the normothermic animals with normothermic tumors did not affect the growth of tumors (crosses). Lower: After a single injection of 50 mg/kg of FU the body weight of normothermic tumor-free (full dots) or normothermic tumor-bearing animals (crosses) continued to increase normally. The body weight of hypothermic hamsters with normothermic tumors (open circles) regressed somewhat after injection of FU, a fact observed in all control animals after deep body cooling.[38,39,43]

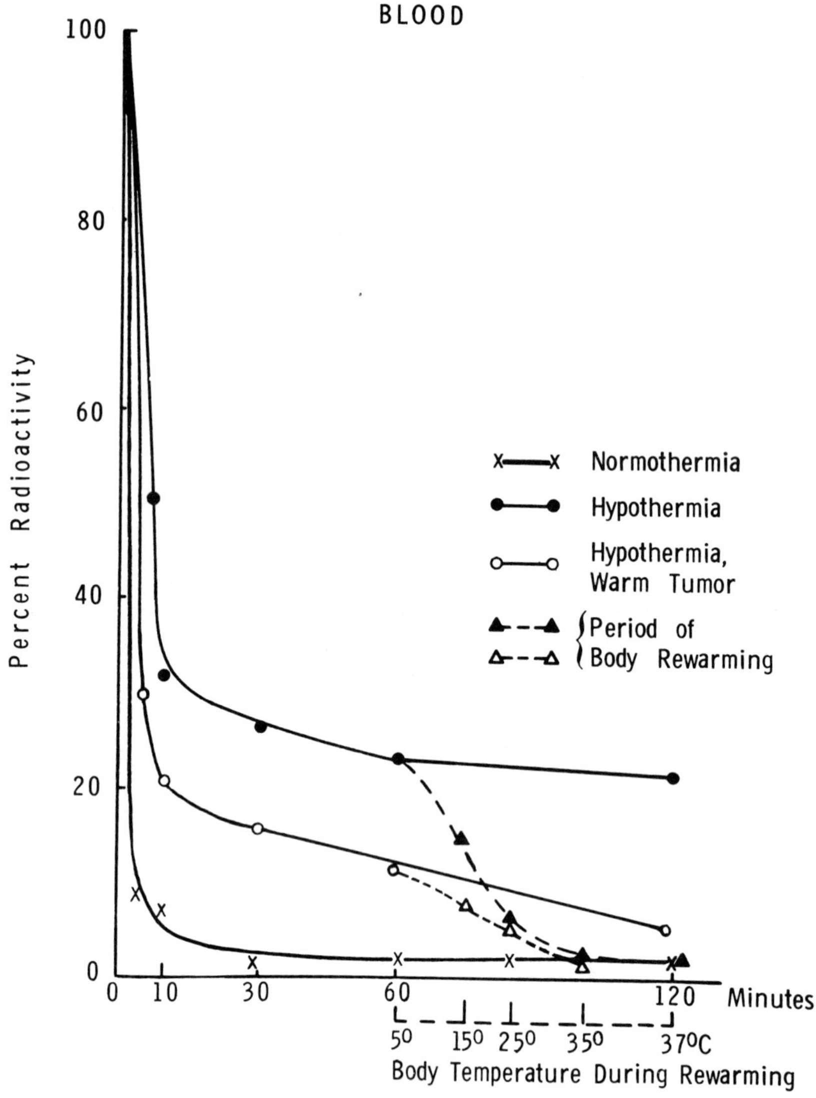

Fig. 9-4. The radioactivity of blood of hamsters after injection of 50 mg/kg of fluorouracil-2-^{14}C. Solid line (mean values): experiments in which the body temperature of the animals was unchanged. Dashed line (mean values): experiments in which the animals were rewarmed after 1 hour of hypothermia. Percentage of radioactivity (*y* axis) refers to percentage of injected radioactivity.

diminished excretion of the drug, or a combination of both. The effect of this phenomenon would be similar to that of a prolonged tissue perfusion by blood with a high FU concentration.[25,30,31,45]

One can merely speculate about the mechanisms causing tumor disappearance after differential hypothermia and 5-fluorouracil. It appears that the enhanced effectiveness of a chemotherapeutic agent when combined with differential hypothermia could be associated with several physiological changes created by differential cooling. These changes are (1) decreased utilization of the drug by cold healthy tissues. The systemic toxicity of drugs, during hypothermic phase, is very low. (2) Decreased usage of the drug by cold tissues keeps the concentration of the drug in the blood and body fluids at a high level for an extended period of time. The warm tumors can utilize this highly concentrated drug longer than when the animals are normothermic. (3) Because of vasodilation of blood vessels caused by differential tumor warming, blood circulation through warm tumors, and consequently the supply of the drug to tumors, is much greater than it is in the cold tumors in hypothermic animals. (4) Due to a high utilization of the drug in warm tumors the concentration of the drug is decreased at the end of 1 hour of differential hypothermia. Rewarming in this case does not bring the detrimental effects of systemic toxicity as it would if the drug were injected in normothermia.[46]

The drug administered to a hypothermic animal is not used by cold tissues and it is not excreted by the kidneys. Thus the concentration of the drug in the body stays at a high level throughout the experiment, that is, until rewarming of the whole body is initiated.[20,43] It is possible that besides a damaging effect of high concentration of the anticancer drug on tumors, the thermogenic changes affect the tumor irreversibly.

In other experiments instead of cooling a large experimental animal, only one organ or organ system was kept hypothermic while a small part of tissue or tumor was kept at a temperature of 38 to 40 C. The heating was done by electromagnetic or ultrasound energy (Figs. 9-5, 9-6,[67] and 9-7[46,47]). This localized differential hypothermia technique was applied to one lung of a slightly hypothermic thoracotomized dog. The lung was either kept collapsed and surface cooled with ice-cold saline or intraalveolarly cooled with ice-cold fluorocarbons (by means of a Carlins cannula[31]). In another type of experiment the entire leg of a normothermic dog was cooled to 5 to

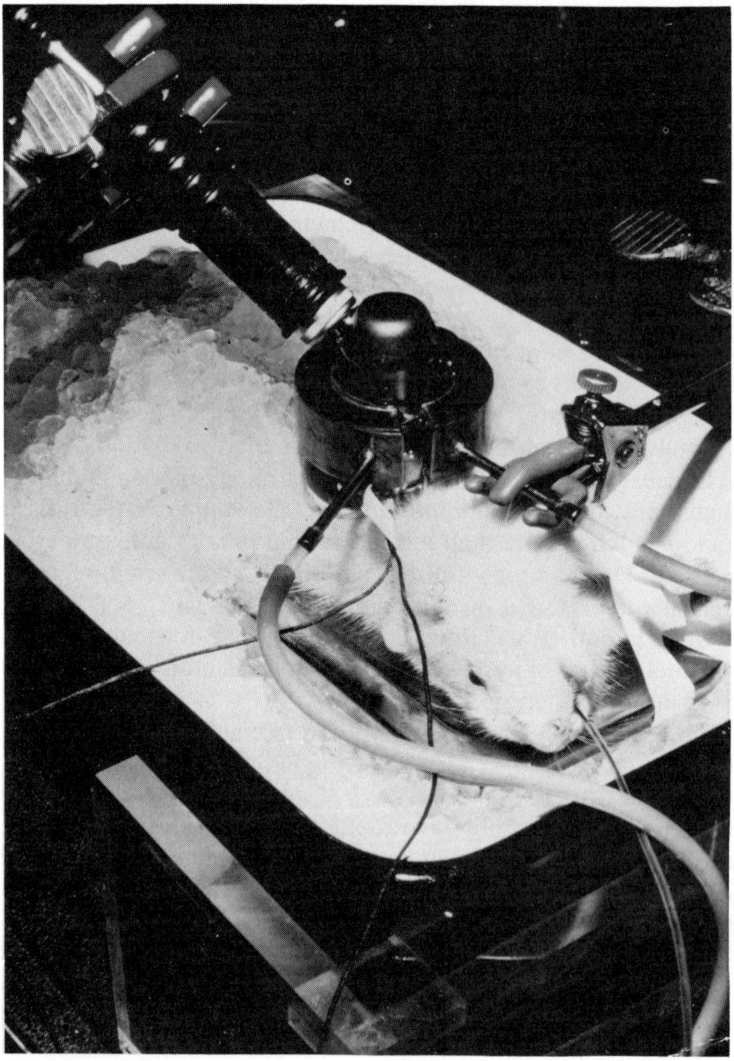

Fig. 9-5. Ultrasonic heater (Mettler Company, Pasadena, California) for warming of tumors in deeply cooled animals. Similar heaters were used to warm tumors to 38 to 40 C in deeply cooled organs or organ systems.

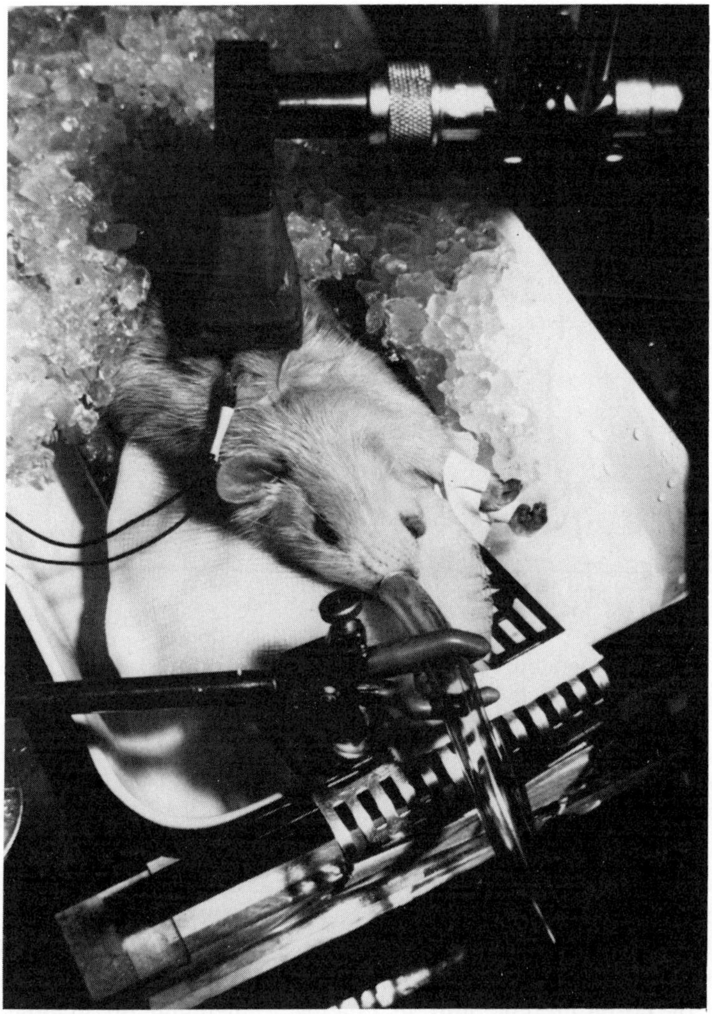

Fig. 9-6. Microwave heating of tumors in deeply cooled animals.[67]

10 C while the muscle gracilis was kept at a temperature of 38 to 40 C by electromagnetic heating. In both cases this procedure led to an increased circulation (6–37 times, determined by Sapirstein's technique[48]) through the warm part of the lung or leg while the circulation through the rest of the cold tissues was decreased.[34–36] Yttrium-loaded microspheres (injected into the femoral artery), in

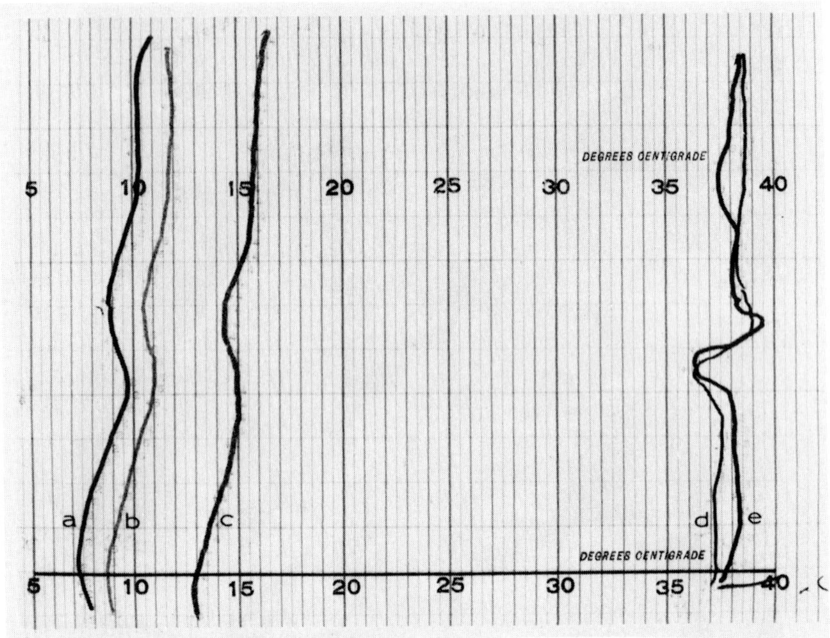

Fig. 9-7. Temperatures of different parts of the body of a mouse during 1 hour of differential hypothermia: (a) deep colonic; (b) intraperitoneal; (c) thoracic; (d) deep tumor; (e) surface tumor. The FU was injected where the heavy horizontal line is drawn. The experiment was terminated where lines are interrupted at the upper part of the recording chart. Spacing between two horizontal lines represents 15 minutes.[46,47]

combination with differential hypothermia, induced 8 times smaller embedding of ^{90}Y microspheres in profoundly cooled hind leg of dogs than in warm muscle gracilis (at a temperature of 37–38 C). This resulted in a pronounced damage or even a complete destruction of normothermic muscle gracilis (depending on loading of microspheres) while leaving undamaged all other muscle tissues that were protected by cold.[31] Therefore, the study of the circulatory parameters in differential hypothermia has shown that the circulation through the rewarmed tissues is enhanced as compared to the rest of the cooled organ system (or the cooled whole body). This led to the induction of selective embedding of the yttrium exactly in the desired tissues (sharply delineated by the increased temperature).

Thus differential hypothermia appears to be a suitable tool for the preferential embedding of medical radionuclides (or medical pharmaceuticals) whenever a selective catheterization of tumors or of other tissues is not possible.

The technique of differential hypothermia has been clinically used in several cases. Recurrent gliomas of the brain were successfully treated with only differential hypothermia or in combination with chemotherapy.[23] Hyperthermic regional perfusion of the abdominal, visceral, or pelvic areas with an alkylating agent showed an enhanced drug action when in combination with general hypothermia to protect bone marrow outside the perfused area.[51,53] Pain relief was reported by the majority of patients after the perfusion.[52] Nausea and vomiting were not observed after large systemic doses of nitrogen mustard.[14] In similar experiments on dogs hypothermic perfusion on pelvic bone marrow provided significant protection to the hematopoietic system while the sternal bone marrow kept at a normal temperature underwent a profound depression.[13] Radioactive indicator mixing curves revealed a significant degree of isolation of the upper and lower circulatory systems.[66]

Differential hypothermia proved to be beneficial in the case of actinic keratosis.[31] Actinic keratosis, defined as dermatosis commonly limited to sun-exposed surfaces, occurs after middle age and is apparent as areas of adherent hyperkeratosis. Actinic keratosis also occurs after exposure to pitch and products of coal distillation, and after ionizing radiation. These hyperkeratotic areas are usually seen on the face, the forearms, and the dorsum of the hands. If left untreated, actinic keratosis may develop into squamous cell cancer of the skin. 5-Fluorouracil (FU) has been used often for the treatment of this condition. However, FU is less effective for actinic keratosis of the hands and arms than for that of the face, which could be associated with differences in the skin temperature of the extremities and the temperature of the face, the temperature of the extremities usually being lower. This temperature difference led to the idea that the effectiveness of chemotherapy for actinic keratosis on the extremities might be increased by local warming. Patients with multiple actinic keratosis of the arms and hands were treated with FU combined with a 1-hour ultrasound warming of the lesions (surface temperature 45 C). All patients showed good remission, cessation of actinic activity (microscopic examination of punch biopsy specimens), and in some cases a complete disappearance of lesions.[31] In control groups (ultrasound heating only, FU therapy only) remission of lesions was observed in only a few cases with a concomitant continuation of actinic activity in all of the remainiing cases. Disappearance of the lesions was never observed.

Summary

Recently the technique of differential hypothermia has been developed and applied to the treatment of tumors. In this case the entire experimental animal is cooled profoundly, while the tumor is kept at the precooling (normothermic) level. This technique combined with chemotherapy induces complete disappearance of transplanted tumors, and significant regressions in chemically induced or spontaneous mammary tumors in C_3H mice. If this same chemothermotherapy is administered to normothermic animals, or to hypothermic animals with cold tumors, the drug is ineffective. Differential hypothermia with or without chemotherapy was used successfully in clinical situations. Mechanisms and possible application of this new method were discussed.

BIBLIOGRAPHY

1. Bory L: De l'action du froid sur les tissus normaux et cancereux. Prog Med 88:75–79, 1960
2. Cavaliere R, Ciocatio EC, Giovanella BC, et al: Selective heat sensitivity of cancer cells. Cancer 20:1351–1381, 1967
3. (Dr.) Chase's Family Physician, Farrier, Beekeeper, and Second Receipt Book. Toledo, Ohio, Chase Publishing Co. 1874
4. Costachel O, Grigoresco S, Tranco A: Influence de l'hypothermie sur les tumeurs greffees chez le rat. Proceedings of the 15th International Congress on Military Medicine and Pharmacy (Symposium on Hypothermia), 1957, p 378
5. Cremer JE: Body temperature and responses to drugs. Br Med Bull 25:299–306, 1969
6. Donhoffer S, Farkas M, Haug-Laszlo A, et al: Das Verhalten der Warmeproduktion und der Korpertemperatur der Ratte bei lokaler Erwarmung und Kuhlung des Gehirnes. Pfluegers Arch 268:273–280, 1958/59
7. Fay T, Henny GC: Correlation of body segmental temperature and its relation to the location of carcinomatous metastasis. Surg Gynecol Obstet 66:512–524, 1938
8. Grollman S, Crass MF III: Effects of cold on the Walker carcinosarcoma 256 in the albino rat. J Appl Physiol 21:1201–1206, 1966

9. Hara T: Temperature dependency of anti-cancer chemotherapeutic effect. Kumamoto Med J 22:140–149, 1969
10. Harris JJ, Jones WC, Woolley GW: The effect of temperature on tumor growth. Proc Am Assoc Cancer Res 3:326, 1962
11. Heine U, Sverak L, Kondratick J, et al: The behavior of HeLa-S_3 cells under the influence of supranormal temperatures. J Ultrastruct Res 34:375–396, 1971
12. Klimpel L, Gerstmann W, Friedriech H: Thermoelectric cooling probe for vaginal hypothermia. Zentralbl Gynaekol 94:631–633, 1972
13. Lee JM, Lesage AM, Sealy WC, et al: Differential perfusion hypothermia. Its use in selective bone marrow protection during the administration of nitrogen mustard. JAMA 179:435–436, 1962
14. Leone LA, Soderberg CH, Colbert M, et al: Chemical treatment of advanced neoplasms: Hyperthermic regional pelvic and abdominal perfusion with nitrogen mustard under general hypothermia. Cancer Chemother 20:127–135, 1962
15. Levine EM, Robbins EB: Differential temperature sensitivity of normal and cancer cells in culture. J Cell Physiol 76:373–380, 1970
16. Love R, Soriano RZ, Walsh RJ: Effect of hyperthermia on normal and neoplastic cells in vitro. Cancer Res 30:1525–1533, 1970
17. Lyman CP, Fawcett DW: The effect of hiberation on growth of sarcoma in the hamster. Cancer Res 14:25–28, 1954
18. Magdon E: Experimentelle Untersuchungen zur Wirkung lokaler Erwarmung bei der Tumortherapie mit Zytostatika in Hypothermie. Wissenschaftliche Chirurgentagung der DDR 1381–1385, 1965
19. Mahaley MS Jr, Woodhall B: Effect of temperature upon the in vitro action of anti-cancer agents on VX-2 carcinoma. J Neurosurg 18:269–272, 1961
20. Masironi R, Popovic V: Differential hypothermia-normothermia as a new tool to enhance the activity of anti-cancer drugs. Radioisotope study. Acta Isotop 7:289–298, 1967
21. Mito M, Tamaki A, Kon T, et al: Experimental studies on differential hypothermia of the liver. J Surg Res 5:207–212, 1965
22. Niazi SA, Lewis FJ: The effect of hypothermia on malignant growth in rats. Surg Forum 6:408–411, 1956
23. Nishimoto A, Nobuto H, Tabuchi I, et al: Treatment of malignant glioma by differential hypothermia. Proceedings of the 28th Neurosurgical Conference, Prague, June 1971, pp 228–231
24. Picha E: Hypothermia in the treatment of gynecologic carcinoma. Wien Klin Wochenschr 82:633–636, 1970
25. Popovic P, Popovic V: Protective effects of differential hypothermia, in Musacchia XJ, Saunders JF (eds): Depressed Metabolism. New York, Am Elsevier, 1969, pp 499–524
26. Popovic P, Sybers H, Popovic V: Permanent cannulation of blood vessels in mice. J Appl Physiol 25:625–626, 1968
27. Popovic V: Lethargic hypothermia in hibernators and nonhibernators. Ann N Y Acad Sci 80:320–331, 1959
28. Popovic V: Survival time of hypothermic white rats (15°C) and ground squirrels (10°C). Am J Physiol 199:463–466, 1960
29. Popovic V: Physiological characteristics of rats and ground squirrels during prolonged lethargic hypothermia. Am J Physiol 199:467–471, 1960

30. Popovic V: Tissue perfusion in hypothermia. in Malinin TJ, Zeppa R, Gollan F, Callahan RA (eds): Reversibility of Cellular Injury due to Inadequate Perfusion. Springfield, Thomas, 1972, pp 422–425
31. Popovic V: Regulatory Biology; Depressed Metabolic States, Holton EM (ed). NASA TM-X-69354, 1973, pp 158–177
32. Popovic V, Baughman JE, Worthington J, et al: Effect of 5-fluorouracil on DMBA induced normothermic tumors in hypothermic rats. Fed Proc 29:717, 1970
33. Popovic V, Kent KM: Factors limiting survival in hypothermic animals. Proceedings of the International Microcirculation Conference, Cambridge (England), 1966, pp 63–64
34. Popovic V, Kostolny I, Larose JH, et al: Enhanced perfusion in microwave heated part of hypothermic lung. J Physiol (Paris) 63:386–389, 1971
35. Popovic V, Kostolny I, Larose JH, et al: Selective embedding of I^{131} albumin in microwave heated part of hypothermic lung. Proceedings of the Institute of Experimental Surgery, Slovak Academy of Science, 1971, pp 247–253
36. Popovic V, Kostolny I, Novicic D, et al: Selective embedding of $I\text{-}^{131}$ albumin in microwave heated part of hypothermic lung. Abstract, Fourth International Hibernation and Hypothermia Symposium, 1971, pp 21–22
37. Popovic V, Masironi R: Disappearance of euthermic tumors after 10-hour generalized hypothermia. Life Sci 4:533–543, 1965
38. Popovic V, Masironi R: Enhancement of 5-fluorouracil action on normothermic tumors in generalized hypothermia. Cancer Res 26:2353–2356, 1966
39. Popovic V, Masironi R: Effets de medications anticancereuses sur les tumeurs normothermiques chez les animaux en hypothermie. J Physiol (Paris) 58:594–595, 1966
40. Popovic V, Masironi R: Disappearance of normothermic tumors in shallow (30°C) hypothermia. Cancer Res 26:863–864, 1966
41. Popovic V, Masironi R: Effect of generalized hypothermia on normothermic tumors. Am J Physiol 211:462, 1966
42. Popovic V, Masironi R: Use of hypothermia in cancer chemotherapy; animal studies. Riv Biol 64:3–14, 1971
43. Popovic V, Masironi R, Lehr R: Distribution of fluorouracil-2-C^{14} in hypothermic animals with normothermic tumors. Cryobiology 6:87–92, 1969
44. Popovic V, Sahovic X: L'influence de l'hypothermie sur la prise et l'evolution du sarcome transplante. Glas Acad Serbe Sci 202:99–106, 1951
45. Popovic V, Sybers HA, Popovic P: Mechanisms of tumor regression after chemotherapy and differential hypothermia, in Stacker A (ed): Chemo- und Immunotherapie der Leukosen und Malignen Lymphome. Vienna, Bohmann Verlag, 1969, pp 404–405
46. Popovic P, Sybers HA, Popovic V: Regression of spontaneous mammary tumors in C_3H mice after 5-fluorouracil and differential hypothermia. Minerva Chir 24:1145–1147, 1969
47. Popovic P, Sybers HA, Popovic V: Regression of spontaneous mammary tumors in C_3H mice after 5-fluorouracil and differential hypothermia. Panminerva Med 13:523–526, 1971
48. Sapirstein LA: Regional blood flow by fractional distribution of indicators. Am J Physiol 193:161–168, 1958

49. Schmahl D, Druckrey H: Beitrage zum Wirkungsmechanismus von N-oxyd-lost. Naturwissenschaften 43:199, 1956
50. Shingleton WW: Selective heating and cooling of tissues in cancer chemotherapy. Ann Surg 156:408–416, 1962
51. Shingleton W, Parker RT: Abdominal perfusion with hypothermia and hyperthermia. Cancer Chemother Rep 10:35–38, 1960
52. Shingleton WW, Parker RT: Abdominal perfusion for cancer chemotherapy using hypothermia and hyperthermia. Acta Union Int Contre Cancer 20:465–468, 1964
53. Shingleton WW, Parker RT, Mahaley S: Abdominal perfusion for cancer hemotherapy with hypothermia and hyperthermia. Surgery 50:260–265, 1961
54. Shingleton WW, Reeves JW, Keppel RA, et al: Studies on abdominal organ perfusion for cancer chemotherapy. Ann Surg 151:741–749, 1960
55. Shingleton WW, Smith AG: Hypothermia against lethal dose of mechlorethamine. Arch Surg 82:400–404, 1961
56. Silberman R: The marrow protective effect of external thoracic cage cooling. S Afr Cancer Bull 11:4–13, 1967
57. Silberman R, Hofmeyer JJC: Protection of thoracic bone marrow by external hypothermia during administration of nitrogen mustard in dogs. Ann Surg 163:60–66, 1968
58. Simard R, Bernhard W: A heat-sensitive cellular function located in the nucleolus. J Cell Biol 34:61–76, 1967
59. Tabuchi K, Arimori M, Yoshizu H, et al: Ultrastructural findings of adenovirus type 12-induced tumor cells treated by differential hypothermia. Gann 63: 725–730, 1972
60. Von Ardenne M: Prinzipien und Konzept 1973 der "Krebs-Mehrschritt-Therapie" mit Optimaldistanz-Nachtherapie. Ther d Gegenw 113:48–60, 1974
61. Weiss L: Sensitivity of hypothermic mammals to X-irradiation (a review). Br Med Bull 17:70–73, 1961
62. Wolin LR, Massopust LC: Selective cooling of the eye. Arch Ophthalmol 76:723–728, 1966
63. Woodhall B, Hall K, Mahaley S Jr, et al: Chemotherapy of brain cancer: Experimental and clinical studies in localized hypothermic cerebral perfusion. Ann Surg 150:640–651, 1959
64. Woodhall B, Pickrell KL, Georgiade ND, et al: Effect of hypothermia upon cancer chemotherapy; application to external cancers of head and face structures. Ann Surg 151:750–758, 1960
65. Woodhall B, Reynolds DH, Mahaley S Jr, et al: The physiologic and pathologic effects of localized cerebral hypothermia. Ann Surg 147:673–683, 1958
66. Young WG, Lesage AM, Dillon ML, et al: Chemotherapy of intrathoracic neoplasms employing differential pelvic perfusion hypothermia. Ann Surg 154:372–382, 1961
67. Zimmer RP, Ecker HA, Popovic V: Selective electromagnetic heating of tumors in animals in deep hypothermia. IEEE Trans Microwave Theory Technique 2:238–245, 1971

10

Hibernation

A strange chip!

The moon is bright,
The skies are clear,
The stars are twinkling
But the winter is near.

A young chipmunk
Stares at the sky,
In the quiet forest
Nearby.

"You must go to sleep
As all others"
The worried mother said
"Your grandma and grandpa
Your sister and brothers
Even your father
Just went to bed!"

"I don't want!
Why not the beaver?
Why not the cat?
I am still warm:
Simple as that!"

The heavy clouds approached
Dressed in winter coats.
One exception makes not the rule:
This are my thoughts.

DEFINITION

Hibernation is a syndrome of seasonal adaptations found in some homeothermic organisms, to escape from the cold of the winter season and from the scarcity of food by decreasing their body temperature and their metabolism. The term hibernation should not be applied to any poikilotherms in winter torpor nor to any nonhibernators artificially cooled. Although some Russian authors still use the phrase "artificial hibernation" for induced hypothermia, this unfortunate term is slowly disappearing. There is little justification in ascribing to nonhibernators any hibernating properties. Hibernation is quite different from induced hypothermia, even in the same animal. To talk about a "hibernating mouse"[8] or any other "hibernating" nonhibernator does not make much sense.

ACTIVE HIBERNATORS

There are many hibernators, and most of them are mammals (rodents, insectivores, and bats),[47,53] although there are also a few birds.[59] Several review articles describe hibernators in depth.[22,28,35,38,39,48] Some hibernators enter torpor even during the summer season; they are called aestivators.[31] During the summer months active hibernators do not differ physiologically from nonhibernators. Their body temperature is regulated in the same way. Body temperature, eating, drinking, sleeping, and waking are controlled by the hypothalamus in both nonhibernators and hibernators. Furthermore, the circulation, respiration, and other physiological characteristics of hibernators are the same as in nonhibernators. The active hibernators fight the low environmental temperatures quite well, often better than nonhibernators.[65] But when the cold months come, hibernators—at their choice of time and place—suddenly lose homeothermic characteristics, their body temperature drops close to that of the environment, and they spend several weeks or several months in hibernating torpor. Satinoff[94] calls these changes "some of the largest and most drastic fluctuations seen in any physiological regulation." This decrease in body temperature and torpor have led many investigators to believe that hibernators become poikilotherms during winter months.[39] However, hibernators when in hibernation are quite different from poikilotherms in winter torpor. While a harmful stimulus (except low external temperature) induces prompt arousal of hibernating animals to homeothermy, poikilotherms do not react even if their lives are in jeopardy. A surgical procedure on a hibernating animal leads to arousal in a few minutes, to struggling, exaggerated movements, and interruption of the operative procedure, while the same animal when artificially cooled, or a nonhibernator that is artificially cooled, will not react. A number of years ago this fact was used to suggest that physical anesthesia of cold can replace chemical anesthesia in surgery.[11,23]

It is interesting to note that the black bear is not a hibernator as some very courageous investigators have shown with direct measurements of rectal temperature (mercury manometer) of these animals during the winter sleep. At this time of the year the body temperature of bears is close to the normal homeothermic level and their oxygen consumption is only slightly diminished.[27] Furthermore, the birth of young takes place in early January, the coldest month of the year.

Study of the ontogenesis of temperature regulation in newborn ground squirrels has shown that chemical thermoregulation (increase of heat production during a moderate cold exposure) is present from the moment of birth, indicating that hibernators are not primitive animals as far as temperature regulation is concerned.[105] However, the physical temperature regulation develops in these animals more slowly than in nonhibernators of similar size.

ENTERING HIBERNATION

How do hibernators enter hibernation? Unfortunately, the mechanisms for entering hibernation are still unknown.[60] External cold might be one of the permissive factors, and usually is. But ground squirrels, even when kept at a temperature of thermal neutrality (30 C) enter hibernation as well.[81]

Before entering hibernation, hibernators "prepare" for hibernation. They eat much more than in the spring and summer months and become extremely obese. This gain in body weight during the prehibernating period is often very great. In a single week some hibernators gain up to 30 percent of body mass,[108] an increase that would correspond to a gain in weight of 50 pounds for a man of average weight (Fig. 10-1). Eighty to 90 percent of the lipids that are accumulated prior to hibernation are in an unsaturated form.[95,96] The amount of fat that a ground squirrel gains in the fall (as compared to all the fatty tissue the same animal had at the beginning of fall) is 300 or more percent. The hibernators become so fat that they can be compared with nonhibernators who become hyperphagic after induced lesions to hypothalamic ventromedial nucleus.[55] It is

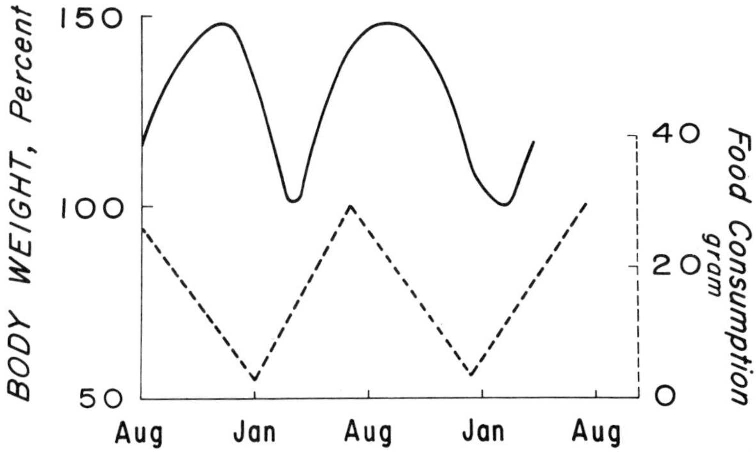

Fig. 10-1. Seasonal changes of body weight (upper curve) and daily food consumption of ground squirrels (idealized after work of Pengelley and Fisher[60]).

possible that a tremendous increase in body fat is one of the prerequisites for a successful entrance into hibernation and maybe even for arousal.[58] Fat formation is not the consequence of excessive eating only. In the fall even when on the same regimen as during the summer months the animals become fat because they are less active and even more because their metabolic rate is greatly decreased.[65,68]

Though little is known about the role of the brain in hibernation, there are some data to indicate its importance. For instance, animals with lesions in the anterior hypothalamus enter hibernation (or is it only hypothermia?) but cannot wake up, and die in torpor. It is also possible that a decrease in the function of central adrenergic fibers[17] is necessary for entrance into hibernation. Hoffman[29] believes that induction into hibernation takes place because of rapid, major modifications in functions of the central nervous system. It might be that hibernators stand cooling better because of greater glucose utilization in their brain as compared to nonhibernators. ATP synthesis in the brains of hibernators is greater too. The hypothalamus might be involved in some of the newly acquired adaptation processes that make hibernators unique in withstanding low body temperature. After induction of lesions in the posterior hypothalamus, hamsters do not hibernate.[51,52,92,93] Thus it is possible that the posterior hypothalamus participates in pituitary–adrenal response and leads to inability to hibernate.[56] A better understanding of these mechanisms, whatever they are, might indicate how to handle hypothermia better and to use all the benefits it offers. These mechanisms, especially the process of entering hibernation and of the early beginning of arousal, might be very illuminating.

Involution and the decrease in endocrine function[3,21,75] appear to be prerequisites for entering into hibernation. The pituitary gland,[13] adrenals,[61,111] thyroid,[44] and reproductive system follow this trend. How the pituitary function is inhibited is still unknown. Hoffman[29] suggested differential vasoconstriction of the pituitary region or a possible absence of the synthesis of hypothalamic releasing factors.

It has been shown that after adrenalectomy ground squirrels or hamsters cannot enter hibernation.[36,106,107] But if cortical hormones are administered or if a small piece of adrenal cortex is transplanted into the anterior chamber of the eye of adrenalectomized ground squirrels, the animals hibernate during the winter season.[73,83–85] It is important to point out here, however, that normal thermoregulation is disturbed even in nonhibernators that are deprived of their adrenal glands.[90,91] Hibernators can hibernate without the thyroid gland, but injection or feeding of thyroid hormones prevents hibernation.[73,75] This last fact might be the consequence of an increased BMR observed after the treatment. However, thiouracil does not change the tendency to hibernate, indicating that the mechanism of hibernation is probably not limited by the thyroid gland alone.

Endocrine glands that are not directly controlled by the hypophysis do not show this striking anatomical and physiological change. On the contrary, they show an increased activity during this time of preparation for hibernation.[29]

Some of these hypotheses dealing at least with "blood borne" factors as mechanisms of hibernation[14–16] can now be tested. It has been said previously that "everyone who has attempted to make experiments on hibernating animals has encountered a major difficulty: when touched, the hibernator awakens with great ease."[41] A recently developed technique of permanent cannulation of the aorta and the right ventricle of the heart[80,82] now offers the opening of some of the closed shutters of the endocrine and blood-borne secrets of hibernation. Employing this technique one can withdraw the blood from hibernating animals without disturbing hibernation, one can inject drugs of hormones, or make parabiotic studies between a hibernating and an active animal or between two hibernating animals. A miniaturized pump oxygenator[62,63] and a miniaturized dialyzer[54] recently developed in our laboratory, also permit an in-depth evaluation of blood-borne factors of hibernation.

After the whole complicated process of preparation is accomplished, the time comes when the hibernator enters hibernation by somehow "resetting" its hypothalamic thermoregulator. Then even while maintaining an unchanged body temperature, the metabolism, oxygen consumption, heart rate, cardiac output, respiration rate, and other physiological processes suddenly decrease to a much lower hibernating level. Therefore, it appears that hibernation starts at a normothermic body temperature and is characterized with sudden shift to different metabolic pathways. A decrease in the metabolic rate causes a decrease in body temperature which in turn creates a further decrease in metabolism. Instead of bringing into play thermoregulatory mechanisms and a much increased heat production, environmental cold leads now to profound cooling. However, hiberators will hibernate even at much higher external temperatures as previously mentioned. Even when kept at an external temperature of 30 C (temperature of thermal neutrality) ground squirrels will hibernate.[71,81] In a Herter system where an active hamster can go from one room to another searching for the external temperature it likes, an active animal prefers a warm external temperature even during the winter months, but chooses a cold corner when ready to enter hibernation.[25]

The ECG studies show that ground squirrels enter hibernation while awake.[94] The theory of "test drops" (stepwise and gradual entering of hibernation that might last several days) was widely accepted earlier,[99–101] but it appears now that very few hibernators (for instance, *Citellus beecheyi*) enter hibernation this way.

PHYSIOLOGICAL CHANGES DURING HIBERNATION

Each bout of hibernation does not last more than several days but is necessarily interrupted with a periodic arousal. Each periodic arousal lasts only a few hours.

In hibernation the oxygen consumption and the metabolic rate of hibernators depend linearly on environmental and body temperature.[71] At a body temperature of 4 to 6 C the oxygen consumption of hibernating hamsters,[46] ground squirrels,[70] or other hibernating animals is about the same, 20 ml/kg/hr. When the oxygen consumption of hibernating animals is compared with the oxygen consumption of normothermic animals at the same external temperature, the ratio is 1 or 2 to 100.

During hibernation the metabolic rate is related to total weight,[37] and not to surface areas as in all other homeotherms. Furthermore, it appears that hibernators do not regulate their body temperature when in hibernation.[26] That is to say that central nervous control of temperature regulation ceases in hibernation. When the environmental temperature—and consequently body temperature—decreases below 1 C, a hibernating animal dies in hibernation, without trying to wake up.[81] The low external and consequently a dangerously low body temperature overcomes the animal. This is because its respiratory (ventilatory) movements eventually cease.

In hibernating animals the heart is active even at a temperature close to the freezing point, while in artificially cooled nonhibernators the heart stops pumping at a body temperature between 8 and 20 C.[32] Thus an adequate capillary blood flow keeps a deeply cooled hibernator (and a very young animal) alive. Inadequate blood flow kills the nonhibernating animals that venture into profound hypothermia. It is important to realize, however, that mechanical devices built during the last 20 years can be used to convert a cooled nonhibernator into a kind of semisuccessful hibernator by restarting its blood flow after a circulatory cessation of 1 to 2 hours.

In hibernation there is little if any sympathetic tone. The heart accumulates glycogen in hibernation. It has been suggested that there is lowering of energy barriers for enzymes of the heart[29] and maybe of other enzymatic systems in the body. This might lead to functional differences in the entropies of the same enzymes in hibernators. Therefore, it appears that an entirely different enzymatic system does not exist in hibernators[88,97] as once was postulated.

In hibernation the heart rate, stroke volume, and cardiac output are decreased to 1 to 2 percent of normothermic value (Fig. 10-2).[77] The arterial blood pressure is very low, 40 to 45 mm Hg, while the central venous pressure remains unchanged (Fig. 10-3).[49,77] Any increase of the arterial pressure above this value leads to electrical

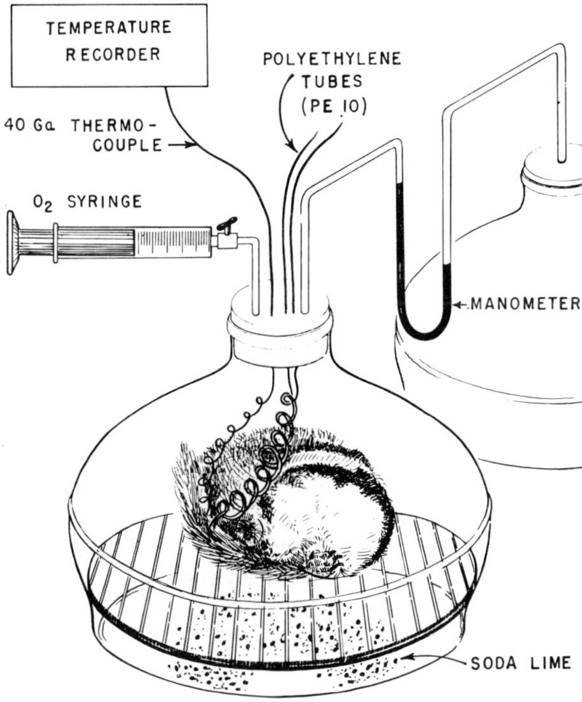

Fig. 10-2. Metabolism chamber (temperature compensated, right chamber) that permits continuous measurement of O_2 consumption, ECG, arterial and right ventricular pressure, and cardiac output of hibernating ground squirrels.[77]

and mechanical cessation of cardiac action lasting 30 to 40 seconds or longer, that is, as long as the arterial blood pressure needs to return below this critical value of 40 to 45 mm Hg (Fig. 10-4). Thus in hibernation one observes resetting of baroreceptors, something that is badly lacking in the artificially induced hypothermic state. In hibernation a very low arterial blood pressure, concomitant with increased permeability of capillaries, does not lead to edema. In hypothermia, a much higher arterial blood pressure and a cold-induced increase in capillary permeability lead to cold swelling and edema which eventually limit the safe survival time of deeply cooled nonhibernators.

Several changes in blood constituents and blood chemistry are

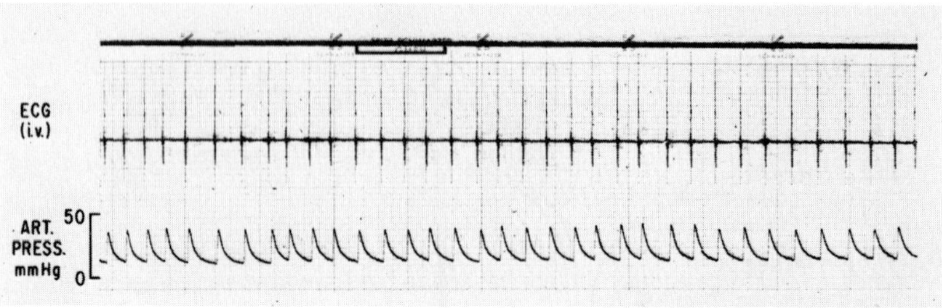

Fig. 10-3. Intraventricular ECG (obtained by means of implanted aortic and right ventricular cannulas) and arterial blood pressure of a hibernating ground squirrel. Upper line, boxed area: 1 minute.

seen in hibernation. The number of reticulocytes is decreased, and blood glycemia is very low.[2,4,6] Blood cell volume appears to be unchanged.[34] The pH of the blood,[49] Mg level,[19,87] and coagulation time are increased. The increased Mg concentration might be of importance. Even in nonhibernators an increased Mg concentration helps the animals to stand lowering of the body temperature better. But what appears to be especially important is the profound he-

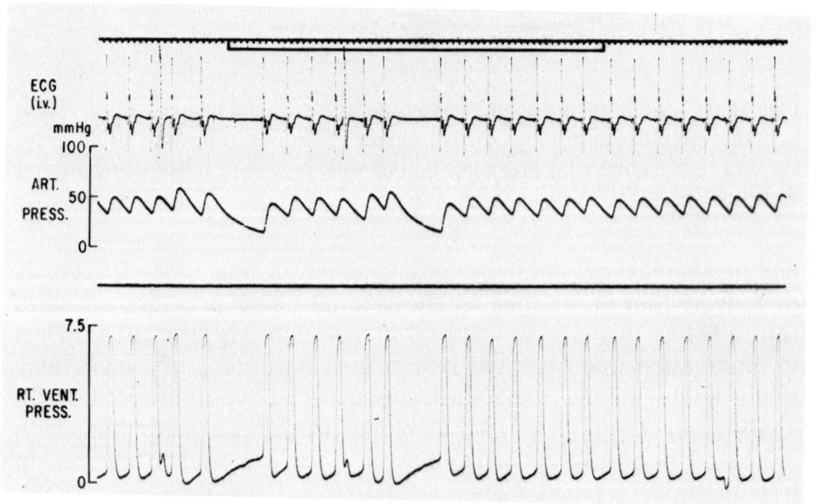

Fig. 10-4. When the arterial pressure reaches a critical point (above 45–50 mm Hg) the heart action is interrupted for a few seconds and the arterial pressure decreases to the normal low value. During the long diastole the right ventricular pressure is increased.

modilution observed in hibernating animals.[77] This hemodilution decreases the blood viscosity which must be rather high at this low temperature and at this very low velocity of blood flow. The lifespan of red blood cells is prolonged from 100 days to an estimated value of 1 to 7 years.[45]

Other physiologic functions are changed too. The activity of peripheral nerves and of the brain in hibernators is observed at a much lower temperature than in nonhibernators. However, brain cortical activity is completely suppressed during extended periods.[50,89] There is one report, however, which describes continuous coritcal activity in hibernation.[98] In hibernation animals show both kinds of sleep, "slow wave sleep" and "paradoxical sleep."[92,93] In hibernation one observes increased glutamic decarboxylase activity of the brain tissue.[43] The RNA content of the hypothalamus is decreased.[86] Neurosecretion that increases during the fall is very intense during hibernation.[103]

In hibernation there is an intense breakdown of fats in brown fat tissue[42] and it appears that fats are oxidized preferentially. The digestive system is profoundly involuted in hibernation,[2,5] and liver glycogen is increased.[7] Kidney function and respiratory movements are greatly decreased. The regeneration of liver and other tissues is greatly extended also. These and other similar findings brought forth the stories of 100 times extended lifespan in hibernation.

Hibernating ground squirrels are very insensitive to a decrease in pO_2 in the inspired air. While oxygen consumption of active hibernators, as well as oxygen consumption of nonhibernators, begins to decrease when the pO_2 in the inspired air is decreased to 90 to 100 mm Hg, the oxygen consumption of hibernating animals is not affected even when the pO_2 is decreased to a value of 40 mm Hg. During this decrease of pO_2 of 40 mm Hg, the hibernating animal begins to wake up and then instead of decreasing its O_2 consumption, as would be seen in any other animal species, one observes an increase of O_2 consumption at least initially.[66,67,72] This very significant resistance to a decreased pO_2 has never been observed in any other homeothermic animal.

Hibernation protects from x-irradiation as well.[9,57] In another detrimental situation, oxygen poisoning, the protective role of hibernation was demonstrated. Exposed to 6 ATA of pure oxygen, hibernating ground squirrels live 40 times longer than normothermic animals.[78]

AROUSAL

Hibernation is always interrupted by periodic arousals.[6] Sometimes the animals do not become fully aroused and reach a body temperature of only 25 to 30 C. It seems that a sojourn longer than 2 to 3 weeks in hibernation must end in death. The hibernating animal must wake up from time to time, even if only for an hour or two to stay alive. A hibernating animal wakes up at any time of the day or night, thus circadian rhythm might be absent in hibernation[40,41] or at least reset during induced arousals.[79]

During arousal the hibernating animal makes a tremendous energetic effort using fats preferentially as the fuel,[7] and liver glycogen is depleted too.[2] In the early part of the arousal—at a body temperature that is still practically *unchanged*—one witnesses a large increase in O_2 consumption (Fig. 10-5).[74] This kind of life machine is unseen in other animals, either poikilotherms or homeotherms.

It is known that during arousal a hibernator always urinates. Is this urge to urinate the cause of arousal? Is the accumulation of water what makes hibernators wake up periodically? Is hyperketonemia the "trigger" for arousal,[10] or does the accumulation of acid metabolites endanger life? Such an accumulation could make a cold animal drown very fast after a critical point is reached,[24] but not everyone accepts this hypothesis.[110]

Another possibility is that profound body cooling induces a slow breakage of the blood–brain barrier in hibernation as it does in hypothermia,[109] thus permitting cyclic AMP to enter the brain tissue (after a number of days) to induce arousal from hibernation. This hypothesis is very attractive because it takes care of the fact that at a somewhat higher body temperature of the brain, arousals will be more frequent.

It appears that the anterior hypothalamus is needed for successful arousal from hibernation. Without the anterior hypothalamus the animals die after 10 days in hibernation (or is it in hypothermia?). Injected epinephrine, many trophic hormones, adenosine, adenine nucleotides, and AMP lead to arousal of hibernating animals. Thus, it is possible that most of these agents which cause the conversion of ATP to cyclic AMP might play a role in the process of arousal.

After adrenalectomy hibernating ground squirrels are able to arouse to normothermic life.[107] Because of the length of the opera-

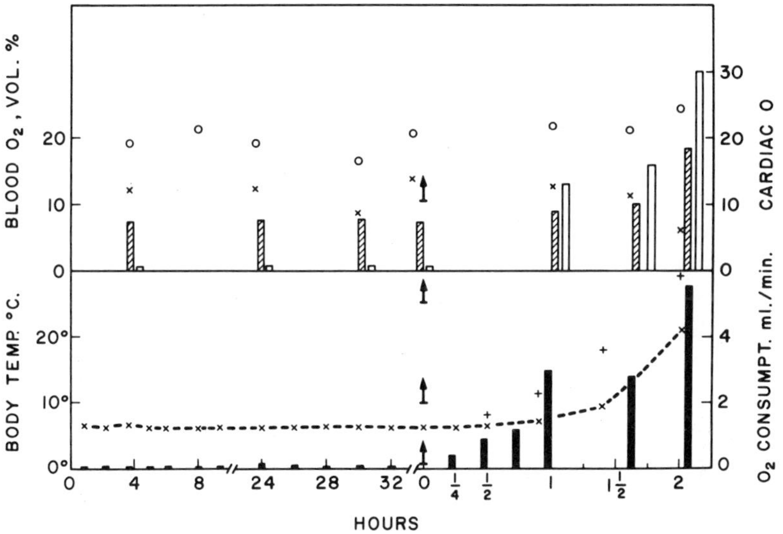

Fig. 10-5. Oxygen consumption (black boxes in the lower part of the figure), body temperature (dashed line, lower part of the figure), cardiac output (open boxes, upper part of the figure), and AV difference of oxygen contents (shaded boxes, upper part of the figure) of a hibernating ground squirrel and of the same animal that began to wake up (right part of the figure) during a period of 2.5 hours. Open circles in the upper part of the figure represent arterial oxygen content, crosses represent venous oxygen content.

tive procedure (at least several minutes) it is possible that the adrenal hormones were already released into circulation before adrenal glands were removed. To avoid this problem hibernating adrenalectomized ground squirrels with cortical implants in the anterior chamber of one eye were suddenly deprived of the implant. These animals were still able to arouse normally to normothermia.[82] However, one observes blockade of arousal from hibernation after inhibition of norepinephrine synthesis.[20] Thus it appears that while the cortical part of adrenals might be necessary for entering hibernation, the presence of the medullar part (and a small sympathetic release) is imperative for successful arousal from hibernation.

During arousal a hibernating animal shivers violently. It has been suggested that differential venoconstriction, shunting the blood toward the heart and anterior region of the body, takes place during hibernation. This process leads to a tremendous temperature difference (10 or even 15 C) between the anterior and posterior parts of the body. It is striking to see a ground squirrel arousing from hibernation that is able to run with its frontal pair of legs while the posterior legs are still completely paralyzed by cold. Within a half-hour the posterior legs are as active as the frontal part of the body, once the temperature has equalized.

The mandatory arousals are extremely uneconomic and during each arousal the hibernators lose a tremendous amount of energy. One single arousal is energetically equivalent to 10 days in hibernation. Thus, this combination of energetic thriftiness in hibernation on one side and energetically expensive arousals on the other side does not appear to be a sound partnership. But whatever it is, and whatever the reasons for it, arousal is definitely neither "dehibernation" nor "recovering" from it.[27] On the basis of all data currently collected, arousal appears to be an active process of extreme intensity, beginning with a fully active life at a still low body temperature.

Some tissues appear to have a more important role in the process of arousal than others. We have already mentioned endocrine glands, especially adrenal cortex. The brain appears to have some role in arousal too. Satinoff[94] believes that arousals are programmed during a hibernating bout by the initial amount and by the rate of dissipation of a central inhibitory transmitter.

In hibernators, the existence of large deposits of brown adipose tissue (brown fat) is found. It occurs to a lesser degree in some nonhibernating animals as well.[18,33] This so-called hibernating gland appears to have an important role especially in rewarming and contributes 10 or more percent of energy during hibernation as well.[30] The brown fat is full of mitochondria which might be involved in the formation of ADP from ATP. However, the brown fat is not an endocrine gland as we previously thought. Even during hibernation one witnesses a large circulation in this tissue.[12] During the tremendous effort to rewarm the body as fast as possible, the brown fat of a hibernator[96] warms up ahead of other tissuess except the heart, indicating that brown fat is one of the main sources of heat production during arousal.[104] In this respect it is interesting to note that newborn and young animals have relatively more of this brown tissue than adult animals, and that young animals withstand profound and long-lasting hypothermia better than adult animals.[64]

The tremendous, expensive energetic efforts for periodic arousals[1] during hibernation cost hibernators (most of them do not eat during the winter season) 30 or more percent of body weight. Thus, in the spring after final arousal, the active hibernator has already found the way to get rid of large deposits of lipids that would make the animal slow, sluggish, lazy, and an easy prey to many predators.

ARTIFICIALLY COOLED HIBERNATORS

An artificially cooled active hibernator enters hypothermia and not hibernation. The difference between the hypothermic state in a hibernator and the hypothermic state in a nonhibernator is quantitative, not qualitative. A hibernator withstands a longer profound hypothermia than a nonhibernator. For instance, a hypothermic ground squirrel cooled to a body temperature of 10 C lives 110 hours, whereas a rat cooled to a body temperature of 15 C lives only 10 hours.[76] However, at the end, both artificially cooled animals die if not rewarmed externally. At the same body temperature the oxygen consumption, heart rate, cardiac output, and mean arterial pressure are much higher in a hypothermic ground squirrel (and in artificially cooled nonhibernators) than in a hibernating animal.[69] A hibernating animal will die also if, for some reason, it cannot arouse itself from hibernation after 240 to 360 hours. Thus it appears that hydrogen ions and other acid metabolites might lead the cold animal to drowning. This hypothesis is appealing not only as an explanation for periodical arousal from hibernation but it can be used to explain the possible cause of death in hypothermia as well.

APPLICATION OF HIBERNATION RESEARCH TO OTHER FIELDS

It should already be obvious to the reader of this chapter that an extreme degree of caution is needed for evaluation of the mechanisms and observed manifestations of the hibernation phenomenon. The study of hibernators and of hibernation might also be very useful for understanding many other physiological processes better. The tremendous plasticity of morphological and physiological characteristics of hibernators offers a very fertile ground for many fruitful physiological investigators. This plasticity encompasses a big increase in the body weight of the animals (300% or more), the decreased metabolism (to 1% of normal value), many profound endocrine and circulatory changes, and the complete return to their respective normal states—all this in the span of several months.

The importance of hibernation research to present and furture hypothermia studies has been stressed throughout this chapter and is summarized in the next section. Here are some other physiological fields of endeavor which might benefit from the study of hibernation.

Hibernators are a wonderful tool in brain research. Because of naturally induced changes, changes not brought about by ablation of parts of the brain or by brain lesions, hibernation appears to offer an especially favorable situation to this kind of scientific endeavor. Furthermore, one tends to repeat with Strumwasser,[102] "In many respects, hibernation is an ideal type of phenomenon to study in order to gain insight into the mechanisms by which the central nervous system elaborates a long term change in behavioral state." Furthermore, hibernation research might also help to better understand the processes of sleep and wakefulness.

In clinical medicine, besides helping to understand the physiological characteristics of profound, long-lasting hypothermia and extension of clinical death, hibernation research might help in studies of frostbite, protective effects of cold for extension of survival after bilateral adrenalectomy, cessation of tumor growth, and other pathologic situations.

Hibernation research might also help in cardiovascular studies, especially those dealing with shock. The problem of how to endure symptoms of shock without entering into the positive feedback loops and return to normal circulatory parameters is something about which only hibernators might enlighten us.

A drug might have a much greater, the same, or much smaller effect when administered to a hibernating animal. Thus it is apparent that a new area of pharmacology, cryopharmacology, is already born. It is also apparent that the study of new properties of a drug administered in hypothermia or in hibernation might give some extra light upon the various mode of actions of this drug.

Hibernation research might also be useful for a better understanding of nutrition processes. Instead of using hypothalamic lesions, one can use intact hibernators, without hypothalamic ablations or lesions, to study the problem of obesity.

HYPOTHERMIA AND HIBERNATION, PERSPECTIVES

It is clear now that hypothermia and hibernation are two different physiological states. While it would be impossible to expect induction of hibernation in man or other nonhibernator, hibernators might enable us to understand some important physiological adaptations that were acquired during their long phylogenesis. These physiological adaptations applied to nonhibernators might minimize dangers to life at a profoundly decreased body temperature and extend safe and profound hypothermic periods. Due to research done during the last few years, we are aware of some of these characteristics that make hibernators so fit for dormant life. Let us mention some that appear important at the present time.

Profound hemodilution is observed in hibernating animals and appears to be extremely beneficial in profound and extended hypothermia. Though there are some contradictory reports, this seems now to be a well-accepted fact.

Fast cooling and fast rewarming are observed in most hibernators. Fast cooling and fast rewarming appear to be beneficial for successful profound cooling in nonhibernators as well.

A very low arterial blood pressure is seen in deep hibernation. Similarly, maintenance of a low perfusion pressure during profound extracorporeal cooling extends the survival time of nonhibernators in profound hypothermia.

Hypercapnia might be of importance for hypothermia. Its possible significance in hibernation has not yet been proved.

Hypervolemia of the fast rewarming anterior part of the body, where vital organs are situated, is the consequence of differential heating observed during arousal from hibernation. Similarly, hypervolemia induced during the last part of rewarming from profound and extended hypothermia permits nonhibernators to overcome easily and without any ill consequences an extended circulatory arrest at a body temperature close to the freezing point.

Periodic arousals, periodic short-lasting rewarmings, are a necessity of life for successful hibernation. Cooled nonhibernators also appear to need "periodic arousal" or artificial rewarming to extend the period of safe profound hypothermia. It has been observed that when a nonhibernator is rewarmed even for a short period of time (interrupting the hypothermic exposure) the duration of safe profound hypothermia can be almost doubled.

Increased level of magnesium is found in hibernating animals and seems to be beneficial for hypothermic animals.

Summary

Hibernation is a seasonal adaptation. It requires physiological preparation during normothermic conditions for entering into torpor as well as preparation during torpor for periodic and eventually permanent (for that year) arousal into active life.

It appears now that hibernation is not a dead-end alley in development of temperature regulation. Hibernation appears to be a new step in adaptation. The hypothalamus might be involved in some of the newly acquired adaptation processes that make hibernators unique in withstanding low body temperature. Or some humoral factors might be involved in the preparation and entering into hibernation as well as in arousal processes. A better understanding of these mechanisms, whatever they are, might indicate how to safely induce profound and long-lasting hypothermia with all the benefits and protective roles hypothermia offers to biology and medicine.

BIBLIOGRAPHY

1. Adolph EF, Richmond J: Rewarming from natural hibernation and from artificial cooling. J Appl Physiol 8:48–58, 1955
2. Agid R, Ambid L: Effects of corporeal temperature on glucose metabolism in a homeotherm, the rat, and a hibernator, the garden dormouse, in Musacchia X, Saunders J (eds): Depressed Metabolism. New York, Am Elsevier, 1969, pp 119–158
3. Agid R, Gabe M, Martoja M: Modifications histologiques des glandes endocrines au cours des reveils periodiques du Lerot hibernant. C R Soc Biol (Paris) 161:459–462, 1967
4. Agid R, Popovic V: Variation de la glycemie, du glucose et de glucogene hepatiques chez le spermophile hibernant. Effet de l'administration de glucagon. J Physiol (Paris) 49:7–9, 1957
5. Agid R, Sicart R: Role de la thyroide dans l'involution et la restauration du tube digestif d'animaux hibernants. C R Acad Sci, 269:1866, 1969

6. Ambid L, Agid R: Variations cycliques de la glycemie et du glycogene hepatique au cours des reveils periodiques d'un hibernant, le Lerot (*Eliomys quercinus L.*). J Physiol (Paris) 59:326, 1967
7. Ambid L, Laporte P, Agid R: Evolution saisonniere de la lipemie et des lipides hepatiques chez un hibernant (*Eliomys quercinus L.*). J Physiol (Paris) 55: 185–186, 1963
8. Axelrod LR: Hibernation—A biological timeclock. Prog Biomed Res 10:1–4, 1964
9. Barr RE, Musacchia XJ: Postirradiation hibernation and radiation response of ground squirrels: Telemetry surveillance. Radiat Res 51:631–637, 1972
10. Baumler J, South FE, Ferren L, et al: A possible basis for periodic arousals during hibernation: Accumulation of ketone bodies. Life Sci 10(II): 463–467, 1971
11. Bigelow WG, Lindsay WK, Greenwood WF: Hypothermia: Its possible role in cardiac surgery. An investigation of factors governing survival in dogs at low body temperature. Ann Surg 132:849–866, 1950
12. Bullard RW, Funkhouser GE: Estimated regional blood flow by rubidium 86 distribution during arousal from hibernation. Am J Physiol 203:266–270, 1962
13. Cushing H, Goetsch E: Hibernation and the pitutiary body. J Exp Med 22:25–47, 1915
14. Dawe AR, Spurrier WA: Hibernation induced in ground squirrels by blood transfusion. Science 163:298–299, 1969
15. Dawe AR, Spurrier WA: The blood-born "trigger" for natural mammalian hibernation in the 13-lined ground squirrel and the woodchuck. Cryobiology 9:163–172, 1972
16. Dawe AR, Spurrier WA, Armour JA: Summer hibernation induced by cryogenically preserved blood "trigger." Science 168:497–498, 1970
17. Draskoczy PR, Lyman CP: Turnover of catecholamines in active and hibernating ground squirrels. J Pharmacol Exp Ter 155:101–111, 1967
18. Edwards BA, Munday KA: The function of brown fat in the hedgehog (*Erinaceus europaeus*). Comp Biochem Physiol 30:1029–1036, 1969
19. Edwards BA, Munday KA: Electrolyte metabolism in the hibernating hedgehog (*Erinaceus europaeus*). Comp Biochem Physiol 31:329–335, 1969
20. Feist DD: Blockade of arousal from hibernation by inhibition of norepinephrine synthesis in the golden hamster. Life Sci 9(I):1116–1125, 1970
21. Gabe M, Agid R, Martoja M, et al: Donnees histophysiologiques et biochimiques sur l'hibernation et le cycle annuel chez Eliomys quercinus. Arch Biol 75:1–87, 1964
22. Giaja J: Les oxydations dans l'hibernation et la poikilothermie experimentale. Bull Soc Chim Fr 36:446–453, 1954
23. Giaja J, Popovic V: Reaction de l'hibernant et du non-hibernant refroidi aux agressions operatoires. C R Acad Sci (Paris) 237:1360–1362, 1953
24. Gollan F: The adequacy of anemic and hypoxemic perfusion, in Malinin J, Zeppa R, Gollan F, Callahan AB (eds): Reversibility of Cellular Injury due to Inadequate Perfusion. Springfield, Thomas, 1972, pp 407–425
25. Gumma MR, South FE, Allen JN: Temperature preference in golden hamsters. Anim Behav 15:534–537, 1967
26. Hammel HT, Dawson TJ, Abrams RM, et al: Total calorimetric measurements of *Citellus lateralis* in hibernation. Physiol Zool 41:341–357, 1968

27. Hock, RJ: Seasonal variations in physiologic functions of arctic ground squirrels and black bears. Bull Mus Comp Zool (Harvard) 124:155–171, 1960
28. Hoffman RA: Terrestrial animals in cold: Hibernators, in Dill DB, Adolph AF, Wilber CG (eds): Handbook of Physiology, Adaptation to Environment. Washington, American Physiological Society, 1964, pp 379–403
29. Hoffman RA: The hibernator as a tool in biological research. Fed Proc 27:999–1007, 1968
30. Horwitz BA, Smith RE, Pengelley ET: Estimated heat contribution of brown fat in arousing ground squirrels (*Citellus lateralis*). Am J Physiol 214:115–121, 1968
31. Hudson JW, Bartholomew GA: Terrestrial animals in dry heat: Estivators, in Dill DB, Adolph EF, Wilber CG (eds): Handbook of Physiology, Adaptation to Environment. Washington, American Physiological Society, 1964, pp 541–550
32. Johansson BW: Heart and circulation in hibernators, in Fisher KC, Dawe AR, Lyman CP, Schonbaum E, South FE (eds): Mammalian Hibernation III. New York, Am Elsevier, 1967, pp 200–218
33. Johansson B: Brown fat: A review. Metabolism 8:221–240, 1959
34. Kallen FC: Plasma and blood volumes in the little brown bat. Am J Physiol 198:999–1005, 1960
35. Kalabukhov NI: Comparative ecology of hibernating mammals, in Lyman CP, Dawe AR (eds): Mammalian Hibernation. Bull Mus Comp Zool (Harvard) 124:45–75, 1960
36. Kayser C: Le sommeil hivernal et les glandes surrenals. Etude faite sur le hamster ordinaire (*Cricetus cricetus*). C R Soc Biol (Paris) 151:982–985, 1957
37. Kayser C: Les echanges respiratoires du hamster ordinaire (Cricetus cricetus) et du lerot (Eliomys quercinus) en hibernation. Bull Mus Comp Zool (Harvard) 124:1–29, 1960
38. Kayser C: Stoffwechsel und Winterschlaf. Helgol Wiss Meeresunters 9:158–186, 1964
39. Kayser C: Hibernation, in Mayer WV, Gelder RG (eds): Physiological Mammalogy. New York, Academic Press, 1965, pp 179–296
40. Kayser C, Heusner A, Stussi T: Y a-t-il conservation du rythme nycthemeral de la depense d'energie pendant le sommeil hivernal? C R Soc Biol (Paris) 158:1140–1144, 1964
41. Kayser C, Malan A: Central nervous system and hibernation. Experientia 19:441–496, 1963
42. Konttinen A, Rajasalmi M, Sarajas HSS: Fat metabolism of the hedgehog during the hibernating cycle. Am J Physiol 207:845–848, 1964
43. Kristoffersson R, Broberg S: Glutamic decarboxylase acitivity in the brains of hibernating and non-hibernating golden hamsters and hedgehogs. Ann Acad Sci Fenn 4:1–8, 1967
44. Lachiver F, Petrovic V: Activite thyroidienne comparee de deux hibernants: le Lerot (Eliomys quercinus) et le Spermophile (Citellus citellus) et d'un homeotherme: le rat, au cours de l'exposition au froid pendant l'ete. C R Acad Sci (Paris) 250:3883–3885, 1960
45. Larsen B: Red cell life span in hibernating hedgehogs (*Erinaceus europaeus L*). Acta Univ Bergensis, Rer Nat 6:1–8, 1968

46. Lyman CP: The oxygen consumption and temperature regulation of hibernating hamsters. J Exp Zool 109:55, 1948
47. Lyman CP: Metabolic adaptations of hibernators. Fed Proc 17:1057–1060, 1958
48. Lyman CP: Hibernation in mammals. Circulation 24:434–445, 1961
49. Lyman CP: Circulation in mammalian hibernation, in Hamilton WF, Dow P (eds): Handbook of Physiology, Circulation III. Washington, American Physiological Society, 1965, p 1967–1989
50. Lyman CP, Chatfield PO: Hibernation and cortical electrical activity in the woodchuck (*Marmota monax*). Science 117:533–534, 1953
51. Malan A: Suppression de l'hibernation par lesions hypothalamiques posterieures chez le hamster d'Europe (*Cricetus cricetus*). J Physiol (Paris) 58:565, 1966
52. Malan A: Suppression de l'hibernation et modification de la thermoregulation par lesions hypothalamiques chez le hamster d'Europe (*Cricetus cricetus*). C R Soc Biol (Paris) 160:1497–1499, 1966
53. Menaker M: Hibernation–Hypothermia: An annual cycle of response to low temperature in the bat *Myotis lucifugus*. Cell Comp Physiol 59:163–173, 1962
54. Miller DA: An efficient, simple dialyzer suitable for small animals. J Appl Physiol 28:689–694, 1970
55. Mrosovsky N: The performance of dormice and other hibernators on tests of hunger motivation. Anim Behav 12:454–469, 1964
56. Mrosovsky N: Hibernation and the Hypothalamus. New York, Appleton, 1971, p 287
57. Musacchia XJ, Barr RE: Survival of whole-body-irradiated hibernating and active ground squirrels, *Citellus tridecemlineatus*. Radiat Res 33:348–356, 1968
58. Panuska JA: Weight patterns and hibernation in *Tamias striatus*. J Mammal 40:554–566, 1959
59. Pearson PP: Torpidity in birds. Bull Mus Comp Zool (Harvard) 124:93–103, 1960
60. Pengelley ET, Fisher KC: The effect of temperature and photoperiod on the yearly hibernating behavior of captive golden-mantled ground squirrels (*Citellus lateralis tescorum*). Can J Zool 41:1103–1120, 1963
61. Petrovic VM, Rajcic O, Hudnik-Plevik T: Etude comparee de l'action du froid et de l'ACTH sur le taux des acides nucleiques et des proteines dans la surrenale et le foie chez le rat et le spermophile. J Physiol (Paris) 58:590, 1966
62. Popovic P, Horecky J, Popovic V: Circulation extracorporelle chez le rat blanc en hypothermie. J Physiol (Paris) 58:594, 1966
63. Popovic P, Horecky J, Popovic V: Hypothermic cardiopulmonary bypass in white rats. Ann Surg 168:298–301, 1968
64. Popovic P, Popovic V: Survival of newborn ground squirrels after supercooling or freezing. Am J Physiol 204:949–952, 1963
65. Popovic V: L'energetique de l'hibernant en etat de veille avant le sommeil hibernal. Glas Acad Serbe Sci 196:113–121, 1950
66. Popovic V: La tension de l'oxygene et le sommeil hibernal. Glas Acad Serbe Sci 200:121–136, 1951

67. Popovic V: La tension de l'oxygene et la respiration de l'homeotherme refroidi. Glas Acad Serbe Sci 200:199–214, 1951
68. Popovic V: Thermogenese des spermophiles a l'etat de veille pendant l'hiver. Glas Acad Serbe Sci 200:215–223, 1951
69. Popovic V: L'hibernation artificielle du spermophile (*Citellus citellus*). Arch Sci Biol (Belgrade) 4:37–43, 1952
70. Popovic V: Contribution a l'etude de la thermogenese de l'homeotherme refroidi. Monogr Acad Serbe Sci 199:1–156, 1952
71. Popovic V: L'effet de la temperature de millieu sur l'intensite de la consommation d'oxygene pendant l'hibernation. Glas Acad Serbe Sci 208:43–52, 1953
72. Popovic V: Influence de la diminution de la tension de l'oxygene sur les oxydations dans l'hypothermie profonde et dans le sommeil hibernal. Arch Sci Biol (Belgrade) 5:161–170, 1953
73. Popovic V: Role de la glande thyroide dans le sommeil hibernal. Arch Sci Biol (Belgrade) 7:25–37, 1955
74. Popovic V: La calorification du reveil de l'hibernant. Arch Sci Physiol (Paris) 11:29–35, 1957
75. Popovic V: Endocrines in hibernation. Bull Mus Comp Zool (Harvard) 124: 105–129, 1960
76. Popovic V: Survival time of hypothermic rats (15°C) and ground squirrels (10°C). Am J Physiol 199:463–466, 1960
77. Popovic V: Cardiac output in hibernating ground squirrels. Am J Physiol 207:1345–1348, 1964
78. Popovic V, Gerschman R, Gilbert DL: Effect of high oxygen pressure on ground squirrels in hypothermia and hibernation. Am J Physiol 206:49–50, 1964
79. Popovic V, Kent BB: Alternation of activity rhythm after induced arousal from hibernation. Rassegna Neur Veget 23:27–36, 1969
80. Popovic V, Kent KM, Popovic P: Technique of permanent cannulation of the right ventricle in rats and ground squirrels. Proc Soc Exp Biol Med 113: 599–602, 1963
81. Popovic V, Popovic P: Sur les limites de temperature de sommeil hibernal. C R Soc Biol (Paris) 150:1439–1440, 1956
82. Popovic V, Popovic P: Permanent cannulation of aorta and vena cava in rats and ground squirrels. J Appl Physiol 15:727–728, 1960
83. Popovic V, Vidovic V: Les glandes surrenales et le sommeil hibernal. Arch Sci Biol (Belgrade) 3:3–17, 1951
84. Popovic V, Vidovic V, Vidovic V: L'influence des hormones corticales sur l'hibernant adrenalectomise au cours du sommeil hibernal. Abst 20 Congr Int Physiol 736–737, 1956
85. Popovic V, Vidovic V, Vidovic V: L'effet du cortizone et du DOCA sur le spermophile surrenalectomize. C R Soc Biol (Paris) 151:1738–1739, 1957
86. Protic S, Minic-Petrovic B, Milhailovic L: RNA and protein content in various brain structures of ground squirrels arousing from hibernation. Yugosl Physiol Pharmacol Acta 6:226–228, 1969
87. Riedesel ML: Serum magnesium levels in mammalian hibernation. Trans Kans Acad Sci 60:99–141, 1957

88. Roberts JC, Chaffee RJ: Suppression of mitochondrial respiration in hibernation and its reversal in arousal. Environ Physiol 101–107, 1972
89. Rohmer F, Hiebel G, Kayser C: Recherches sur le fonctionnement du systeme nerveux des hibernants. Les ondes cerebrales pendant le sommeil hibernal et le reveil. Etude sur le spermophile. C R Soc Biol (Paris) 145:747–752, 1951
90. Sahovic X, Popovic V, Anaf M: Transplantation des glandes endocrines. I. Transplantation des glandes surrenales. Role du transplantat dans la thermoregulation. Glas Acad Serbe Sci 204:79–85, 1951
91. Sahovic X, Popovic V, Anaf M: Contribution a l'etude de la thermoregulation. Role de cortex de la glande surrenale. Glas Acad Serbe Sci 204:99–124, 1951
92. Satinoff E: Aberrations of regulation in ground squirrels following hypothalamic lesions. Am J Physiol 212:1215–1220, 1967
93. Satinoff E: Disruption of hibernation caused by hypothalamic lesions. Science 155:1031–1033, 1967
94. Satinoff E: Hibernation and the central nervous system, in Steller E, Sprague JM (eds): Progress in Physiological Psychology III. New York, Academic Press, 1970, p 204
95. Smalley RL, Dryer RL: Brown fat in hibernation, in Fisher KC, Dawe AR, Lyman C, Schonbaum E, South FE (eds): Mammalian Hibernation III. New York, Am Elsevier, 1967, pp 325–345
96. Smith RE, Horwitz BA: Brown fat and thermogenesis. Physiol Rev 49:330, 1969
97. South FE: Hibernation, temperature and rates of oxidative phosphorylation by heart mitochondria. Am J Physiol 198:463–466, 1960
98. South FE, Breazile JE, Dellman HD, et al: Sleep, hibernation and hypothermia in the yellow-bellied marmot (*M flaviventris*), in Musacchia XJ, Saunders JF (eds): Depressed Metabolism. New York, Am Elsevier, 1969, pp 277–312
99. Strumwasser F: Factors in the pattern, timing and predictability of hibernation in the squirrel, *Citellus beecheyi.* Am J Physiol 196:8–14, 1959
100. Strumwasser F: Thermoregulatory, brain and behavioral mechanisms during entrance into hibernation in the squirrel, *Citellus beecheyi.* Am J Physiol 196:15–22, 1959
101. Strumwasser F: Some physiological principles governing hibernation in *Citellus beecheyi.* Bull Mus Comp Zool (Harvard) 124:285–320, 1960
102. Strumwasser F, Smith JE, Gilliam JJ, et al: Identification of active brain regions involved in the processes of hibernation. 21 Int Zool Congr 2:53, 1965
103. Suomalainen P, Nyholm P: Neurosecretion in the hibernating hedgehog. Bertil Hanstrom Zool papers in honor of his sixty-fifth birthday, Lund, 1956
104. Suomalainen P, Saarikoski PL: The content of non-esterified fatty acids and glycerol in the blood of the hedgehog during the hibernation period. Experientia 23:457–458, 1967
105. Vidovic V, Popovic V: L'evolution de la thermoregulation au cours de l'ontogenese chez le spermophile Citellus citellus. Arch Sci Biol (Belgrade) 1:137–155, 1949
106. Vidovic V, Popovic V: The role of the adrenals and the thyroid during wintersleep of the ground squirrel. Arch Sci Biol (Belgrade) 5:171–189, 1953

107. Vidovic V, Popovic V: Studies on the adrenal and thyroid glands of the ground squirrel during hibernation. J Endocrinol 11:125–133, 1954
108. Wade O: Rapid fat production in ground squirrels preceding hibernation. Chicago Academy of Science, Natural History Museum 28:1–3, 1948
109. Wells LA: Blood-brain barrier system in hibernation and hypothermia. Cryobiology 9:306–307, 1972
110. Willis JS, Goldman SS, Foster RF: Tissue K concentration in relation to the role of the kidney in hibernation and the cause of periodic arousal. Comp Biochem Physiol 39A:437–445, 1971
111. Zimny ML: Histological studies of the ground squirrel adrenal following hibernation and cold exposure. Anat Rec 135:279–284, 1959

Author Index

The numbers in parenthesis refer to the chapter in which the author's name appears. The other numbers refer to the reference number.

Subject Index

a
4 b
5 c
6 d
7 e
8 f
9 g
0 h
1 i
8 2 j